ADELLE DAVIS

Adelle Davis was one of the country's best-known nutritionists. She studied at Purdue University, graduated from the University of California at Berkeley, and took postgraduate work at Columbia University and the University of California at Los Angeles before receiving her Master of Science degree in biochemistry from the University of Southern California Medical School. Throughout her career, she worked with physicians, beginning in New York with dietetics training at Bellevue and Fordham hospitals and her first job at the Judson Health Clinic.

Later, in Oakland, California, and then in Los Angeles, she worked as a consulting nutritionist with physicians at the Alameda County Health Clinic and the William E. Branch Clinic in Hollywood as well as seeing patients referred to her by numerous specialists. After planning individual diets for more than 20,000 people suffering from almost every known disease, she gave up consulting work to devote her time to her family, writing, and lecturing.

Adelle Davis was the author of four best-selling books, *Let's Cook It Right, Let's Have Healthy Children, Let's Get Well,* and *Let's Eat Right to Keep Fit.* In the light of new developments in nutritional science and the steady decline in our national health, Miss Davis revised LET'S EAT RIGHT TO KEEP FIT. The revised hardcover edition is published by Harcourt Brace Jovanovich, Inc.

Let's Eat Right To Keep Fit

Newly Revised and Updated

ADELLE DAVIS

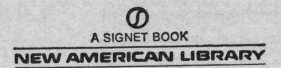

A SIGNET BOOK

NEW AMERICAN LIBRARY

Publisher's Note

The ideas, procedures, and suggestions contained in this book are not intended as a substitute for consulting with your physician. All matters regarding your health require medical supervision.

SIGNET TRADEMARK REG. U.S. PAT. OFF. AND FOREIGN COUNTRIES
REGISTERED TRADEMARK—MARCA REGISTRADA
HECHO EN CHICAGO, U.S.A.

SIGNET, SIGNET CLASSIC, MENTOR, ONYX, PLUME, MERIDIAN AND NAL BOOKS *are published by NAL PENGUIN INC.,* *1633 Broadway, New York, New York 10019*

FIRST SIGNET PRINTING, SEPTEMBER, 1970

38   39   40   41   42   43   44   45   46

PRINTED IN THE UNITED STATES OF AMERICA

Dedicated

to

The Perfection That Is You

FOREWORD

ADELLE DAVIS IS THE ONLY AUTHOR I KNOW WHO CAN present authoritative, accurate information concerning vital, complicated human nutritional processes in such an interesting and fascinating manner. I could hardly leave the manuscript at my first reading. Even as a physician especially informed and interested in human nutrition I learned much from this book, as I have from hearing the author lecture on many occasions.

Each chapter has such a personal impact and meaning for the reader that he will stop and ponder as to how the facts and knowledge gained specifically apply to himself. This happened to me. Many chapters will be reread several times. The book is well documented and is an excellent source of reference material.

Here is the book for the physician and technically trained person as well as for the layman. Non-medical people are constantly asking for more and more reliable technical knowledge expressed in direct yet simple understandable language. This is it as far as food, diet, and human nutrition are concerned. It will serve as a good review for even the physician and will bring the nutritionist up to date.

How I wish I could have read this book before or during my medical school education. In medical college, the students tend to get lost among the trees of technical knowledge. It is difficult for them to grasp the broader perspectives. They are taught the sound principle of specific therapy for the specific disease. In my opinion, we all suffer from malnutritional disease with resultant physical and mental deterioration. However, the human being probably never develops just a single nutritional lack. Only in animals that we place in pens and feed food lacking in a single nutrient can we produce specific nutritional diseases. Can you imagine a diet for the human being which lacks only a single nutrient? It has occurred to me gradually that one nutritional deficiency meant others, and if one tissue was harmed, others were also.

Undoubtedly many vitamins and other food elements have not yet been discovered. Every year new ones are found that are essential for life or health. How many more are there yet to be isolated in the next 10 years; the next 100 years? We cannot get adequate nutrition even to sustain life from synthetic foods and vitamins. They will only help, and they may lull us into a false sense of security. We must get our real sustenance from our food, from good food, as the author explains.

So many factors militate against our receiving the good health that our food should bring us. First, our soils today are mostly mediocre or poor, and hence the plants do not contain proper or frequently even the essential nutrients. The animals that eat these plants cannot have the proper food chemicals in their meat, milk, or eggs. Also, the processing or improper cooking of these foods further deteriorates them. And, finally, there are important psychological deterrents which prevent us from feeding ourselves properly.

There is so much psychology involved in the very act of eating. In the oral, first-year stage of our life the actual foundation is laid for most of our eating habits. Most of these are on a subconscious level, and we are not aware of reasons behind our likes and dislikes. We may overeat because of longing for affection. We may fail to eat or to eat properly because of unresolved hostilities. It is common knowledge to psychologists that we all possess unconscious needs and desires to hurt and injure ourselves, the less neurotic punishing themselves only to a lesser degree. Otherwise why do we "learn to like" so much of the devitalized food we eat? Why do we drink so much alcohol? Why do we smoke so much? Why do we overwork or underwork? In some people only adequate psychoanalytical consultation will remove these self-damaging tendencies.

It is well known that husbands and wives cannot easily sell each other, or their children for that matter, on new ideas or needed changes. This is especially so in regard to eating habits which have been a lifetime in building, when they are so deeply rooted in and forgotten by the subconscious. This book can be much help, for instance, to the mother who feels so helpless in trying to promote good nutrition for her family. At the start she should ask her husband to read only one chapter of this book—the second. In fact, almost any single chapter, read alone, seems to be adequate and complete in itself. Therefore, one can profitably read this book even for fifteen or twenty minutes at a time.

If the principles set forth in this book were followed by most people, I believe a greater advancement in health would result than from any other occurrence in the history of mankind. It surely represents the basis of preventive medicine.

W. D. Currier, M.D.
National Secretary, American Academy of Nutrition

1954

CONTENTS

CHAPTER 1

NUTRITION CAN BE A
FASCINATING SUBJECT

NUTRITION IS A PERSONAL MATTER, AS PERSONAL AS YOUR diary or income-tax report. Your nutrition can determine how you look, act, and feel; whether you are grouchy or cheerful, homely or beautiful, physiologically and even psychologically young or old; whether you think clearly or are confused, enjoy your work or make it a drudgery, increase your earning power or stay in an economic rut. The foods you eat can make the difference between your day ending with freshness which lets you enjoy a delightful evening or with exhaustion which forces you to bed with the chickens. To a considerable degree, your nutrition can give you a coddled-egg personality or make you a human dynamo. In short, it can determine your zest for life, the good you put into it, and the fulfillment you get from it.

Nutrition is the study of how foods, after they are swallowed, make you tick. It is often confused with dietetics, the study of foods which should be swallowed. Nutrition can be fascinating because it is about you. If this knowledge is both personal and fascinating, why does not everyone apply it? There are many reasons. Nutrition is a young subject; it has been kicked around like a puppy that cannot take care of itself.

Food faddists and crackpots have kicked it pretty cruelly. They usually have no scientific training, peddle tremendous amounts of misinformation, make unjustifiable claims, and are often out for commercial gain. They not only put people off by their ridiculous recommendations, they make every thinking person necessarily skeptical of the whole subject.

The followers of the food faddists are usually overzealous people. A friend of mine claims they either get "religion" or nutrition. They can dream up the most amazing concoctions to eat. I know; they have fed such foods to me with what I think is sadistic delight. I have eaten liquefied grass which tastes the way a newly filled haymow smells. The smell used to be good; the taste never is. They seem to believe that unless food tastes like Socratic hemlock, it cannot build health. Frankly, I often wonder what such persons plan to do with good health in case they acquire it. The longer I work in nutrition, the more convinced I become that for the healthy person all foods should be delicious.

There is no sense in your eating any food you do not like. It is good sense, however, to realize that you consider many health-building foods delicious, and still better sense to learn to enjoy foods particularly rich in nutrients your body must have to function normally. It can be done by the nibble method. Probably every person who enjoys coffee or bourbon hated the first sip.

Let us suppose you have certain nutritional deficiencies and think perhaps better food might help. You are offered some nauseating glop; it is so revolting that you immediately lose interest and eat as you are accustomed. Eventually your malnutrition makes you so ill that you are not expected to live. Who almost killed you? It seems to me the near-murderer was the person who gave you the unpalatable food. Had he given you delicious food instead, you would have improved your diet and perhaps felt wonderful. To my way of thinking, there should be two standards for selecting any food: it should taste delicious; it should help build health.

Another reason why nutritional knowledge is not applied is that much of our information concerning food comes from advertising. Commercial interests wish us to buy and eat certain foods. Highly refined foods keep better than do natural foods; they are easier to store and ship. They cannot spoil because they cannot support the health of bacteria, fungi, molds, or weevils; certainly they cannot build human health either. Although the few nutrients remaining in such foods are ballyhooed, the removal of many others during refining is kept strictly quiet: the implication is that such foods have great nutritive value. Why bother to improve a dietary which is already excellent?

An additional reason why people understandably shy away from nutrition is that there is a widespread "should-not" philosophy. For example, I once spoke to a certain "health" organization. Before I was introduced, the chairman ranted with astounding fury about "poison white sugar" killing people. Probably each person in the audience had eaten "poison white sugar"; yet most of them appeared to be alive. Had that been my introduction to nutrition, I would probably have felt a surge of nausea thereafter when the subject was mentioned. It would be more constructive to state that some foods have more to offer than others.

A further reason why nutrition is not valued is that people are so gullible. We live in a culture where a headache is "cured" by an aspirin; therefore an ulcer or other abnormality should be "cured" by a vitamin pill. Millions of people take capsules which "contain everything," believing that these preparations can maintain health. Such a capsule could be made, but it would be the size of a baseball. Why not try it? A python can swallow a pig.

Still another reason why nutrition is not applied is that so much information is inaccurate. For example, people frequently tell me, "I'm eating a high-protein diet." When I check the diets of such persons, I usually find their protein intake to be perhaps one-third of that recommended by the National Research Council. As a result of their thinking that they have knowledge when they do not, they fail to improve their nutrition. In the same category are pseudo-information and misinformation, the amount of which seems endless.

A serious reason why nutrition is not applied—quite alarming to me—is that wives often become interested in the subject before their husbands do. When a husband suffers from nutritional deficiencies, a wife who genuinely loves him tries to move heaven and earth to get him to change his eating habits. Any husband not a hopeless Milquetoast resents such maneuvering. Sometimes the reverse is true. A husband, sincerely trying to prevent medical and dental bills and such problems as fatigue and irritable dispositions, appears to be merely criticizing his wife's selection and preparation of food; this apparent criticism understandably antagonizes her. In either case the two reach a deadlock.

If a good fairy were to grant me a wish concerning this book, my wish would be that families might read it aloud together, stopping frequently to discuss their problems. In case you are the only member of your family to read it, my advice is to apply nutrition as best you can but to do it as quietly as possible. When positive improvement follows, your partner cannot help observing it, and he will want what you have achieved.

Perhaps the most important reason why nutrition is not applied is that eating has emotional connotations: to many people it symbolizes pleasure, pain, reward, punishment, and so forth. The person who suffered from poverty during childhood perhaps had nutritious food, but he may associate it with deprivation; less nutritious food, eaten by wealthy persons, becomes a mark of social standing. White bread and sugar often represent purity and cleanliness just as a white operating room once did. To many persons orange juice means castor oil. A psychiatrist tells me that some persons who think they hate milk actually hate their mothers who tried to make them drink milk; guilt feelings prevent them from hating her outright. We all have emotional reasons for hating certain foods and liking others. For example, my father held stern clean-up-your-plate convictions: once he made me eat meat fat which was nauseating; I still hate fat meat. I used to hate brains because we threw them away when we butchered, just as we did entrails; I identified brains with entrails. Theoretically, I hold that we should learn to enjoy all nutritious foods. To put the theory into practice, I once ate a platter of snails in a French restaurant and was violently ill for hours afterward; the snails did not make me ill, but my repugnance to them still makes me squirm. All of us have pleasant or unpleasant associations with food which we do not want to change; even if we tried, it might be impossible. People often think nutrition means giving up those foods we favor emotionally and eating those we hate.

Another factor which prevents nutrition from being applied is that we look to our physicians to guide our health; if the doctor has not revised one's diet, it seems logical to assume that nutrition is unimportant. We often forget that the study of medicine is *a study of medicine*. From the first day of medical school throughout the years of a physician's practice, this study is primarily one of disease rather than health. Many physicians are doing outstanding work in nutrition; their numbers increase yearly. Nevertheless the purpose of medicine is to help the sick person get well or, in the case of serious illness, to keep him alive. The purpose of nutrition is to maintain health and to prevent illness. Even today not one medical school in the United States teaches a course in nutrition, though a smattering of the subject is included in other courses. What little nutrition is taught is usually limited to the recognition and treatment of so-called deficiency diseases, such as scurvy, which rarely occur. The tragic result is that nutrition is tremendously underemphasized, misinformation is given patients, much suffering continues needlessly, and drugs are expected to do what good food could accomplish.

Physicians are often overworked to the point of exhaustion; yet they must constantly keep up with recent developments in antibiotics, hormones, new surgical techniques, treatments for new diseases and new treatments for old diseases. I have worked with physicians for four decades. They are wonderful people; I have yet to meet finer. The criticism implied by the remark, "Why didn't my doctor tell me diet was important?" seems to me to be unfair; it is like expecting me to perform delicate brain surgery. You may find the time to study nutrition; probably he cannot.

Lastly, nutrition often is not applied because of the vast gap, perhaps of 20 or 30 years, between scientific and clinical research. In hundreds of laboratories all over the world, scientists feed experimental animals diets deficient in one nutrient or another and study the effects upon their health. These scientists, however, do not study human beings to find the counterpart of the abnormalities they produce in animals. Their research is merely reported each month in hundreds of expensive scientific publications which the busy physician rarely sees, although if he did he might immediately recognize the symptoms described daily by his patients.

Nevertheless, this knowledge of the means of producing health, gained largely from research with animals, is consistently being found to apply equally to humans. Regardless of how radiant your health, a thorough knowledge of nutrition and its application can usually bring vast improvement. Such application is your insurance of feeling your best, looking your best, and giving your best. As nearly as possible, it is your hope of making a long, active, and rewarding life a reality.

Let us find out how to keep fit.

CHAPTER 2

BREAKFAST GETS THE
DAY'S WORK DONE

FORTY OR MORE NUTRIENTS ARE NEEDED TO BUILD HEALTH. Valuable unrefined foods such as milk might supply all 40 of these nutrients, whereas a highly refined food such as sugar supplies only one. Single nutritional deficiencies, therefore, apparently never occur in humans. A person whose diet is faulty suffers from multiple and overlapping deficiencies simultaneously. The symptoms of a single deficiency resulting when animals are given diets adequate except in one nutrient are far simpler than the symptoms found in people. The discussions of single deficiencies in this chapter and the following ones are therefore unavoidably oversimplified and unrealistic. A single deficiency can, however, predominate over other deficiencies. For example, an undersupply for only a few hours of the amount of sugar furnished your tissues can wreck your day.

You determine how you will feel throughout each day by the type of breakfast you eat. You can produce inefficiency in yourself by eating too little food or too much of the wrong kind of food. Your breakfast establishes how readily your body can produce energy that day or, more specifically, the amount of sugar in your blood. Your energy production, which corresponds to the quality of sugar available, determines how you think, act, and feel. Energy is produced in your body by the burning (oxidizing) of sugar alone or sugar and fat together. Only when the blood plasma contains adequate amounts of sugar can each cell select the quantity it needs. The amount of sugar in the blood is an index of the quantity available to each cell.

Thousands of blood analyses have shown that a normal person who has not eaten for 12 hours has 80 to 120 milligrams of sugar in about ½ cup (100 cc.) of blood. This figure, known as the fasting blood sugar, depends on the kind and amount of food eaten at the previous meal. The average is 90 to 95 milligrams. At this point energy is rather well produced. As the supply of blood sugar is used, energy is produced less readily, and lassitude sets in. When the sugar falls to about 70 milligrams, hunger is experienced, and lassitude gradually becomes fatigue. If the blood sugar drops to about 65 milligrams, a craving for sweets is often noticed and/or "growling" in the intestines. A continued drop in the sugar supply causes fatigue to become exhaustion. Headaches, weakness, and wobbliness often occur; palpitations of the heart may be noticeable; the legs may suddenly give way; nausea and even vomiting are often experienced.

The cells of the nerves and brain can produce their energy only from sugar, never from fat by itself or protein. Even when the amount of sugar available to the cells decreases only slightly, thinking becomes slowed and confused, and nerves become tense. The person whose blood sugar falls below normal becomes progressively more irritable, grouchy, moody, depressed, and uncooperative. Since the brain derives its energy only from sugar, blackouts or fainting may occur if the supply drops dangerously low.

On the other hand, if your food intake is sufficiently adequate to cause your sugar to increase above the fasting level, energy is easily produced; you feel wonderful and full of drive. Your thinking is quick and clear. You have no desire to eat; sweets seem distasteful. Your disposition is at its best, your attitude gracious, cheerful, and co-operative. At this level, life is good.

Many studies have been made of the factors influencing the level of blood sugar. In one such study,[1] for example, 200 volunteers ate various types of breakfasts; each individual's blood sugar was determined before the meal and hourly for three hours afterward. After black coffee alone, the blood sugar decreased, and the volunteers experienced lassitude, irritability, nervousness, hunger, fatigue, exhaustion, and headaches; the symptoms became progressively worse as the morning wore on. Two doughnuts and coffee with sugar and cream caused a rapid rise in blood sugar, but the amount fell within an hour to a low level, again resulting in inefficiency and fatigue. A basic breakfast was selected

[1] E. Orent-Keiles and L. F. Hallman, "The Breakfast Meal in Relation to Blood Sugar Values," U. S. Department of Agriculture Circular No. 827 (1949).

because it was typical of the morning meal eaten by millions of Americans: a glass of orange juice, two strips of bacon, toast, jam, and coffee with cream and sugar. The blood sugar rose rapidly but fell far below the pre-breakfast level within an hour and remained below normal until lunch time. The next breakfast was the same except for the addition of a packaged cereal; again the blood sugar rose, fell quickly, and remained below normal all morning. A fifth breakfast was the basic one plus oatmeal served with sugar and milk; the blood sugar rose rapidly but fell more quickly and to a lower level than after any other breakfast studied. Then 8 ounces of whole milk fortified with 2½ tablespoons of powdered skim milk was drunk with the basic breakfast of orange juice, bacon, toast, jam, and coffee. After this meal the blood sugar rose above normal and stayed at approximately 120 milligrams throughout the morning; unusual well-being was experienced. Two eggs were then served instead of fortified milk; again a high level of efficiency was maintained. The last breakfast was the basic one with eggs or fortified milk and larger amounts of toast and jam; efficiency stayed high once more.

These scientists then studied the effect of the different breakfasts on the well-being of the volunteers throughout the afternoon. Persons who had eaten the different breakfasts were given lunch: a cream cheese sandwich on whole-wheat bread and a glass of whole milk. Blood samples were taken at hourly intervals. In all cases the blood sugar increased soon after lunch. Persons who had eaten eggs or fortified milk for breakfast showed a high blood sugar all afternoon. When the breakfast allowed blood sugar to be low during the morning, the increase after lunch rose to the level of cheerfulness and efficiency for only a few minutes; then it fell to a low level which lasted throughout the afternoon. Your selection of food at breakfast, therefore, can prevent or produce fatigue throughout the day.

A similar study was made at Harvard University by Doctor Thorn[2] and co-workers who determined blood sugar levels for six hours after meals high in carbohydrate (sugar and starch), fat, or protein. A high-carbohydrate breakfast consisted of orange juice, bacon, toast, jelly, a packaged cereal and coffee, both with sugar and milk. The blood sugar rose rapidly but fell to an extremely low level, causing

[2] G. W. Thorn, J. T. Quinby, and M. Clinton, Jr., "A Comparison of the Metabolic Effects of Isocaloric Meals of Varying Compositions with Special Reference to the Prevention of Postprandial Hypoglycemic Symptoms," Annals of Internal Medicine, XVIII (1943), 913.

fatigue and inefficiency. A packaged cereal eaten only with whipping cream formed the high-fat breakfast, after which the blood sugar increased slightly, then remained at the fasting level throughout the morning. The high-protein meal consisted of skim milk, lean ground beef, and cottage cheese; the blood sugar rose slowly to the high level of 120 milligrams and remained there throughout the entire following six hours. To determine the effect of different types of food on energy production, metabolism tests were taken at frequent intervals. The metabolism, or energy production, increased only slightly after the meals high in fat or carbohydrate. After the high-protein meal, however, the metabolism rose more quickly than did the blood sugar and stayed high throughout the entire six-hour study period.

Studies similar to these have been conducted in many universities. The results have been consistently the same: well-being and the level of efficiency experienced during the hours after meals depend upon the amount of protein eaten; the meals which produced a real zest for living also contained some fat and a certain amount of carbohydrate. It is only when there is a combination of sugar, which is the source of energy, and protein and fat, which slow digestion, that sugar is gradually absorbed into the blood, and energy is maintained at a high level for many hours.

The sources of sugar and starch in our American diet are cheap and overabundant; proteins are expensive and scarce. Typical American breakfasts, therefore, consist of fruit or juice supplying natural sugar, cereals, hotcakes, waffles, coffee cake, toast, or other starch quickly changed into sugar during digestion; usually refined sugar is added to cereal and coffee; jam or jelly may be eaten; quantities of sugar pour rapidly into the blood. In a matter of minutes the blood sugar may increase from 80 to 155 milligrams. Any rapid increase stimulates the healthy pancreas into pouring forth insulin; the insulin, in turn, causes the liver and muscles to withdraw sugar and store it as a form of starch, or glycogen, or change it into fat, thus preventing it from being lost in the urine. As the digestion of a high-carbohydrate meal continues, however, sugar keeps pouring into the blood. In effect, it calls to the pancreas, "Send more insulin! More! More!" The pancreas obeys; it is overstimulated; because of its efficiency, it sends too much. The tremendous amounts of sugar defeat the purpose for which sugar is needed: to produce energy efficiently. Too much sugar is withdrawn due to the oversupply of insulin; the result, ironically, is fatigue. The more carbohydrate eaten, the greater the insulin oversupply. For example, in the studies mentioned, the largest amount of sugar was freed during the digestion of the breakfast containing oatmeal.

When three high-carbohydrate meals are eaten daily, the pancreas becomes overefficient, or trigger-happy; too much insulin is produced too quickly. Persons eating such meals often produce actual insulin shock in themselves. This fact is emphasized by a diabetic specialist[3] who observed insulin-shock symptoms among his non-diabetic patients. Since American meals are largely carbohydrate, self-produced insulin shock is probably much more common than is realized. The same symptoms, however, can occur whenever the blood sugar drops far below normal because no food has been eaten and/or because exercise has used up the available sugar.

The cells can store only a little glycogen; any remaining sugar is changed into fat. After digestion is completed, however, the only normal source of sugar is stored glycogen, which is broken down into sugar again; this sugar is soon used up, especially if vigorous exercise is taken. Most of the cells then burn fat alone to supply energy, but fat is not burned efficiently without sugar; it leaves "clinkers" or "ashes" in the form of acetone and two acids, all somewhat harmful to the body. Energy ebbs, and damage is done by the acids. The brain and nerves, however, must have sugar to sustain life; the adrenals send out cortisone, and cells are destroyed so that their protein can be converted in part to sugar. Bad eating habits thus force the nervous system to become a parasite, living off other body tissues. If you allow this destruction to happen often, you will not like the sags and bags you see in your mirror.

On the other hand, if breakfast has supplied a small amount of sugar and fat and moderate protein, digestion takes place slowly; sugar trickles into the blood, giving a sustained pickup hour after hour. Insulin production is not overstimulated. Glycogen storage proceeds normally; no hated fat is formed. Energy urges the body into activity; warmth is produced as needed, or the cooling system functions with equal efficiency if the weather is hot.

Proteins are measured in grams. For example, an egg supplies 6 grams of protein; a quart of whole milk, 32 grams (see table, p. 40). In the studies mentioned, efficiency for three hours after a meal was produced only when 22

[3] E. M. Abrahamson and A. W. Pezet, *Body, Mind, and Sugar* (Henry Holt and Company, 1951).

grams or more of protein were obtained. The meal furnishing 55 grams of protein sustained a high level of energy and a high metabolism for six hours afterward. It now appears that the more protein eaten at any meal, the greater is the efficiency and the longer it is maintained. Lunches and dinners must also supply high protein with some fat and carbohydrate if well-being is to be sustained for hours after the meals. Further studies show that blood sugar levels are lower during hot weather, when little protein is eaten, than in winter, when sharp winds whet the appetite.

Another means of maintaining a high blood sugar level, now studied extensively, is to eat between meals. The objections to this procedure are that nutritious foods are frequently unavailable and non-nutritious ones too readily available. Also people often gain too much. The mid-meals found most effective[4] contain protein, fat, and carbohydrate; of mid-meals studied so far, a glass of whole milk with 100 calories of fresh fruit has produced the greatest efficiency.

If we now consider typical American meals with a critical eye, we see innocent stupidity elevated to an art. Breakfast may supply too little sugar to maintain the blood sugar level or so much sugar that insulin is oversupplied. Lunches are usually sketchy; mid-meals, if taken, are usually coffee, soft drinks, or sweets; thus is inefficiency produced until dinner time. Protein is eaten at dinner but, alas, efficiency does not always follow. The accumulation of the day's fatigue may be too great unless masked by alcohol and/or coffee; so much food may be eaten that drowsiness is induced. The husband may snore in his chair while his wife reflects bitterly that their marriage has gone to pot. If it is a social evening, the time is often passed in desultory, boring conversation. By bedtime, the acetone bodies have been excreted, and the food is largely digested; efficiency is then produced and slept off much as a drunkard sleeps off a binge.

There is nothing new about high-protein breakfasts. For morning meals on our Indiana farm when I was a youngster, we had hot cereal, steaks, ham and/or eggs, huge patties of sausage or fried chicken with country gravy; a large pitcher of milk was regularly on the table. Remember the English novels where buffet breakfasts of fish, meats, eggs, hot cereals, and creamed dishes were described? A friend returning from the Scandinavian countries recently told of

[4] H. W. Haggard and L. A. Greenberg, "Between Meal Feeding in Industry: Effects on Absenteeism and Attitude of Clerical Employees," *Journal of the American Dietetic Association*, XV (1939), 435.

having a smörgasbord with thirty kinds of fish, cheese, and meats served at breakfast. Actually, breakfasts need not be large.

You may say you are not hungry in the morning; this remark means, "I overate last night." Hunger sets in only when the blood sugar drops to about 70 milligrams; 12 hours after a typical American dinner the blood sugar is usually 95 milligrams or even higher. To launch a campaign of efficiency, the best technique is to have a mid-meal in the late afternoon. Dinner should be simple and graciously served: a soup or salad so delicious that everyone wants a second helping, meat or meat substitute, perhaps a low-starch vegetable, milk, buttermilk, or yogurt, and fruit. Appetites can be satisfied and the meal enjoyed without potatoes, gravy, and dessert, provided the afternoon snack is sufficient. Such a meal is easy to prepare, creates less havoc in the kitchen, and allows you eagerness for breakfast the next morning. The objection to small dinners is that husbands have no time to eat a large meal in the morning or at noon. Why eat a large meal at any time? All meals should be simple, filling, and enjoyable. When hungry, one always finds time to eat. I have yet to meet a red-blooded man who did not enjoy a high-protein breakfast.

Many of our national problems can be traced directly to our faulty eating habits. For example, a third of our population is obese; missing breakfast aggravates this problem. Ninety-eight per cent of Americans have tooth decay caused by eating too much sugar; the craving for sweets disappears when the blood sugar is kept high. Lassitude, fatigue, nervousness, irritability, even exhaustion and foggy thinking are widespread indeed. Prevention or remedy are easy; for the essentially healthy person, fatigue can be changed to amazing vitality in a single day. Schoolchildren are difficult to handle and often learn slowly; thus much school-tax money is wasted. Confused thinking in political, public, and private life is all too common. The greater number of automobile accidents occur when the blood sugar is lowest, when thinking is confused and reactions are slow. Our excessive use of coffee, cigarettes, and alcohol is related to our level of blood sugar; they stimulate the production of adrenal hormones which cause the blood sugar to be increased, thereby producing the needed "lift," but insulin is quickly secreted, causing the sugar level to fall again. Irritability resulting from low blood sugar can be a factor in divorces. It now appears that virus infections are usually contracted when the blood sugar is particularly low. Summer heat decreases the appetite for proteins and increases the craving for sugar-filled iced drinks and ice cream; exercise, such as swimming, uses up the sugar available; hot-weather fatigue and crankiness follow.

Blackouts or near-blackouts resulting from low blood sugar are not unusual. For example, I was consulted by a woman who blacked out almost every time she went shopping; on each "dollar day" she came to in the nurse's office of some department store. Her meals customarily were largely carbohydrate. She hated breakfast; when she became hungry, she bought a pound or more of candy and ate it on the spot; approximately an hour later she blacked out. Another example was a student too psychologically upset to eat; for a short period she blacked out many times daily and had to drop college. She had had so many accidents and near-accidents that only her friends were driving her new Buick convertible. Still another was a motorman on a streamliner who had blacked out on the job and had become so frightened that he had taken sick leave; he had been eating huge meals almost entirely of carbohydrate. Persons who have blacked out usually know when to expect a recurrence by the pounding of their hearts; several tell me that at such times they have parked their cars only in the nick of time. My advice is that if you value your car and/or your life, you should not drive when your blood sugar is low. Low-blood-sugar driving is almost as dangerous as drunken driving.

Weakness or faintness, legs giving away and/or a blackout, together with a pounding heart, cause many people to believe they are having heart attacks. Within the last few months, four men have consulted me because of "heart conditions"; three had "heart attacks" in the evening. One had been hunting all day, a packed lunch forgetfully left behind. A second owned a garage, had gone to work without breakfast, and had been too busy to stop for lunch. A third was vacationing in the mountains; he had taken a walk before breakfast, decided to climb a mountain, and had exercised all day without eating. The fourth was following a strict reducing diet; his "heart attacks" usually occurred between 3 and 7 A.M. Physicians could find nothing wrong with these men's hearts, but each man was still severely frightened when I first saw him; each was taking as good care of himself as if he were a premature baby; and the life of each family revolved around "Father's heart condition." Certainly a person experiencing such symptoms should see his physician immediately; if the physician can find nothing wrong with the heart, however, a blood sugar analysis should be requested.

As long as the adrenal glands are healthy, low blood sugar can be immediately corrected merely by avoiding coffee and by eating small but frequent high-protein meals free from refined foods. If the B vitamin pantothenic acid is undersupplied or if the adrenals are exhausted from prolonged stress, these glands cannot produce the hormones necessary to convert body starch (glycogen) into sugar; hence the blood sugar remains low until adequate nutrition restores adrenal function. Furthermore, too little potassium in the cells (p. 190) prevents glycogen from being formed, thus causing the blood sugar to remain chronically low.

When the blood sugar is extremely low, the resulting irritability, nervous tension, and mental depression are such that a person can easily go berserk. If hatred, bitterness, and resentments are harbored, and perhaps a temporary psychological upset causes a person to go on a candy binge or makes it impossible for him to eat or digest food, the stage is set; violence or quarreling can occur for which there may be no forgiving. Add a few guns, gas jets, or razor blades, and you have the stuff murders and suicides are made of. The American diet has become dangerous in many more ways than one.

Maximum well-being and efficiency can and should be produced for every hour we are awake. Your meals can be planned to give efficiency when you need it most. For example, if you are on a swing shift, your meal highest in protein should be eaten before you go to work. The general rule, however, is to eat breakfast like a king, lunch like a prince, and dinner like a pauper.

CHAPTER 3

THE STUFF YOU'RE MADE OF

YOUR BODY IS LARGELY MADE OF PROTEIN: YOUR SKIN, MUS-
cles, internal organs, nails, hair, brain, and even the base of
your bones. Only when protein of excellent quality is supplied can each cell function normally and keep itself in
constant repair. Since your muscles contain a greater amount
of protein than do other body structures, a glance at yourself in the mirror will give you a rough estimate of the
adequacy of your protein intake.

Strong well-nourished muscles automatically hold the
body erect. When muscles have not received the food necessary for their repair, they lose their elasticity, like old rubber
bands, and posture becomes poor. A mother who says to a
child, "Stand up straight," is complaining of her own failure
to provide nourishing food. Without conscious effort a
healthy person holds his head high, his chest out, his shoulders and abdomen flat; he has only a slight forward curve
in the center of the back. The pelvic bone is almost hori-
zontal, supporting the viscera in the way a large salad bowl
holds its contents; the feet have well-defined arches; the step
is rhythmical.

It is almost unbelievable how quickly faulty posture can
improve. Not long ago I planned a nutritional regime for
a sixty-eight-year-old woman. A few weeks later she told me
that for the first time in her life it was easy for her to hold
herself erect; as a young girl her shoulders were so rounded
that she had begged her mother to buy her a brace. It had
always been impossible for her to hold herself erect except
for a few strained moments, but at last her desire had been
achieved. Another case which I found astonishing was that
of a three-year-old boy: his chest was sunken; he had an
enormous pot belly and feet as flat as a tabletop. Three
months later this child had a high chest, beautifully arched

29

feet, and a total absence of protruding abdomen. The rarity of good posture and a rhythmical, graceful stride tells of our widespread protein deficiency.

Since hair and nails are made of protein, this nutrient must be adequate to maintain their health. Like the muscles, hair which lacks elasticity and resiliency and perhaps breaks or refuses to take a permanent will often change to healthy hair after a few weeks of improved nutrition. Nails which break, peel, or crack can likewise change when the diet is improved.

Advantages of an adequate protein intake are that energy is readily produced and sustained, and life is made easier. Although a major cause of fatigue is low blood sugar, there are other causes resulting from protein deficiency which are less quickly corrected: low blood pressure, anemia, and the body's inability to produce the enzymes necessary for the breakdown of foods into energy.

Blood pressure means the push or force of the blood against the walls of the blood vessels. Only when the tissues of the vessel walls are strong can the blood pressure be maintained at its normal level. If these tissues become flabby and weak, they expand, making more room in the vessels. Since the volume of blood remains the same, the blood presses with decreased force against the walls; less blood plasma, carrying all nutrients, is pushed into the tissues. Adequate supplies fail to reach the cells; thus fatigue results. Since relaxation is greatest during the night, the person with low blood pressure finds that he is especially exhausted in the early morning; getting out of bed is a chore, and he is usually irritable and sluggish until his blood pressure has been increased by the stimulus of strong coffee. After a diet has been made adequate, however, low blood pressure usually becomes normal in one to three weeks.

Another cause of fatigue, particularly common among women and children, is anemia, or lack of red corpuscles, which are made almost wholly of protein. Without adequate protein anemia quickly results and persists until the nutrition is made normal. Anemia, however, can result from any number of nutritional inadequacies.

All energy is produced by means of enzymes, organic substances whose principal component is protein. Vitamins are important only because they form part of certain enzymes. When protein is inadequate, however, none of the enzymes can be formed in adequate quantities. Fatigue is only one of many abnormalities which result.

If protein is abundantly supplied and the diet is otherwise

adequate, we can expect high resistance to diseases and infections. Although there are many mechanisms which help to protect the body against infections, two are particularly dependent upon the protein intake: antibodies and white blood cells. Under normal circumstances, the liver produces proteins known as gamma globulins, or antibodies, whose purpose it is to combine with and make harmless various bacteria, bacterial toxins, and presumably viruses. Studies of persons suffering from almost every type of infection, bacterial or viral, show that the gamma globulins of the blood are undersupplied. These globulins might be thought of as a militia guarding your health.

Within recent years, it has become medical practice to take blood globulins from the plasma of healthy persons who have built up immunity and to inject these globulins into malnourished persons; such a treatment has been widely publicized as a means of preventing colds. If your nutrition is adequate, your body can produce all the antibodies it needs and more, but that simple fact is not given publicity. Experimental work has shown that when a low-protein diet is replaced by one high in adequate proteins, the antibody production is increased a hundredfold within a single week.

Another marvelous mechanism which helps to protect our bodies from infections is the production of cells known as phagocytes. *Phago* means to eat; *cyte* means cell. Some of these white blood cells circulate in the lymph and blood. Other phagocytes are stationary and remain in the walls of the blood vessels, in the tiny air sacs of the lungs, and in other tissues where they, like the antibodies, stand constant guard. When bacteria invade the body, the phagocytes mobilize, surround the enemies, and digest them. These valuable cannibals are made of protein and are produced in adequate amounts only when proteins of high quality are obtained in the diet.

Adequate protein is also necessary to maintain normal digestion. Since enzymes, necessary to change food into particles which can dissolve in water and pass into the blood, are made of protein, the stomach, small intestine, and pancreas can pour out enzymes only when adequate protein is supplied. The walls of the stomach and intestine are muscular and, like other muscles, contract and relax alternately, thus mixing foods with digestive juices and enzymes and bringing already digested food into contact with the intestinal wall, where it may pass into the blood. Furthermore, the entire digestive system must be held in a normal position to work efficiently. When proteins are undersupplied, muscular walls and ligaments become flabby, and the "internal posture" suffers: the stomach may sag; the transverse bowel, or colon, may coil in snake-like fashion on the pelvic bone; the uterus or urinary bladder may be tipped; and other internal organs may be displaced. The flabby muscles of intestinal walls no longer contract normally; much food remains undigested. This food, on reaching the large bowel, supports the growth of billions of putrefactive bacteria; gas formation and flatulence result. Because flabby muscles are unable to push waste material from the body normally, constipation often occurs. Laxatives or cathartics may be used, causing food to be forced through the body before the protein it contains can be digested; or enemas may be resorted to, which further break down the worn muscles. Only when the protein intake is entirely adequate does digestion become normal again.

Proteins help to prevent the body fluids from becoming too acid or alkaline; they can combine with and neutralize either acid or alkaline substances. They are the raw material from which most of the hormones are made. Proteins are also necessary in helping blood to clot. They have almost endless other functions without which life would be impossible.

In still another particular way proteins are immensely important in regulating body processes. A protein known as albumin, produced by the liver provided all the building stones are furnished by the diet, makes urine collection possible. As the blood cruises through the capillary beds, the force of the blood pressure pushes the plasma into the tissues; when the blood thus becomes concentrated, the protein albumin attracts fluids from the cells back into the blood. In these fluids are dissolved the waste materials, urea, uric acid, carbon dioxide, and others from the breakdown of tissues within the cells. These wastes are then carried to the kidneys and lungs.

When the diet is so inadequate that sufficient albumin cannot be formed, waste materials are not completely removed from the tissues. Many weeks or months of mild protein deficiency may occur without the accumulated water becoming noticeable; such a person merely thinks he is overweight and often tries to reduce by cutting down still further his protein intake. If the deficiency becomes more severe, the tissues are noticeably puffy, and the entire body is waterlogged. The ankles swell, especially toward the end of the day; swollen face and hands and puffy bags under the eyes are evident in the morning.

This condition is extremely common in persons of all ages. For example, most reducing diets are now fairly high in protein. It is not unusual for a person staying on 1,000 calories a day to lose 8 or 10 pounds during the first week; 3 pounds of this loss may be fat, and the remainder is usually water held because of previous faulty urine collection. Not long ago a young woman for whom I had planned a reducing diet lost 18 pounds the first week. Two women who came with legs and ankles badly swollen from waste-laden liquids lost 18 and 24 pounds respectively in two months, although neither was given a reducing diet.

Unfortunately, water held in the tissues gives the appearance of chubbiness often associated with health, especially in children; thus this abnormal condition may be looked upon as advantageous. Studies of youngsters suffering from pneumonia and other diseases show that the blood proteins, both the albumin and the globulins, or antibodies, are low and have been low long before the onset of the disease. Children entering the hospital with diarrhea or various infections or diseases are frequently so waterlogged that they appear to be fat; when a diet high in protein is given them and normal urine collection is resumed, they can be seen to be extremely emaciated.

It is my belief that only when the role of protein in building and maintaining health is understood will persons make the effort to select food with sufficient care to promote health.

CHAPTER 4

ONE TRICK IN STAYING YOUNG

WHEN ALL PARTS OF THE BODY ARE MAINTAINED BY THE absorption and utilization of adequate food, health and youthfulness are likewise maintained. Conversely, you grow old on the days your diet is inadequate. Since your body structure is largely protein, an undersupply can bring about aging with depressing speed.

The bodies of animals, like our own, are composed largely of protein; meats, fish, and fowl, therefore, are excellent food sources. Other superior sources are eggs, fresh milk, buttermilk, yogurt, powdered milk, cheese, soybeans, and powdered yeast. Nuts, beans, peas, and grains are fair sources. Plants can synthesize their own proteins; we cannot because certain parts of this substance cannot be made in the body.

Proteins are made of amino acids, all containing nitrogen, which other foods lack. Twenty-two different amino acids are known. Just as thousands of words are made from the 26 letters of our alphabet, so are thousands of proteins made from different combinations of amino acids. Not only do the proteins in milk differ from those in soybeans, but the proteins in all parts of your body vary because of different combinations of amino acids which form them. Each protein may contain a combination of several thousand individual amino acids and is thus as complex as would be a word of thousands of letters (heaven forbid).

When proteins are eaten, the digestive processes of a healthy person break them down into amino acids, which pass into the blood and are carried throughout the body. The cells select the amino acids they need and use them in constructing new body tissue and such vital substances as antibodies, hormones, enzymes, and blood cells.

Every instant of life, body proteins are being broken

down by enzymes in your cells, and if your health is to be maintained, amino acids must be available for immediate replacement. Since the waste products are excreted by the kidneys, the urine can be analyzed for nitrogen, which comes only from proteins; the quantity of nitrogen found in the urine shows the amount of body tissue being replaced at any given time. If your diet is adequate, the cells, by the help of enzymes, combine fresh amino acids into new proteins. Food proteins, therefore, are needed continuously from birth until death. If your diet is complete in other respects, you can maintain health whenever all the required amino acids are generously supplied.

When you eat more protein than your body can use immediately, your liver withdraws amino acids from your blood and changes them temporarily into storage protein. As your cells use amino acids, the supply is replenished from the breakdown of stored protein. As long as your diet is adequate, the amount of amino acids in your blood is thereby kept relatively constant. If you ignore your health to the extent of eating insufficient protein, the stored protein is quickly exhausted. From that time on, the less important body tissues are destroyed to free amino acids needed to rebuild more vital structures. Such a process may go on month after month or even year after year. Your body continues to function after a fashion. Unseen abnormalities set in because blood proteins, hormones, enzymes, and antibodies can no longer be formed in amounts needed. Muscles lose tone; wrinkles appear; aging creeps on; and you, my dear, are going to pot.

On the other hand, it is possible, although not probable, that you may eat more protein than your body needs. After the storage depots are filled, the leftover protein is changed by the liver into glucose and fat, the nitrogen portion being excreted in the urine; the sugar and fat may be used immediately to produce energy or may be stored as fat. Proteins are also used to produce energy whenever too few other foods are eaten to meet the calorie requirements, a situation which rarely occurs for the simple reason that protein foods are too expensive to be eaten exclusively.

Most of the 22 amino acids are needed in forming every tissue in the body. All but eight of these acids, however, can be made by the cells from fat or sugar combined with the nitrogen freed from the breakdown of used proteins. The eight which the body cannot make are spoken of as the essential amino acids, a misleading term because all amino acids are essential to health even though it is not essential that 14 of them be obtained from food. These so-called essential amino acids, however, must be supplied in the diet if health is to be maintained; each of them is as important as is any vitamin.

Physicians now use separate amino acids in the treatment of certain disease conditions; since the names frequently appear in the lay press, you should be sufficiently familiar with them to recognize them as amino acids. The ones which cannot be made in the body are tryptophane, lysine, methionine, phenylalanine, threonine, valine, leucine, and isoleucine.[1] Children usually cannot make enough histidine and arginine to support growth, especially during periods of stress; hence these two acids are at times essential to children. The other amino acids, which the body can make, are glycine, alanine, glutamic acid, proline, hydroxproline, aspartic acid, serine, tyrosine, cystine, hydroxyglutamic acid, norleucine, and di-iodo-tyrosine.

The value of any protein depends on the number and amount of essential amino acids it contains. Proteins containing the eight essential amino acids in generous amounts are called complete or adequate. If enough of any complete protein, such as milk, is taken alone, it can support health. A protein lacking one or more essential amino acids or supplying too little of an essential amino acid to support health is spoken of as an incomplete or inadequate protein.

Since essential amino acids are supplied in greatest abundance in egg yolk, fresh milk, liver, and kidneys, these foods have the highest protein value. Proteins from muscle meats, used in roasts, steaks, and chops, are complete but contain fewer of some essential amino acids than do glandular meats and are therefore less valuable. On the whole, animal proteins, such as meat, fish, eggs, milk, and cheese, contain more essential amino acids in greater abundance than do vegetable proteins; hence they have superior value. Of the animal proteins egg white and gelatin alone lack essential amino acids.

Proteins from brewers' yeast, certain nuts, soybeans, cottonseed, and the germ of cereals are complete proteins. The proteins of peas, lentils, most varieties of beans, and cereals and flour with the germ removed lack some of the essential amino acids; they are therefore incomplete and cannot support life alone. There are many proteins on the borderline between complete and incomplete. For example, the protein from peanuts can support growth and mainte-

[1] W. C. Rose, "Amino Acid Requirements of Man," *Federation Proceedings*, VIII (1949), 546.

nance but not reproduction. Furthermore, the amino acid lysine is harmed when the nuts are roasted or milk is treated with heat during canning or drying, thus changing the protein from a complete to an incomplete form.

If two or more incomplete proteins are eaten at the same meal, one may supply the amino acids lacking in another, and together they may make a valuable contribution to health. For example, most grains lack the amino acids lysine and threonine, whereas beans supply these acids but lack methionine; the proteins of baked beans and corn bread together could supplement each other, and the body could form complete proteins by combining the amino acids of the two. Dr. Cannon[2] has shown, however, that if half the essential amino acids are eaten at a certain time and the other half taken only one hour later, the body does not build protein from them. Formerly it was believed that if cereal and toast were eaten at breakfast, the amino acids from the digested protein would lounge about waiting for the missing amino acids to catch up, perhaps after the next meal. It appears now that the standards of the liver are so high that only complete proteins are held in storage. Since protein food is expensive, it becomes important to obtain all the amino acids at every meal to prevent their being wasted.

A tremendous amount of research is being done with both animals and humans to find the specific symptoms of ill health which occur when certain amino acids are lacking. For example, when the diet of animals or babies lacks tryptophane, methionine, or isoleucine, the liver cannot produce the blood proteins albumin and globulin (antibodies), and urine can no longer be collected normally; swelling, known as edema, and susceptibility to infections result. Methionine has been found to be particularly deficient in the diets of children with chronic rheumatic fever[3] and of women suffering from the toxemia of pregnancy.[4] In animals a lack of tryptophane or methionine causes the hair to fall out; a lack of histidine, phenylalanine, or any one of several other amino acids causes the eyes to become bloodshot and/or cataracts to form. An undersupply of arginine causes animals to become sterile and brings about

[2] Paul R. Cannon, *Recent Advances in Nutrition* (Lawrence, Kansas: University of Kansas Press, 1950).

[3] Anthony A. Albanese, "The Effects of Amino Acid Deficiencies in Man," *Journal of Clinical Nutrition*, XLIV (1952), 1.

[4] N. W. Philpot, M. Hendelman, and T. Primrose, "The Use of Methionine in Obstetrics," *American Journal of Obstetrics and Gynecology*, LVII (1949), 125.

a decrease in the formation and mobility of sperm in men,[5] whereas too little tryptophane causes the animals' testicles to degenerate (atrophy) or females to lose their young. A deficiency of methionine allows fat to be retained in the liver of both animals and humans. Only future research can give an understanding of the role each amino acid plays in building and maintaining the body. It is known, however, that all the amino acids are used together and that taking one or two alone can never build health.

Both the quality (or the number and abundance of amino acids supplied) and the quantity of proteins eaten, determined in grams per day per person, must be considered if health is to be maintained. The greatest hindrance to good health in this respect is ignorance. Many surveys of thousands of persons having enough money to eat as they choose have shown that about 60 per cent get far less protein than is adequate. Since the complete proteins most enjoyed are expensive, persons with low incomes almost invariably suffer from protein deficiency. Yet adequate protein can be obtained even when the budget is extremely limited. It is my opinion that health cannot be built until persons learn the amount of protein they need and the grams supplied by ordinary foods. You should know these quantities so thoroughly that you can estimate in a second your protein intake for the day.

The Food and Nutrition Board of the National Research Council recommends the following amounts of protein, in grams, daily:

CHILDREN				ADULTS	
Under 12 years		Over 12 years			
1-3	40	Girls 13-15	80	Men	70
4-6	50	16-20	75	Women	60
7-9	60	Boys 13-15	85	Pregnancy	85
10-12	70	16-20	100	Lactation	100

The National Research Council, however, has attempted to set up standards which they hope will be practical for our entire population, including millions of families whose income cannot buy foods necessary for optimum health. These figures, therefore, are generally considered to be too low. If you wish to maintain your attractiveness, vigor, and youthfulness as long as is humanly possible, it is probably wise to eat considerably more protein than the Board recom-

[5] L. E. Holt, Jr., and A. A. Albanese, "Observations on Amino Acid Deficiencies in Man," *Transactions of the Association of American Physicians*, LVIII (1944), 143.

mends and/or to count only the grams of adequate protein you eat. Whenever the diet has been deficient in protein for some time, an intake of 150 grams or more daily is probably advisable for a month or more. Such large amounts are also needed in the treatment of various disease conditions.

You should thoroughly familiarize yourself with the approximate quantities of protein in ordinary foods listed in the table on the following page.

There are, of course, many foods not listed in this table which supply protein but which, in my opinion, are not worth bothering with. Gelatin, for example, lacks two essential amino acids and is almost entirely lacking in three others; hence its protein value approaches nil. Similarly, many vegetable proteins are so incomplete that it is misleading to emphasize their protein content. Most cereals aside from pure germ are not only deficient in lysine and threonine but often contain almost no protein. For example, rice flakes and puffed wheat supply only one gram of poor-quality protein per cup. Prepared cereals are largely pure starch which is changed into sugar; allowing a child to eat them is like passing him the sugar bowl and saying, "Help yourself." The latter would be less troublesome and expensive.

Until a person knows enough about nutrition to estimate his daily intake by counting protein grams easily and to distinguish between complete and incomplete proteins, he almost invariably believes he consumes a far better diet than he does. Thousands of persons think they get adequate protein from one egg at breakfast and meat for dinner; their actual intake may be 26 grams or less, although their requirement is perhaps many times that amount. Since a quart of milk supplies 32 to 35 grams of protein, one usually finds that the person who drinks a quart daily has a fairly adequate protein intake, whereas the person who avoids milk is almost invariably deficient.

If milk, cheese, or eggs are disliked or unobtainable, getting adequate protein becomes a serious matter indeed. When the complete proteins of wheat germ, soybeans, brewers' yeast, and nuts are eaten, it is possible to obtain sufficient amounts of essential amino acids, provided the diet is planned with utmost care. Some of the world's leading athletes and scholars have been vegetarians. Unless a vegetarian is trained in nutrition, however, he usually becomes an unhealthy vegetarian.

Of all proteins available, the most concentrated and least

Sources of proteins	Amounts	Completeness	Grams of protein
soybean flour, low fat	1 cup	com.	60
cottonseed flour	1 cup	com.	60
whole-wheat flour	1 cup	inc.	8 to 12
white flour	1 cup	inc.	6 to 10
wheat germ	½ cup	com.	24
brewers' yeast, powdered	½ cup	com.	24
powdered skim milk			
instant	⅔ cup	com.	18
non-instant	⅔ cup	com.	35
egg	1	com.	6
milk, whole or skim, buttermilk	1 qt.	com.	32 to 35
cottage cheese	½ cup	com.	20
American or Swiss cheese	2 slices	com.	10 to 12
soybeans, cooked	½ cup	com.	20
peanut butter	2 tbsp.	inc.	9
cooked cereals	¾ cup	inc.	10 to 18
prepared cereals	1 cup	inc.	1 to 3
navy or lima beans	1 cup	inc.	6 to 8
macaroni, noodles, rice	¾ cup	inc.	3 to 4
bread or bacon	1 slice	inc.	2
nuts *	½ cup		14 to 22
meat, fish, fowl	¼ lb. or 1 serving	com.	
boned or with little bone or fat †	¼ lb.		18 to 22
with moderate bone and/or fat ‡	¼ lb.		15 to 18
with much bone and/or fat §	¼ lb.		10 to 15

* The protein in certain nuts is complete; in others incomplete.

† Such as liver, tongue, rump roast, round steak, or soup meat; roast leg of lamb; veal chops, cutlets, or stew; boned rabbit or rabbit thigh or breast of chicken or turkey; halibut and other fresh fish; fresh corned beef, canned chicken, tuna, sardines, salmon, or mackerel.

‡ Such as hamburger, rib roasts or steaks, loin steaks or stew meat; lamb chops or shoulder roast; ham or pork chops; frankfurters; heart or kidney; canned corned beef or shrimps; liver sausage and other luncheon meats; less bony pieces of rabbit, chicken, or other fowl; cod, haddock, lobster, crab, or fresh shrimps.

§ Picnic ham, link sausages, or spareribs; brains or sweetbreads; corned-beef hash; bony parts of chicken or other fowl; herring, clams, oysters, and scallops.

expensive are brewers' yeast,[6] powdered skim milk, wheat germ, soy flour, and cottonseed flour.[7] The use of these foods makes it possible to obtain protein on an extremely limited budget and can change a diet low in protein to one high in protein with little thought or effort.

To obtain too little protein is a mark of carelessness or ignorance; to obtain too much is foolish and expensive; to obtain an adequate amount is to stay young for your years.

[6] See recipe for fortified milk, pp. 219-220.
[7] Hundreds of recipes using these foods are to be found in the writer's *Let's Cook It Right* (Harcourt Brace Jovanovich, Inc., 1962).

CHAPTER 5

DO NOT UNDERESTIMATE
THE FAMILIAR

THE THING TO REMEMBER ABOUT NUTRITION IS THAT EACH nutrient is equally important. A lack of fat can—and probably does—cause as many abnormalities as a deficiency of any other nutrient. Its principal use is to supply calories, but some 35,000,000 unhappy Americans can testify that obtaining calories is not a problem.

More vitally important is the type of fat used as part of the structure of every body cell. The nerves and brain, to be normal, must be supplied with even larger amounts of certain fats and fat-like substances. The hormones of the adrenal cortex and sex glands are made of particular kinds of fat. Also important to health is fat which must be available to valuable bacteria in the intestinal tract before they can multiply. Any old fat can supply calories; only certain types of fat can serve the foregoing purposes.

When fats are eaten, they are broken down during digestion to glycerin (glycerol) and fatty acids. These acids, each differing from the other, have names, and scientists have pried into their private affairs. Even if no fat is eaten, the body can make most of these acids from sugar. But three of them the body cannot make. One, linoleic acid, is absolutely essential to life itself.[1] Another fatty acid, called arachidonic acid, can pinch-hit for linoleic acid fairly well, and still another, linolenic acid, can pinch-hit to the extent of supporting growth but not health. These three are spoken of as essential fatty acids. The bodies of persons and well-fed animals contain large amounts of linoleic acid. If ani-

[1] George O. Burr, "The Role of Fat in the Diet," in *Dietotherapy: Clinical Application of Modern Nutrition* (Philadelphia: W. B. Saunders Company, 1945), pp. 62–83.

mals are put on a diet lacking it, this fatty acid cannot be withdrawn from the tissues even when the supply in the blood falls far below normal and the deficiency becomes so severe that it causes death. One cannot carry sacks of cement from a warehouse after the cement has been used in the structure of the building. It now appears that we must have linoleic acid or one of its pinch-hitters to form the sex and adrenal hormones, valuable intestinal bacteria, and the fat-containing portion of every cell's structure.

The principal sources of essential fatty acids are natural vegetable oils. Corn, soybean, and cottonseed oils contain from 35 to 70 per cent linoleic acid,[2] whereas safflower oil furnishes 85 to 90 per cent. Margarine, hydrogenated cooking fats, animal fats, such as cream, butter, fish-liver oils, fat meats, and the fat in egg yolk, supply little. Natural lard is the richest animal source, containing 5 to 11 per cent. Since so many vegetable fats are hydrogenated and animal fats contain little unsaturated fatty acid, the only dependable sources are salad oils and mayonnaise, nuts, and unhydrogenated nut butters. Avocados, almonds, and olive oil contain little linoleic acid, coconut and palm oils none.

Fatty acids are often spoken of as chains; some are long, some short. Just as a charm bracelet may have certain links where the charms can be attached, essential fatty acids have certain links where other substances can easily be added. If oxygen is added, the fat becomes rancid; if hydrogen is added, the fat becomes more solid. The body must have these unfilled links, or unsaturated fatty acids, which can combine with other nutrients, help to transport them, and, together with them, be used in building cell structure.

When you eat more sugar and/or starch than your body needs immediately, the excess is changed into fat made up only of fatty-acid chains which cannot be added to. These chains make a compact fat, for which we who gain easily can say a hearty "Thank heavens!" The body, however, as we have seen, cannot produce the fatty acids essential to sustain health. Although sugar can be changed into fat, the fat cannot be changed back into sugar.

According to Dr. George O. Burr, former director of physiological chemistry at the University of Minnesota, rats lacking these acids drink water in excessive amounts which is held in the body. The hair of these animals soon becomes extremely dry and thin, and the skin thick, dry, scaly, and

[2] Franklin Bicknell and Frederick Prescott, *The Vitamins in Medicine* (London: William Heinemann Medical Books, Ltd., 1948), p. 790.

scurfy, especially on the face. In females, the ovaries are so damaged that ovulation, reproduction, and lactation are interfered with; males become sterile and refuse to mate. The animals develop eczema. If the deficient diet is given to the young, growth is markedly retarded. The deficiency causes early death, and on autopsy 100 per cent of the animals show damaged kidneys.

The counterpart of these abnormalities in humans has scarcely been studied. Dr. Burr and a co-worker produced eczema in themselves by staying on a diet deficient in essential fatty acids. Numerous physicians have reported eczemas being accidentally produced by low-fat diets; these skin conditions were cured when vegetable oils were given. Persons with eczemas have also been found to have abnormally small amounts of essential fatty acids in their blood.

In my opinion, deficiencies of these acids are more common than is appreciated. For example, babies are rarely given vegetable oils until old enough to eat mayonnaise. I recall a boy of three whom I first saw at eighteen months of age. His father had been an All-American football player and wanted an athletic son more than anything else in the world. Instead, this pathetic child was smaller than most one-year-old children and had been covered with severe eczema since he was three weeks old. The boy was lethargic and seemed dim-witted. A diagnosis of "allergy" had been made, and thousands of dollars had been spent seeking correction. After a few minutes' conversation with the mother, I placed the boy in a high chair and offered him a tablespoon of soybean oil. At the first taste, the child became alive as if electrified. He leaned across the tray, mouth wide open, and even a moment's delay caused him to scream for more. He must have had six or eight tablespoons of oil before his mother, fearing he would be ill, made me stop. I suggested that she give him several tablespoons every hour if he wanted it and seemed to tolerate it well. Within three days, the eczema was almost gone, and in a week his skin was beautiful. After that the child bloomed. His bone development became particularly excellent; he grew muscular and has now achieved normal size and weight. If there is one man in this world willing to die for me, it is probably this boy's father. I strongly suspect that such eczemas, appearing so soon after birth, are caused by mothers avoiding fats during pregnancy, being unaware of their need for linoleic acid.

Linoleic acid has been shown to help prevent or cure eczemas resulting from a lack of any one of several B vitamins, possibly because this fatty acid stimulates the growth

DO NOT UNDERESTIMATE THE FAMILIAR

of intestinal bacteria which can produce these vitamins. Even the stubborn eczema-like condition known as psoriasis usually disappears rapidly when salad oils and lecithin (p. 47) are added to the diet.

From cases I have seen, I believe that deficiencies of essential fatty acids are widespread; I have interviewed many persons who, though adhering to fat-free diets which otherwise appear to be fair, show abnormalities produced in animals lacking linoleic acid. For years I have been puzzled by overweight persons whose ankles, legs, and even thighs remained swollen with edema; yet their intake of adequate protein was high; when two tablespoons of salad oil were added to their daily diet, they lost pounds. Persons on seemingly adequate diets except for oil have reported increased sex interest after dietary improvement; menstrual difficulties have disappeared, and longed-for (as well as unlonged-for) conception has taken place. Only recently a Powers model who had wanted a baby for years conceived soon after oil was added to her diet, an item she had carefully avoided because her work depended on her figure. Time and again I have seen dry, lifeless hair take on a glossy luster and rough, parched, and scaly skin become soft and lovely; the only important addition to the diet was salad oil. If you pet lovers want beautiful animals, do not fail to give salad oil to your dogs, cats, and other pets.

For three reasons, eating too little fat is probably a major cause of overweight. First, many seemingly fat persons are only waterlogged; an adequate diet including salad dressing daily often causes them to lose pounds. Second, it has been proved by what is known as the respiratory quotient that when the essential fatty acids are insufficiently supplied, the body changes sugar to fat much more rapidly than is normal; Dr. Bloor points out that it would seem as if the body were speedily trying to produce the missing nutrients. This quick change makes the blood sugar plunge downward, causing you to be as starved as a wolf; the chances are that you overeat and gain weight. Third, fats are more satisfying than are any other foods. If you forego eating 100 calories of fat per meal, you usually become so hungry that you eat 500 calories of starch and/or sugar simply because you cannot resist them; unwanted pounds creep on.

A certain amount of fat is necessary to stimulate the production of bile and the fat-digesting enzyme, lipase. Only when fat enters the intestine does the gall bladder empty itself vigorously. Without fats, too little bile is formed, and the gall bladder holds its reserve bile. This faulty emptying may be a factor contributing to the formation of gall stones. If a fat-free diet is continued long, the gall bladder eventually shrivels, or atrophies. Yet vitamins A, D, E, and K, as they occur naturally, cannot be absorbed from the intestines into the blood without the presence of fat and bile. Deficiencies of these vitamins can be produced either by fat-free diets or by bile failing to reach the intestine.

Fatty acids cannot pass into the blood without first combining with bile salts. After they enter the intestinal wall, they recombine with glycerin to form neutral fats which are carried as tiny droplets in the blood and lymph. Each of the billions of body cells withdraws essential fatty acids for structural replacement and fat to be used for immediate energy. Some fat is held in the liver to be returned to the blood later as a source of energy. The remainder is stored, usually where you want it least.

A small amount of stored fat is advantageous. Fat around the kidneys supports them. A thin layer of fat under the skin protects the muscles and nerves and helps to maintain body temperature. A reserve of fat becomes a valuable source of energy during illnesses or at any time when insufficient food is eaten. Fat stored in excess is, of course, undesirable.

Mineral oil is sometimes used for frying or making salad dressing or is taken as a laxative. Since this oil cannot be digested, it is not a food. Studies have shown, however, that approximately 60 per cent of the mineral oil reaching the intestine passes into the blood. As this oil circulates through the body, vitamins A, D, E, and K are absorbed into this mineral oil, are held captive, and are later excreted in the feces; thus deficiencies of these vitamins are produced. Although the harm done by mineral oil has been known for over 40 years and medical journals have repeatedly warned physicians not to recommend it, many persons still use it as a laxative. I personally would be afraid to use this oil even in baby oils, cold creams, and other cosmetics.

Unrefined vegetable oils furnish vitamin E, whereas such animal fats as butter, cream, and egg yolk are carriers of vitamin A, and fish-liver oils supply both A and D. Animal fats also contain a cousin of the fat family known as cholesterol, which can be produced by the liver. Studies have shown that approximately 800 milligrams of cholesterol are obtained daily from a diet high in animal fat; a normal adult liver produces 3,000 milligrams or more per day. Cholesterol forms the raw material from which vitamin D, the sex and adrenal hormones, and bile salts are made. The fact that cholesterol is concentrated in such vital tissues as the brain and nerves indicates that it serves valuable unknown functions in maintaining health.

Another cousin of the fat family, lecithin, is supplied by all natural oils and by the fat of egg yolk, liver, and brains. Lecithin is an excellent source of the two B vitamins cholin and inositol; if health is to be maintained, the more fat eaten, the larger must be the intake of these two vitamins. This substance can be made in the intestinal wall provided cholin, inositol, and essential fatty acids are supplied. Lecithin appears to be a homogenizing agent capable of breaking fat and probably cholesterol into tiny particles which can pass readily into the tissues. There is evidence that coronary occlusion (p. 117) is associated with deficiencies of linoleic acid and the two B vitamins cholin and inositol, and perhaps with a lack of lecithin itself. Huge particles of cholesterol get stuck in the walls of the arteries; they might be homogenized into tiny particles if sufficient nutrients were available for the normal production of lecithin. When oils are refined or hydrogenated, lecithin is discarded.

The vitamin E supplied by unrefined vegetable oils is an antioxidant which prevents rancidity. When allowed to remain in food, vitamin E keeps oxygen from combining with and destroying carotene and vitamins A, D, and K. In the body, it still protects these vitamins from oxygen and similarly prevents the destruction of adrenal and sex hormones, thus greatly decreasing the need for oxygen. Unfortunately, oxygen quickly destroys vitamin E itself, which is completely lost when oils are refined or hydrogenated.

The eating of rancid fats can induce serious vitamin deficiencies. Vitamin E is quickly destroyed by rancidity whether in food, in the intestine, or in the blood itself. Vitamins A and K and several B vitamins can likewise be destroyed at any of these points. Your first reaction may be that you would never eat rancid fat, but if you watch for it, you may be amazed at how often slightly rancid foods are served. All of us have probably been guilty of serving slightly rancid ham, sausage, bacon, mayonnaise, or butter. The reason children so frequently dislike wheat germ is that mothers unknowingly serve it after it has become rancid. A common source of rancidity results from keeping a can of bacon drippings near the range, often week after week, and using it for sautéing. Packaged piecrust and cake mixes, potato chips, corn chips, popcorn, salted nuts, ground nuts, and similar foods, held too long in markets, are frequently rancid. The nut and popcorn dispensers in public places, kept heated to give the illusion of freshness, are potentially so dangerous that they should be removed from the market.

When fats are hydrogenated, the hydrogen is added to the unfilled chains of the essential fatty acids; thus their health-building value is destroyed. Such fats can supply calories but nothing more; they cannot become rancid; neither can they support life of bug or beast. Each year the list grows longer: margarine, hydrogenated cooking fats, processed cheeses, and now peanut butter, formerly such an excellent food for children, and even lard. If lucky, however, you can still find an occasional market where peanuts are put into a grinder, and untinkered-with peanut butter comes out before your eyes. Old-fashioned cheeses and some natural lard are still available. French dressing, mayonnaise, and salad oils appear to be the only good sources of essential fatty acids left. Oils untreated by heat and still containing some vitamin E can be purchased at health-food stores.

Since butter contains little essential fatty acid and vitamin A is added to margarine, the two may be equally valuable in most respects. Summer butter, however, if made of un-pasteurized cream, contains a vitamin known as the Wulzen factor which prevents an arthritis-like disease in animals.

Aside from obvious sources of fat, there are many more or less hidden fats: cheese, egg yolk, bacon, avocados, nuts, peanut butter and "lean" meats, fish, and fowl. No one knows the amount of fat needed by any individual; it varies with activities, size, climate, and many other factors. The person who enjoys salad dressings and whose weight is normal is likely to obtain all he needs. Persons who intentionally restrict their fat intake probably get too little of the essential fatty acids to sustain health.

The American intake of fats, mostly saturated and refined, has doubled during this century. One result has been an all-time record of heart disease, obesity, and related illnesses; and the life expectancy of American men has fallen from 11th place among nations in 1949 to 37th place in 1966. Younger and younger men are dying of heart attacks each year; and because of the tremendous amounts of greasy hamburgers and potatoes fried in hydrogenated fats consumed in the past two decades, we can soon expect such deaths to occur in the thirty- and even twenty-year-olds.

To maintain health, a few general rules should be followed: avoid hydrogenated fats such as hydrogenated peanut butter, processed cheeses, and solid cooking fats and the French-fried foods cooked in these solid fats; limit the solid, or saturated, animal fats obtained mostly from beef and lamb and increase your intake of fish and fowl having less saturated fat; eat no food containing coconut or palm oils, both saturated vegetable fats used in imitation cream, filled milk, and even infant formulas; have at least one to three teaspoons of vegetable oil daily. Use unrefined, or cold-pressed, oils and keep them refrigerated after they have been opened. If a fat is treated so that it cannot become rancid, do not buy it; if any fat does become rancid, throw it away.

CHAPTER 6

CAN WE PREVENT BEING DELUGED?

I WAS RECENTLY TAKEN TO A FAMOUS RESTAURANT IN A CITY famous for its restaurants. The meal consisted of salad, steak, potatoes, lima beans, hot biscuits, honey, coffee, and a choice of French pastries. The salad was small. The steak would have been flattered by an estimated 15 grams of protein; it was perched on toast to give a misleading elevation. A deluge of sugar was supplied by the starch from potatoes, toast, lima beans, biscuits, pastry, and the sugar itself of the honey and dessert; one might have added more to coffee. Our group planned to work during the evening; yet no one could be on the beam after such a meal. Three of us trained in nutrition ate the steak and salad, nibbled at the other food, and ordered a glass of milk each.

Our American diet has become largely one of sugar. To me it seems that the survival of every person unaware of nutrition is at stake: caught in this tide, the innocent victim is flooded by waves of sugar every time he entertains or is entertained, every time he eats at a restaurant, and often at every home meal and mid-meal. Sugar is an essential nutrient just as is water, but an ocean is too much. This situation is not usually realized because many sugars are hidden. Persons may consume one or even two cups of sugar daily and still believe they have eaten "no sugar at all."

Besides the obvious sugar added to such foods as cereals, coffee, and fruits or consumed in candy, jam, or jellies, as much as one or two tablespoons or more of granulated sugar is obtained in each small glass of fruit ades, ginger ale, cola drinks, cider, Manhattans, and highballs; every serving of cake, pie, gelatin dessert, ice cream, pudding, custard, or canned fruit with juice; or even a single cookie.

Almost every food we eat supplies natural sugar or potential sugar in one form or another. For example, all fruits contain fructose, or fruit sugar; sucrose, or ordinary table sugar; and glucose, the type of sugar in blood. Honey and the solid part of grapes are almost entirely fructose and glucose. These sugars are also found in sweet potatoes, fresh corn, beets, onions, and other vegetables. Dates contain 78 per cent sugar, and raisins 64 per cent, whereas a chocolate bar may be only 54 per cent; the sugar in dried fruits adheres to the teeth more than the sugar in candy and therefore may cause them to decay more quickly.

Glucose and fructose both pass into the blood unchanged and can even be absorbed through the stomach wall. The sugar from orange juice, for example, when taken at breakfast, reaches the blood within three or four minutes after it is swallowed. There are two other sugars, galactose and mannose, which pass into the blood unchanged but which must be converted into glycogen before they can be used for energy.

The most valuable sugar is lactose, which occurs only in milk. It digests less readily than other sugars and apparently sometimes not at all; for this reason lactose is not fattening. If absorbed, it is first broken down into glucose and galactose. Babies fed breast milk are rarely fat, whereas infants given formulas containing an equal amount of other sugar often become flabby butterballs. Powdered skim milk is 56 per cent lactose; powdered whey, about 95 per cent. Lactose serves as food for valuable intestinal bacteria, which change it into lactic acid. Too much milk sugar, however, can be harmful to persons who eat no fat (p. 94).

Ordinary table sugar, sucrose, occurs naturally in many fruits and vegetables, such as apples, pineapples, carrots, and peas. The sugar in maple and cane syrups and molasses is largely sucrose. Commercial sugar has at times been prepared from apples, grapes, ordinary beets, and a number of other foods. The overcooked substance amusingly known as "raw sugar" is sucrose together with a few molecules of iron and other minerals. It has all the disadvantages of refined sugar in that it can cause tooth decay, overstimulate insulin flow, and ruin appetites. Perhaps it builds mental health by instilling a sense of virtue in its users, but I personally prefer the first-to-thine-own-self-be-true philosophy.

During digestion, table sugar is changed into glucose and fructose. A similar sugar, maltose, is obtained from malt. During the digestion of starch, maltose is formed momentarily in the intestine and broken down still further to glucose.

Starch is our major source of hidden sugar. Ample starch to meet our needs could be obtained from fresh fruits and vegetables such as bananas, apples, corn, peas, lima beans, yams, potatoes, and squashes. Instead we are deluged at almost every meal by sugar coming from cheap, starchy foods: refined cereals, breads, and every variety of breadstuffs; macaroni, noodles, or spaghetti; dried beans, lentils, peas, rice, or tapioca; and cake, pies, cookies, and other varieties of pastry. If you doubt that such starches can deluge you, try eating at a school cafeteria for a few weeks and see how vigorous you feel. In case you wish to curtail your sugar intake, visualize all refined starchy foods as servings of sugar.

There are still other sources of sugar. Since animals store sugar as the starch glycogen, we obtain sugar in this form from liver and other meats, fish, scallops, and abalone. Like any starch, glycogen is changed into glucose during digestion. All fats are approximately 10 per cent glycerin, which can be converted into sugar in the body. Citric acid from orange juice, lactic acid from buttermilk, and malic acid from apples can be changed into glycogen in the body and later used as sugar.

For some reason not fully understood, glucose, a sugar in honey and many fresh fruits, appears to be less harmful than table sugar, or sucrose. When volunteers were kept on an adequate but chemically pure diet in which glucose was the sole source of calories, the blood cholesterols fell to an average of 140 milligrams. Later ordinary table sugar was given instead of glucose; although no other change was made in the diet, the blood cholesterols quickly soared to the danger zone. Many investigators believe that eating too much refined sugar rather than solid or saturated fats causes problems from cholesterol deposits.

Sugar is a body requirement equal in importance to any other, but if health is to be achieved, sugar should be obtained from unrefined, natural sources. Even then it has only one purpose: to be used to produce energy when a supply of energy is demanded. Otherwise it may be stored as fat for the duration of your life. It cannot build body tissue or improve general health and attractiveness.

CHAPTER 7

WHICH APRICOT?
GROWN WHERE?

ONE COULD DEFINE VITAMINS AS CHEMICALS ESSENTIAL FOR the normal function of cells. Usually they cannot be made by the body. Vitamin A is a colorless substance found only in animal foods. It is formed in the animal or human body from a yellow pigment, carotene, found in carrots, apricots, yams, all green vegetables, green pasture crops, and seaweeds, the quantity roughly paralleling the intensity of the color. We get vitamin A itself from such animal foods as liver and fish-liver oils; egg yolks, butter, and cream supply both carotene and vitamin A.

Mild deficiencies of vitamin A are so common that you have probably experienced them. A slight deficiency impairs vision. A substance containing vitamin A, visual purple, is formed in the eyes; any light reaching the eyes breaks down part of the visual purple, and the products of this purposeful breakdown set up nerve impulses which tell the brain what the eyes see. More visual purple is formed and again destroyed. This cycle of regeneration and breakdown continues through life. Vitamin A is therefore somewhat like the film in a camera in that it photographs what you see but the "film" is used up.

Both day vision and night vision require vitamin A, but night vision depends on the vitamin-A mechanism entirely; therefore a subtle vitamin-A deficiency first causes difficulty in seeing in the dark. You can test your vitamin-A adequacy any time you drive at night. The lights of on-coming cars destroy vitamin A in your eyes; if your ocular fluid contains ample vitamin, you can see again almost immediately; if you are deficient, you will be blinded, the length of time depending on the severity of your deficiency. Tests have

shown that persons having auto accidents at night are patho-
logically deficient in this vitamin. When better lighting of
highways results in fewer accidents, it is because day vision
rather than night vision is used and vitamin A is less relied
upon.

There are varying degrees of night blindness. The person
with a mild deficiency believes his vision to be normal but
sees more efficiently in daylight. With a slightly greater deficiency, he experiences eye fatigue after watching television, for example, but he usually assumes that others have
similar difficulty. If his need for vitamin A is still greater,
he may suffer pain in his eyes, especially after long use, and
experience nervousness, headaches, and visual fatigue. A
severe deficiency can cause such discomfort and eyestrain
that he may refuse to drive at night.

Such a person is sensitive to bright light during the day
and feels more comfortable wearing dark glasses; thus less
light reaches his eyes and less vitamin is destroyed. The majority of people who wear dark glasses eat too little vitamin
A to allow normal vision. I recently interviewed a woman
whose eyes were so sensitive to light that she wore dark
glasses even in the house; a month after dietary improvement
she experienced no discomfort in intense sunlight.

People who work in bright light, which destroys vitamin
A quickly, or dim light, which requires night vision entirely,
use relatively more vitamin A than do persons working in
moderate light. Typists and bookkeepers who face the glare
of light on white paper frequently suffer from eyestrain preventable by diets richer in vitamin A; persons who sew, read,
or watch television a great deal, miners working in dim light,
welders facing flashing fire, photographers working both
with bright lights and in darkrooms, and people living on
the desert or beach, where the sunlight is reflected by white
sand, often have visual difficulties because their need for
vitamin A is unusually great. Perhaps no glare is so destructive to the vitamin A in the eyes as sunlight on clean
snow; trappers, hunters, and skiers are often too familiar
with this vitamin deficiency.

When the lack becomes severe, burning, itching, and inflamed eyelids, eyestrain, perhaps severe pain in the eyeballs
themselves or frequently occurring sties are experienced in
addition to nervousness and exhaustion. Mucus may accumulate in the corners of the eyes; ulcers or sores sometimes
appear on the covering of the eye, or cornea. Severe deficiencies of this vitamin have been thought to occur only in
such countries as India or China, but a survey of low-income

families in New York City[1] revealed corneal ulcers in almost half of the cases studied.

Although eye symptoms may be the first to be noticed in a mild vitamin-A deficiency, even earlier changes take place in the skin. Cells in the lower layers of skin die and slough off. They plug the oil sacs and pores, thus preventing oil from reaching the surface; the skin may become so dry and rough that the entire body sometimes itches. The pores plugged with dead cells cause the skin to have the appearance of "goose pimples" although they are unaffected by temperature changes. This roughness usually occurs first on the elbows, knees, buttocks, and back of the upper arm. Pores enlarged by an accumulation of dead cells and oil are spoken of as whiteheads or blackheads. If these cells become infected, pimples may result. The skin is likewise susceptible to such infections as impetigo, boils, and carbuncles. These abnormalities can usually be corrected by increased amounts of vitamin A, provided the diet is adequate in other respects.

Through the years I have been consulted by dozens of girls whose faces are covered with pimples; often they tell me they have never had skin trouble until recently. Invariably I find they are doing office work, usually under fluorescent lights, and the continuous use of their eyes, together with the glare and reflection from white paper, has greatly increased their need for vitamin A. I can often tell them how long they have been in their jobs—approximately four months previous to the onset of the pimples.

When vitamin A is undersupplied, the hair becomes dry and lacks sheen and luster. Dandruff usually accumulates on the scalp. The nails may be affected and peel easily or become ridged.

Simultaneously with the visual difficulties and the changes in the skin, a vitamin-A deficiency allows abnormalities to occur in the tissues spoken of as mucous membranes. These tissues line the body cavities such as the throat, nose, sinuses, middle ears, lungs, the gall bladder, and the urinary bladder. If the diet is adequate in vitamin A, these membranes continuously secrete a liquid, or mucus, which covers the cells and prevents bacteria from reaching them and also cleanses the surface. Furthermore, bacteria cannot live in mucus. Worn tissues are digested by enzymes, and the wastes are removed; therefore healthy tissues contain no accumulation of dead cells. Because of substances known as antien-

[1] H. D. Kruse, "The Ocular Manifestations of Avitaminosis A," *Public Health Reports*, LVI (1941), 1301.

zymes which counteract the effect of the enzymes produced by bacteria, live cells can protect themselves from bacterial destruction. Millions of bacteria find their way to these healthy tissues but cannot reach the cells because of the mucus covering or are made ineffective by the mucus; they are offered no food and/or are rendered harmless by the antienzymes. Since they cannot get a foothold, no infection occurs.

Individuals deficient in vitamin A allow conditions ideal for bacterial growth to be set up in their bodies; bacteria can grow only when they are provided with warmth, moisture, and food. Dr. Wolbach of the Harvard School of Medicine points out that during vitamin-A deficiency the cells of the mucous membranes grow more rapidly than usual but quickly die. These cells are crowded forward by other rapidly growing cells which likewise die until there accumulates a cheesy-like surface of layer upon layer of packed, dead cells. Since dead cells cannot secrete mucus or produce antienzymes, their surface is no longer washed and their self-protective mechanisms are gone. Heat, moisture, and a continually replenished food supply combine to set up conditions ideal for bacterial growth; bacteria themselves are ever present. Infections are usually the result.

Changes in the mucous membranes occur early in the bronchial tubes and lungs, where air sacs may be completely plugged with dead cells, and in the middle ears, sinuses, kidneys, urinary bladder, and prostate gland. What has been described as an "accumulation of profuse debris" may cause irritation or obstruct narrow ducts, such as those from the salivary glands or the pancreas; the mouth may become dry; the pancreatic juices may fail to reach the intestine. Dead cells from the uterus and vagina may slough off, causing leucorrhea, often accompanied by profuse menstruation. Cysts may be formed around the accumulated dead cells in almost any part of the body.

Studies have been made of the mucous membranes of animals fed different amounts of vitamin A. It was found that harmful bacteria were always present. The animals deficient in this vitamin had millions of bacteria feeding off their dead cells, however, and 98 per cent showed infections; those fed adequate vitamin A harbored few bacteria and showed no infections. Microscopic studies of the mucous membranes of hundreds of humans dying from accidental death or infection show similar correlations; there is freedom from an accumulation of dead cells and from infections; or the number of dead cells parallels the severity of the infections. Furthermore, the liver tissue of adults meeting accidental death has been found to average 20 times more vitamin A than that of persons dying from infections or infectious diseases.

The absorption of adequate vitamin A will correct deficiency symptoms, the length of time depending on the amount of vitamin given, the severity of the deficiency, and the tissues affected. Studies have shown that improvement in mild eye symptoms has occurred in as little as one hour after 50,000 to 100,000 units of vitamin A have been given. On the other hand, when the deficiency is severe and the vitamin dosage small, normal night vision may not be recovered for weeks or even months. In correcting mild visual abnormalities, the vitamin need merely be absorbed into the blood and carried to the ocular fluid. Recovery from corneal ulcers or changes which have occurred in the skin and mucous membrane, however, means that new tissue must be grown to replace the unhealthy tissue produced during the deficiency. It has been reported that the dryness of skin has disappeared and the lubricating oils have returned in as short a time as two weeks after dietary improvement; it has been my experience, however, that a longer interval is needed for recovery.

Some years ago a physician referred to me a woman whose face was covered with hundreds of large warts. A number of reports had pointed out that warts often disappeared when the diet was made adequate in vitamin A. I therefore planned a nutrition program for her, making it as adequate in all nutrients as I possibly could, and suggested that she take 100,000 units of vitamin A daily. When her skin showed no change after four months, we both became discouraged. A week later she came to see me, greatly excited. Not a wart remained, nor has one returned since then. This case convinced me that it takes approximately four months for unhealthy tissue to be replaced by healthy tissue, although probably wide individual variations should be expected.

Aside from helping to maintain normal vision and resistance to infections, adequate vitamin A is essential to the development of bones and the tooth enamel, good appetite, normal digestion, reproduction, lactation, and the formation of both red and white blood corpuscles. It appears to delay the onset of senility and to promote longevity. Vitamin A also has a profound influence upon development before birth.[2]

The National Research Council has recommended that an adult have 5,000 units of vitamin A daily to maintain health. A table of food analysis would show that the richest sources of carotene, averaging about 12,000 units per serving (100 grams), are green leaves such as chard, kale, spinach, and other greens. Even one serving of string beans, broccoli, carrots, yellow squash, apricots, sweet potatoes, or yams would supply 5,000 units, all one supposedly needs for a day. A serving of tomatoes, peas, unbleached celery, lettuce, and asparagus averages nearly 2,000 units. Except for apricots, most yellow fruits offer little more than 400 units per serving. Vegetables which have lost their color or have never been green lack this vitamin.

Such a table would show that liver may be extremely rich in vitamin A and that kidneys and sweetbreads contain appreciable amounts. Since this vitamin is not stored in muscles, such meats as roasts, chops, and steaks lack vitamin A. Eggs and butterfat contain it, the amount depending upon the animals' food. Whole milk varies from 500 to 7,000 units per quart but usually averages 2,000 units. Most of the vitamin A may be destroyed by oxygen when milk is homogenized, although this problem appears not to have been studied. Winter butter, produced when the cows are given dry feed, may contain only 2,000 units per pound, whereas summer butter averages 12,000 units. Butter substitutes usually have 12,000 units of the vitamin added per pound.

Fish-liver oils are the richest commercial sources of vitamin A. The vitamin content of liver, however, depends on the animals' food and age. Aside from polar-bear liver, the richest source ever determined was the liver oil of a python estimated to be 100 years old when killed in a London zoo. Halibut-liver oil is richer in vitamin A than is cod-liver oil because halibut is elderly when marketed, whereas cod is a mere adolescent; the halibut has had more years to eat green sea algae. For the same reason beef and mutton liver usually contains more vitamin A than do calf and lamb liver.

Scientists as well as laymen have been led to the conclusion, from studying tables of food analysis, that we easily obtain all the vitamin A we need from foods. Surveys in which thousands of persons have kept records of foods eaten for a month or more, however, show that three-fourths of our population obtain only about 2,000 units of vitamin A

[2] Adelle Davis, *Let's Have Healthy Children*, rev. ed. (Harcourt Brace Jovanovich, Inc., 1959).

daily. In these surveys the assumption has been that all the vitamin A obtained from food is absorbed into the blood.

Unfortunately, there is many a slip between the lip and body cells. Vegetables analyzed in a laboratory perhaps grew on excellent soil and received the optimum amount of rain and sunshine; possibly they contained a hundred times more vitamin A than those grown under less ideal conditions. Carrots, for example, have been analyzed which contain no carotene whatsoever. Losses of the vitamin occur during shipping, storage, freezing, canning, and cooking. Milk from cows feeding on a luxuriant growth of alfalfa has been found to lack vitamin A; the alfalfa, when analyzed, was found to contain no vitamin E, necessary to prevent the destruction of vitamin A in the body. Furthermore, nitrates from chemical fertilizers destroy carotene and vitamin A in our growing foods, in our bodies, and in animals we use for meat.

Even if vegetables are rich in carotene, there is no insurance that it will be absorbed. The carotene in vegetable foods is held inside cell walls made of cellulose, a substance which cannot be digested by humans. Carotene cannot dissolve in water; therefore it cannot pass through these walls. Only when the cell walls have been broken by cutting, chopping, cooking, or chewing is it freed to pass into the blood. Approximately 1 per cent of the carotene from raw carrots has been found to be absorbed,[3] whereas cooking increases the absorption from 5 to 19 per cent.[4] Studies show that the absorption of carotene from most vegetables averages from 16 to 35 per cent; the softer the texture, the larger the amount of carotene which reaches the blood. Presumably all the carotene is absorbed when vegetables are liquefied or juiced, but if the juice is not drunk immediately, much of the vitamin is destroyed by oxygen.

In the small intestine, both vitamin A and carotene must combine with bile salts before they can pass into the blood. If the diet is low in fat, little or no bile reaches the intestine, and 90 per cent of both carotene and vitamin A may be lost in the feces. Not all the carotene which reaches the blood is changed into vitamin A. Unless the vitamin-E intake (p. 148) is adequate, any Vitamin A reaching the blood is destroyed, and any already stored is quickly used up. Vita-

[3] H. C. H. Graves, "The Vitamin A Value of Carotene in Vegetables," *Chemistry and Industry*, LXI (1942), 8.

[4] M. Kreula and A. I. Vitranen, "Absorption of Carotene from Carrots in Humans," *Nutrition Abstracts and Reviews*, X (1940-41), 394.

min A cannot be stored if the B vitamin cholin is under-supplied. When one considers all of these points, one wonders how people have obtained enough vitamin A to stay alive.

If you plan carefully, however, you can probably buy 50 times more vitamin A with the same amount of money this week than you did last; some of it will certainly be absorbed, and there may even be an excess for storage. Select your fruits and vegetables for their yellow or green color. Serve liver, kidneys, cheese dishes, or an egg soufflé more often than roasts, chops, and steaks. Use storage butter and eggs rather than winter products. Grow carotene-rich vegetables in your garden and freeze them for winter.

Since carotene and vitamin A dissolve in fat, and since fat can be stored in the body, this vitamin is stored, provided an excess is absorbed and not destroyed. The vitamin is stored largely in the liver; the amount can be doubled if the intake of vitamin E is adequate. This stored vitamin A can be called upon to meet your needs whenever your diet is inadequate. Experimental animals, given an excess of vitamin A, store a hundred times more than is necessary to produce all appearances of good health. Analysis of human livers indicates that the same is true of people. Animal experiments show that a generous storage of vitamin A is advantageous during both health and disease.

Amounts of vitamin A greater than 50,000 units daily can be toxic if continued for a long period and can cause headaches, blurred vision, itching skin, thinning hair, sore lips, bruising, nosebleeds, painful joints, and tenderness and swelling of the long bones. These symptoms disappear in a few days after the vitamin has been withdrawn.[5] Even when toxic doses are taken, the damage can be prevented or corrected by an increased vitamin-C intake (ref. 2, p. 43). The only natural food known to contain a toxic amount of this vitamin is polar-bear liver, but toxicity has resulted from the use of vitamin-A concentrates.

There is little if any evidence that vitamin-A deficiencies can be more quickly overcome by taking amounts larger than 100,000 units daily; much research indicates that no more than 50,000 units per day can be well utilized. The addition of vitamin E in amounts of 100 units (or milligrams) daily has been found to double the curative effect of vitamin A. Doses of vitamin A are also more effective if taken in small amounts twice or three times daily rather

[5] R. W. Hillman, *American Journal of Clinical Nutrition,* IV (1956), 603.

than at one time. The Council on Pharmacy and Chemistry of the American Medical Association[6] has approved the following therapeutic doses: 25,000 units three times daily for prolonged or chronic deficiency; 25,000 units twice daily for two months for general treatment. They have not approved any single dose larger than 25,000 units.

The amount of vitamin A needed by healthy persons varies widely with each individual. Adults require more vitamin A than do children because the vitamin is needed in proportion to body weight; men usually require more than do women. Aged persons often utilize their food less well and therefore appear to need more of most vitamins than do younger adults. The requirements also vary with intensity of light, use of eyes, season, source, amount absorbed, and intake of vitamin E. One individual may thus require two or three times more than another of the same weight and degree of health. Moreover, when the vitamin is supplied by carotene, twice as much is needed as when it is supplied by vitamin A itself. Obviously no exact rules can be laid down. Since an excess can be stored to great advantage and only massive doses are toxic, it seems wiser to err by obtaining slightly too much rather than too little.

Dr. Henry C. Sherman, when at Columbia University, carried on experiments to determine the amount of vitamin A used advantageously by animals. A certain quantity of the vitamin allowed the animals all the appearances of good health. When that quantity was doubled, tripled, and quadrupled, signs of greater health, greater resistance, and greater vigor were evident, and with each increase the life span was lengthened. Beyond that point, increases brought no further improvements. Based on these experiments, Dr. Sherman recommends 20,000 units of vitamin A daily for adults, or four times the amount which usually gives the appearance of good health.

Considering that the vitamin-A content of foods varies widely and that it is readily destroyed by nitrates from chemical fertilizers and food preservatives, I see no way by which one can be reasonably sure his vitamin-A intake is adequate without taking a supplement. I believe that recurring symptoms of vitamin-A deficiency can be expected in the majority of persons who fail to take this precaution. Any fish-liver-oil concentrate should be taken immediately after the meal containing the largest amount of fat. The

[6] Council on Foods and Nutrition, "Vitamin Deficiencies, Stigmas, Symptoms and Therapy," *Journal of the American Medical Association*, CXXXI (1946), 666.

quantity of vitamin E needed to prevent the destruction of vitamin A is not known; I have usually recommended a minimum of 100 or 200 units of vitamin E, or d-alpha tocopherol acetate, for each 25,000 units of vitamin A. For adults, I prefer capsules supplying 25,000 units of vitamin A together with 2,500 units of vitamin D, both from fish-liver oils. Because of insufficient fat, babies and small children cannot well absorb vitamins A and D from concentrates or capsules. In my opinion the best source of vitamins A and D for children is old-fashioned cod-liver oil, provided it is always refrigerated and given daily with at least 50 units of vitamin E.

Tables of food analysis cannot be accurate because foods grown on different soils and under different conditions, harvested, handled, and processed by different methods contain different amounts of nutrients. Whenever I read the statement that apricots or other foods are rich in such nutrients as vitamin A, iron, and copper, my only reaction is: Which apricot? Grown where?

CHAPTER 8

THE PAUPERS WERE BETTER OFF

THE 15 OR MORE B VITAMINS ARE SO MEAGERLY SUPPLIED IN our American diet that almost every person lacks them. Dr. Norman Jolliffe has pointed out that a few generations ago even the paupers received a diet rich in these vitamins. They were better off than the wealthiest are today.

The reasons for this drastic decrease are numerous. Formerly every bite of bread, cereal, and foods prepared from grain supplied B vitamins. Since there was no refrigeration or canning and there were few fruits and vegetables, the mainstay of the diet was breadstuffs. In 1862 machinery was invented which refined grains in such a way that most of the nutrients were discarded. Molasses, rich in certain B vitamins, was once the only sweetening. No refined foods and few sweets of any kind were available. Now the consumption of sugar has increased tremendously; all the original nutrients are discarded; it quickly destroys the appetite and greatly augments the need for certain B vitamins. Whereas no nutrients were formerly discarded, two-thirds of our calories are now supplied by foods from which the original nutrients are largely or wholly discarded. Furthermore, we lead such sedentary lives that our food intake is small compared with that of our grandparents. Seventy years ago, men consumed approximately 6,000 to 6,500 calories daily; women 4,000 to 4,500. Today the average is 2,400 to 2,800 for men and 1,800 to 2,200 for women.

The advantage of using whole-grain breads and cereals was shown during World War I, when shortages caused the Danish government to forbid the milling of grains; nutrition in Denmark was so improved that during the war years the death rate fell 34 per cent. The incidence of cancer, diabetes, high blood pressure, and heart and kidney diseases dropped markedly, and evidences of positive health greatly

63

increased. Much the same improvement occurred in England during and after World War II, when grains were only slightly milled. Although the English diet was deficient in many respects, surveys showed that the national health did not suffer during this period.

Now that our breadstuffs are refined, no food rich in the B vitamins is ordinarily eaten daily. In fact, there are only four good sources of these vitamins: liver, brewers' yeast, wheat germ, and rice polish. A few foods are high in one or two B vitamins, but to obtain our daily requirement of all of them from such foods is impossible.

A source of B vitamins perhaps more important than any other is that synthesized by valuable bacteria in the intestine; the amount from this source cannot be easily measured. Studies of B vitamins found in the blood and urine of persons on diets lacking these vitamins show that intestinal bacteria can produce large amounts of certain B vitamins, which disappear from the blood and urine if the bacteria are destroyed. For reasons not understood, other persons on a B-vitamin-deficient diet have been found to have little or none of these vitamins in their blood and urine.

It appears that these bacteria grow best on milk sugar and cannot grow unless fat is supplied them; milk-free and/or fat-free diets, therefore, may be dangerous. The taking of sulfonamides and antibiotics, such as streptomycin and aureomycin, completely destroys these valuable bacteria; symptoms of multiple B-vitamin deficiencies may quickly appear unless food which promotes the growth of desirable intestinal bacteria, such as yogurt, is eaten. This food, sometimes spoken of in America as a fad, has been eaten for centuries in countries from Turkey to Lapland, Iceland to China. A study made by Dr. Seneca[1] of the College of Physicians and Surgeons of Columbia University points out that when yogurt is eaten over a long period, no other bacteria except those from yogurt are found in the stools.

The B vitamins appear to be needed equally by every cell in the body. For example, if a well-fed animal is killed and its tissues are analyzed separately, these vitamins are found to be evenly distributed throughout the tissues. Conversely, when animals are kept on a deficient diet, then killed, and separate tissues are analyzed, each tissue is uniformly deficient. Most of the other vitamins are needed more by cer-

[1] H. Seneca, E. Henderson, and A. Collins, "Bactericidal Properties of Yogurt," *American Practitioner and Digest of Treatment*, I (1950), 1252.

tain tissues than by others. Dr. Roger J. Williams[2] has pointed out that because these vitamins are needed equally by all cells, a deficiency can produce severe damage before the condition can be noticed. The damage is nevertheless real. Instead of one organ showing abnormalities, as do the eyes during a vitamin-A deficiency, the entire body degenerates into a one-hoss-shay collapse. This overall abnormality is difficult to recognize in an adult, but severely stunted growth makes it markedly noticeable in the young.

Dr. Williams also points out that only when the deficiency becomes quite severe does one group of cells show greater damage than another. For example, when a person feels below par, he automatically decreases his activity and may spend much time sleeping; thus most of his cells do less work, and their need for B vitamins decreases. The heart, however, works continuously from birth until death; even though the deficiency is already severe and every cell has been equally damaged up to this point, the first deficiency signs may now appear in the heart.

It has become increasingly clear that since the B vitamins occur together in food, no person is deficient in any one B vitamin without being deficient in all of them. There are, however, as many degrees and variations of B-vitamin deficiencies as there are different individuals. Formerly the disease beriberi was thought to be caused by a deficiency of vitamin B_1, and pellagra by lack of the B vitamin niacin. When human volunteers have stayed on diets lacking vitamin B_1 or niacin, however, neither beriberi nor pellagra has been produced. These diseases actually result from multiple deficiencies of all the B vitamins, the lack of vitamin B_1 or niacin being only more prominent.

In a general way you can tell how adequate your intake of B vitamins has been by looking at your tongue.[3] It should be moderate in size, an even pink in color, and smooth around the edges without coating or indentations showing where it has rested against your teeth. The taste buds should be uniformly small and cover the entire surface and edges. If you can find a healthy child, you may see what the normal tongue should look like.

When the B vitamins are undersupplied, many changes take place in this organ. The first change appears to be enlargement of the buds at the front and sides of the tongue.

[2] R. J. Williams, "Chemistry and Biochemistry of Pantothenic Acid," *Advances in Enzymology,* III (1943), 253.

[3] *Clinical Nutrition,* ed. by Norman Jolliffe, F. F. Tisdall, and Paul R. Cannon (Paul B. Hoeber, Inc., 1950).

Later these buds become small or even disappear, making the tip and sides smooth, whereas the buds farther back will progressively enlarge. These buds have a flat appearance, like button mushrooms. As the deficiencies of these vitamins become more severe, clumps of taste buds fuse and grow together, pulling apart from other clumps and thus forming grooves or fissures. The first groove usually forms down the center of the tongue. In a severe B-vitamin deficiency, the tongue may be so cut by grooves and fissures that it looks like a relief map of the Grand Canyon and the surrounding territory or a flank steak run through a tenderizing machine.

When the deficiencies are still more severe, the taste buds literally disappear. First the tip and edges become smooth and shiny; then the buds disappear progressively from front to back. This extreme condition is found most often in elderly persons whose diets have been inadequate for years; they complain that their food has little flavor. In some cases such tongues are intensely sore. In other cases, persons having extremely abnormal tongues are surprised to find that they differ from normal.

The size of the tongue also indicates deficiencies of these vitamins. The tongue may be large, beefy, and full of water (edematous). Often such a tongue shows scallops around the edges where it has rested against the teeth. The beefy tongue is so named because it has the appearance of beef and is usually an intense deep red. On the other hand, it may become too small, or atrophied. Other tongues may have a purplish, or magenta, cast, and still others may be a brilliant red. Often the tongue shows a combination of colors with perhaps a red tip and magenta center. The color and texture vary depending upon which B-vitamin lack is most prominent. For example, a magenta tongue (the color seen most often) indicates that a deficiency of vitamin B_2 predominates over the other B-vitamin deficiencies. A beefy tongue is thought to show that pantothenic acid is particularly undersupplied. When deficiencies of vitamin B_{12} and folic acid are most prominent, the tongue becomes strawberry red and smooth at the tip and sides; it is often shiny and not coated. If the deficiency is predominantly the B vitamin niacin, the tongue may be fiery red at the tip and may appear to be either too small or too large and so coated that it is fuzzy with debris. The heavy coating is caused by the growth of undesirable bacteria; it usually indicates much putrefaction in the intestine. Since valuable bacteria in the intestine produce B vitamins, such coating probably never occurs if bacteria growth is normal.

I asked a professor in medical school if he thought it wise to include a description of abnormal tongues in this book; I feared that people would worry excessively about their tongues. To my amazement he answered, "You never see them anyway. I'd omit it." He does not see them because he does research, but I have examined hundreds of tongues and have found only three normal ones in two years. I still chuckle every time I remember an occasion when, lecturing before a small group, I was requested to examine the tongue of everyone present; not one normal tongue had come to the lecture. The group sat like so many panting collies, astonished at one another's deficiencies. When the diet is made adequate, however, the tongue gradually becomes normal again, the recovery time depending upon the severity of the deficiency and the completeness of absorption.

Studies indicate that 60 to 100 per cent of the persons showing severe tongue changes are unable to produce sufficient amounts of hydrochloric acid in their stomachs; their output of digestive enzymes is far below normal. In such cases, digestion is so faulty that unless tablets of hydrochloric acid and digestive enzymes are taken temporarily (p. 227), much gas, flatulence, digestive disturbances, and discomfort may be experienced. In fact, if your digestion is so faulty that you have intestinal gas after you add foods rich in the B vitamins to your diet, you can be sure you have been deficient in these vitamins.

All the B vitamins dissolve in water and for this reason cannot be stored in the body. Just as a sponge can be slightly moist or dripping wet, however, so can the cells hold little or much of each B vitamin, depending on the amount offered. To maintain ideal health, the offering of B vitamins should be sufficient for each cell to take all it can use to advantage. Any B vitamins not needed are excreted in the urine.

It appears that all B vitamins work together; this cooperation is called the synergistic action of the B vitamins. The taking of one or more B vitamins increases the need for the others not supplied, probably because any one B vitamin alone can increase the activity of each body cell. The group in its entirety can be obtained only from such foods as liver, yeast, and wheat germ.

To discuss deficiencies of the B vitamins separately is unrealistic; they exist alone only in an experimental laboratory. A deficiency of one, however, often predominates over others. If the first symptoms of that deficiency are recognized, they can serve as a warning that unless your nutrition is improved, greater deviations from health can be expected.

CHAPTER 9

IT IS ONLY AN ASSUMPTION

SO MUCH IS KNOWN OF THE B VITAMINS THAT ENTIRE volumes could be written about them. If these known facts were universally applied, the improvement in health would be beyond imagination. Yet of some of this group of a dozen or more vitamins, collectively spoken of as the B complex, relatively little is known; three of these are the antistress vitamins.

These antistress vitamins appear to be unnecessary under normal conditions or to be needed in such small amounts that they can be made in the body or perhaps by bacteria in the intestines. Even though a diet contains all previously known nutrients and is adequate to support health under normal conditions, it can still be inadequate during conditions of stress unless these antistress vitamins are supplied. Stress is anything which puts an extra load on the body. Conditions of stress are produced by drugs, chemicals, infections, surgery, noise, excessive fatigue, psychological upsets, resentments, hatreds, and hundreds of other factors. All nutrients are needed in larger amounts during stress than under normal circumstances.

When animals on seemingly adequate diets are subjected to stress, widespread damage occurs in their bodies. If these animals, however, are given fresh or dried liver or a crude liver concentrate, little harm is done. For example, when the strength of animals was tested by making them swim in ice water, the animals on "normal" diets could swim only three to ten minutes before drowning; animals given the same diet fortified with liver swam two hours or longer and lived to swim again.

If liver is given, the harmful effects of such stressor agents as atabrine, excessive thyroid, extreme heat or cold, lack of oxygen, X rays, and various drugs have been prevented or decreased. Animals subjected to stress but not given liver often die unexpectedly, apparently of heart failure,[1] although they may have all the outward appearances of good health. Liver of all varieties appears to be the richest source of the antistress vitamins; kidney, soy flour, and brewers' yeast contain some. These vitamins have not been made synthetically, therefore are never available in tablets or capsules. Much more research is needed before their true value can be known.

Several other B vitamins have been insufficiently studied. Both their distribution in foods and the amounts needed remain a mystery, and, if deficiencies occur, they are not commonly recognized.

One such vitamin is biotin, the richest source of which is yeast. Animals lacking biotin develop eczema, or dermatitis; their hair falls out; they are particularly susceptible to heart abnormalities and lung infections. If cancers are transplanted, they grow rapidly in biotin-deficient animals. Growth is extremely stunted in young animals; adults become emaciated; death comes quickly to both.

A substance in raw egg white, avidin, can combine with biotin in the intestinal tract and prevent it from reaching the blood. Biotin deficiencies have been produced in human volunteers by adequate diets to which was added daily ½ cup of powdered but uncooked egg whites. The first symptom noticed was mental depression. In time the subjects developed dry peeling skin, extreme fatigue, muscular pain, nausea, and distress around the heart. The mental depression became so intense that it was described as "panic," and some volunteers experienced suicidal tendencies. All symptoms disappeared in three to five days after biotin was added to the diet.

Such a study would indicate that biotin is a valuable nutrient and that raw eggs should be avoided. Several reports have told of men, mostly laborers who enjoyed uncooked eggs, developing severe eczema which cleared rapidly when biotin was given them and/or raw eggs withdrawn. In a still later study, however, as many as 36 fresh raw egg whites were given daily to volunteers who failed to show any abnormalities. It would appear, therefore, that a few raw eggs daily are safe to eat, provided one has no biotin-deficiency symptoms.

Another of the B vitamins assumed to be adequately sup-

[1] Benjamin H. Ershoff, "Comparative Effects of Liver and Yeast on Growth and Length of Survival of the Immature Thyroid-fed Rat," *Archives of Biochemistry*, XV (1947), 365.

plied in the diet is para amino benzoic acid, or PABA, a vitamin as essential for bacteria as it is for humans. Sulfanilamide, for example, is an effective drug only because it takes the place of PABA in the bodies of bacteria. Similarly, such drugs take the place of the vitamin in human enzymes. Because sulfa drugs can never perform the functions of the vitamin, they produce extreme fatigue, anemia, and eczema. These PABA-deficiency symptoms were often so severe that sulfanilamide was largely discontinued in favor of the less toxic antibacterial agents.

A man whom I used to see frequently suffered from a recurring eczema which disappeared whenever his diet was adequate. On one occasion he was given sulfanilamide; a day later weeping eczema covered his entire body and was so severe that his eyes were swollen shut and his ears were twice their normal thickness. This condition cleared like magic when he took PABA. The number of other eczema cases I have seen improve after taking PABA has led me to believe that deficiencies of this vitamin are not unusual.

PABA was first publicized as an anti-gray-hair vitamin because black animals lacking it became gray. Dr. Benjamin Sieve studied the hair of persons given 200 milligrams of PABA after each meal. Some hair was restored to its natural color in 70 per cent of the cases. Several women who had wanted children for years conceived after this vitamin was added to their diets. Other persons who had suffered from vitiligo, or whose skin had become heavily pigmented in some spots and lacked pigment in others, developed normal skin color and the heavier spots of pigment faded.

Deficiencies of at least four B vitamins, PABA, biotin, folic acid, and pantothenic acid, appear to affect hair color. One scientist who has conducted years of research on these B vitamins and has repeatedly produced gray hair in dark mice, rats, silver foxes, and black dogs even states that all gray hair is probably a symptom of multiple nutritional deficiencies. The color of hair is rarely restored by taking synthetic B vitamins, however, but I have seen many people whose hair returned temporarily to its natural color after they had followed adequate diets especially rich in all the B vitamins.

Because PABA makes sulfa drugs ineffective, the Food and Drug Administration does not allow any supplement furnishing more than 30 milligrams to be sold without a prescription. This action has literally brought all research concerning PABA to a stop; the vitamin has almost disappeared from the market and is even difficult to obtain with a prescription. Yet sulfa drugs are now rarely used. As much as 48 grams (48,000 milligrams) of PABA have been given daily without toxicity.

Prior to its removal from the market, PABA was shown to be especially effective in clearing up certain diseases caused by parasitic organisms transmitted by fleas, mites, ticks, and lice, such as Rocky Mountain spotted fever and typhus. Vitiligo, which is becoming progressively more common, was reported to have cleared up when 1,000 or more milligrams of PABA were taken daily, especially if generous amounts of pantothenic acid and fresh liver, preferably uncooked, were obtained with it. Persons who sunburned readily were also found to tolerate 50 to 100 times more sunshine than previously when they were given 1,000 milligrams of PABA daily. Fortunately, PABA cream or ointment is available, which, if applied to the skin, can protect susceptible individuals from sunburn. Persons using such ointment have been found to tolerate eight hours or more of Florida sun without burning, a godsend to anyone susceptible to skin cancer.

In all probability, persons who sunburn readily, those susceptible to sun-induced skin cancers, and those who suffer from vitiligo have unusually high requirements for PABA. How this need can be fulfilled, however, unless the Food and Drug Administration will rescind its edict to limit the sale of this vitamin, I do not know.

More research should also be done on the B vitamin inositol. In addition to liver, yeast, and wheat germ, its sources are whole-wheat bread, oatmeal, corn, and especially dark, unrefined molasses. Inositol is available in huge quantities as a by-product of cornstarch manufacture, and is added to the gray paint used by our navy.

When animals are put on a diet lacking inositol, their hair falls out. If the vitamin is then added to the diet, their hair grows in again. Male animals lose their hair twice as quickly as do females, indicating that the male requirement is higher than that of the female. A deficiency also causes constipation, eczema (dermatitis), and abnormalities of the eyes. Inositol is particularly concentrated in the lens of the human eye and in the heart muscles, perhaps indicating that it plays some role in normal vision and in heart action. A hundred times more inositol than any other vitamin except niacin is found in the human body.

Separate B vitamins have been given with barium to volunteers, and the contractions of the stomach and intestines studied by fluoroscope; the activity of these organs increases the digestion and absorption of foods, thus preventing gas pain and abdominal distress. Of all the B vitamins, only inositol markedly increased the contractions of the eliminatory tract. Poor appetites became normal, foods were tolerated with greater ease, and previously existing constipation was relieved.

A few years ago I became interested in the possibility that a lack of inositol might be one cause of baldness in men. For a time I recommended inositol together with other sources of B vitamins to all the bald men who consulted me. In almost every case they soon reported that their hair was no longer falling out. Wives or mothers particularly mentioned that, whereas loose hair had formerly covered pillows and washbasins, they now had no loose hair to clean up. In some cases new hair growth was obvious in a month. One man of forty-eight, who had been bald for years, grew hair so thick that it looked like rabbit fur; surprisingly enough, he was extremely proud of it. One white-haired man of sixty-five had a bald spot far back on his head; the entire spot filled in with black hair, and a distinguished streak of black hair in the white appeared above his forehead. One man, who had been bald since he was twenty, grew so much hair that no bald spot remained. Some of the men, however, grew not one encouraging wisp.

Loss of hair often occurs in animals deficient in any one of several B vitamins or certain amino acids. Since I recommended for baldness a teaspoon of pure inositol daily added to a quart of fortified milk (p. 106) unusually rich in all these vitamins and protein, new hair growth may have been brought about by increased amounts of nutrients other than inositol. Hereditary tendencies and other causes of baldness undoubtedly exist. Family albums showing our elderly forefathers with luxuriant hair growth makes me suspect, however, that baldness is becoming more common and is developing at a younger age than it did a hundred years ago.

Inositol has been found to reduce the amount of cholesterol in the blood. This vitamin, together with the B vitamin cholin, is part of the structure of lecithin, a fat-like substance produced daily by the liver provided these vitamins are amply supplied and the diet is otherwise adequate. Lecithin keeps cholesterol in tiny particles which can readily pass into the tissues to be utilized. The brain contains a large amount of lecithin, though its function there is not yet clear. A protective covering over the nerves, the myelin sheath, is formed largely of lecithin; the loss of this sheath appears to be the cause of the disease multiple sclerosis. Lecithin helps to digest, absorb, and carry in the blood fats and vitamins A, D, E, and K, which dissolve in fats; and it is essential to the utilization of fats in the cells themselves. As part of lecithin, both inositol and cholin may serve their most important functions.

The richest sources of cholin are brains, liver, yeast, wheat germ, kidneys, and egg yolk; and pure granular lecithin, separated from soy oil destined to be used for paint. The assumption usually is that cholin deficiencies do not exist because this vitamin can be formed in the body from the amino acid methionine, a part of all complete proteins. First, however, the protein intake must be so generous that "excess" methionine i. available, not needed to build or repair tissues. Secondly, vitamin B_{12} and another B vitamin, folic acid, must be present as part of an enzyme essential in forming cholin from methionine. Any one or all of these three nutrients may be inadequate.

When young animals are given a diet deficient in cholin, the kidneys are so damaged that nephritis is produced. The blood pressure becomes high; albumin and often blood are lost in the urine; and, since lecithin cannot be formed without cholin, the blood cholesterol soars far above normal. Even when the diet is high in protein, young animals are unable to form enough cholin from methionine; hence severe kidney damage can occur in a single week.

In one experiment, for example, four little calves were given a diet adequate except for cholin; they died seven days later, their kidneys hemorrhaging with severe nephritis. When similar calves were given 1,000 milligrams of cholin on the sixth day, kidney repair began almost immediately; "dramatic improvement" was said to have occurred in 24 to 48 hours, and health was quickly regained. Physicians who have studied nephritis produced experimentally in cholin-deficient animals stress that it is strikingly similar to that found in humans. For instance, in animals and humans alike the blood cholesterol reaches abnormally high levels because without cholin lecithin cannot be produced. In children, the blood cholesterol should probably not exceed 140 milligrams, yet in nephritis it averages 570 milligrams.

It is in young, rapidly growing animals, whether rats, calves, or any other, that cholin deficiency is most likely to result in nephritis even on a high-protein diet. When the illness slows their growth sufficiently to reduce their need for protein, more methionine becomes available to be changed into cholin, and they may survive. Similarly, it is

the rapidly growing children who so often develop nephritis.
If their growth is halted by the disease, they usually survive,
although far too many die.

I have never known of a kidney specialist who gave
cholin to patients suffering from nephritis, yet surely it is
impossible to follow the research without being convinced
that this vitamin should be started the very day a diagnosis
of nephritis is made. Cholin is never toxic; I myself have
taken 1,000 milligrams daily in B-complex tablets for years.
Recently I was thrown socially with a physician who special-
ized in children's kidney diseases, a fine, intelligent individual who was raising money for kidney machines. He was
both untrained in nutrition and depressingly intolerant of
it; he gave low-protein, cholin-deficient diets to youngsters
under his care. Without a physician's co-operation, mothers
of young patients, knowing that nephritis is often fatal, are
usually far too frightened to give their ill children anything
except the refined foods which allowed the disease to develop in the first place. If dietary improvement is delayed,
the kidney damage rapidly becomes more severe; all nutrients are then lost so quickly through the damaged kidneys
that repair becomes difficult and sometimes impossible.
A dozen or more parents, however, have written or told me
that their child, slated for a kidney machine, has recovered
soon after being given a high-protein, completely adequate
diet containing large amounts of cholin.

Because high blood pressure is produced in animals by
a cholin-deficient diet, a study was made of 158 persons
whose blood pressure was so dangerously high that several
had suffered strokes and/or hemorrhages in the eyes; others
had nephritis. Each of these individuals had long been on
various medications without improvement; therefore all
drugs were stopped and cholin was given, though otherwise
the diet was unchanged. Headaches, dizziness, ear noises,
awareness of heartbeat, and constipation improved or completely disappeared within five to ten days. By the end of
three weeks the blood pressure had dropped in every case,
in many to a normal level. Other improvements followed
gradually: patients reported sleeping better; water retention,
when it had been present, no longer occurred; visual disturbances were relieved; blood vessels dilated (as they do
when experimental animals are given cholin) and the work
of the heart was greatly decreased. If cholin was discontinued, however, the blood pressure again increased above
normal and the other symptoms recurred.

If a cholin-deficient, low-protein diet is given to grown

animals, excessive fat is deposited in the liver, a condition similar to human cirrhosis; and a large per cent of the animals die of liver cancer. Fatty liver is by far the best-known symptom of a cholin deficiency and the only one many physicians recognize.

Most investigators believe that the fatty liver produced by a cholin-deficient diet is analogous to the liver condition common among alcoholics whose diets are notoriously deficient in proteins, all the B vitamins, and most other nutrients. Large amounts of cholin and methionine given daily to alcoholics with severe liver damage caused marked improvement. The two nutrients alone, however, could not restore health or prevent extensive scarring. When a completely adequate high-protein diet is given and supplemented with 1,000 milligrams or more of cholin and inositol and several tablespoons of lecithin daily, liver damage can be repaired to a truly remarkable degree.

Cholin appears to have many other duties. It is necessary for the synthesis of nucleic acid in the business center, or nucleus, of every cell in the body and for the production of DNA and RNA, which carry the blueprint of heredity. Animals deficient in this vitamin develop stomach ulcers, liver cancer, and hemorrhages in the heart muscles and adrenal glands. Because cholin is part of an enzyme which helps transfer nerve messages, it is essential for normal muscle contraction. A type of muscular dystrophy can be produced by a cholin-deficient diet. Certain insecticides are effective because they inactivate cholin-containing enzymes, causing paralysis of the insects' throat muscles. It now appears that these same insecticides may be one cause of the rapidly increasing disease myasthenia gravis.

The amount of cholin required to maintain health is in proportion to the intake of solid, or saturated, fats in the diet; the more of such fats eaten, the more cholin needed. The exact requirement is not known but has been estimated to be between 3,000 and 5,000 milligrams per day. A serving of liver (¼ pound) supplies 500 to 700 milligrams; ½ cup of wheat germ, 400 milligrams; a heaping tablespoon of granular lecithin, 500 milligrams; an egg, 280 milligrams; a tablespoon of yeast, 40 to 180. Other foods are not rich. A serving of vegetables or meat may furnish only 10 to 50 milligrams of this vitamin.

Because cholin deficiency, by restricting the synthesis of lecithin, allows cholesterol to clog arteries throughout the body, it is vital that this vitamin be adequately supplied in the diet. A high blood cholesterol can be lowered by avoiding the solid, or saturated, fats (coconut oil, the fat of beef, pork, and lamb, and all hydrogenated fats), thus decreasing the need for cholin; or by increasing the cholin content of the diet together with all nutrients necessary for lecithin formation. Fortunately both granular lecithin and vitamin supplements containing 1,000 milligrams of cholin in a day's portion are available.

The vitamins discussed in this chapter are rarely included in preparations claiming to furnish "all the B vitamins." The assumption has been that these vitamins are unimportant or are adequately supplied in the diet. This assumption has already been proved to be incorrect.

CHAPTER 10

I'M AFRAID TO TAKE
THE CHANCE

MOST OF THE B VITAMINS ARE FOUND LARGELY IN LIVER, yeast, wheat germ, and rice polish. Vitamin B_{12}, however, occurs only in animal foods such as milk, eggs, cheese, and most meats. Liver is the richest source.

When a prolonged deficiency of B vitamins prevents the stomach from producing hydrochloric acid and an enzyme known as the intrinsic factor, vitamin B_{12} cannot be absorbed into the blood. Such is the case in pernicious anemia or when the stomach has been removed. Unless vitamin B_{12} is injected, a deficiency develops causing a sore mouth and tongue, nervousness, neuritis, menstrual disturbances, an unpleasant body odor, back stiffness and pain, difficulty in walking, and a shuffling gait. In time the spinal cord degenerates until irreversible paralysis results. Such tragedies occur mostly among vegetarians, although for years it has been known that they could keep healthy by taking a 50-microgram tablet of vitamin B_{12} once each week.

If the diet of the person lacking vitamin B_{12} is otherwise adequate, however, he does not develop anemia. Pernicious anemia results from simultaneous deficiencies of both vitamin B_{12} and folic acid, another B vitamin. Liver, torula yeast, nuts, and green vegetables are rich in folic acid. It is readily destroyed by heat in foods containing acid and, like all B vitamins, is lost if cooking water is discarded. Such drugs as phenobarbital and dilantin destroy folic acid so quickly that they should not be given unless the vitamin is taken with them.

Folic acid is necessary for the division of all body cells and for the production of the substances which carry our hereditary patterns, RNA and DNA. Without it, no growth can take place, not even of a hair, sperm, or fingernail, and no healing can occur. As part of dozens of enzymes in the cells, it is essential for the utilization of sugar and amino acids and the building of antibodies to prevent infections. Yet Dr. Leevy found that folic-acid deficiencies, which affected 45 per cent of hospital patients, were more common than deficiencies of any other vitamin.

Persons obtaining too little folic acid develop a large-cell anemia, fatigue, paleness, dizziness, mental depression, a grayish-brown skin pigmentation, and shortness of breath. Folic acid deficiencies are particularly frequent and dangerous during pregnancy, and can result in hemorrhaging, miscarriage, premature birth, difficult labor, high infant death rate, and infants already anemic at birth. Expectant mothers so frequently show a grayish-brown skin pigmentation that it has become known as "pregnancy cap," though it quickly disappears when five milligrams of folic acid are taken after each meal. Among women who use oral contraceptives, which greatly increase the need for folic acid, such pigmentation has now become common.

The young of animals lacking folic acid are grossly abnormal. Similarly, women given drugs which take the place of this vitamin in the cells (folic-acid antagonists) have given birth to malformed and mentally retarded infants. Yet as little as 1 milligram daily taken both before conception and during pregnancy appears to be adequate, though to correct anemia 5 milligrams of the vitamin 1 to 3 times daily are usually necessary.

Folic acid is not toxic; 450 milligrams have been taken day after day without harm. Yet our Food and Drug Administration allows only 0.1 of a milligram per supplement to be sold without prescription. The reasoning is that if vegetarians, whose diets are already high in folic acid (so named for foliage, or green leaves), were to receive even more of this vitamin from supplements, the discovery of their vitamin-B_{12} deficiencies would be still further delayed simply because they develop no anemia and no fatigue and do not seek medical help; hence more of them would produce lifelong and irreversible paralysis in themselves.

At best, limiting the sale of folic acid to 0.1 milligram per supplement may help a few hundred vegetarians but it dooms thousands upon thousands of other persons who do not eat liver, yeast, or many vegetables to folic-acid deficiencies. No other country in the world restricts the sale of this vitamin. Unless the Food and Drug Administration edict is withdrawn, we can expect more blemished skins, more infections, more exhaustion, more unsuccessful pregnancies, and more mentally retarded and malformed children. I get my personal supply in 1- or 5-milligram tablets of folic acid from Canada. Perhaps if all readers of this book would write the Food and Drug Administration, Washington, D.C., requesting that an adequate amount of folic acid be sold with vitamin B_{12} (to protect vegetarians) it could again become available in the United States.

Both folic acid and biotin are necessary before still another B vitamin, pantothenic acid, can be utilized. This vitamin, usually sold as calcium pantothenate, can be obtained from liver, kidney, heart, yeast, wheat germ and bran, whole-grain breads and cereals, and green vegetables. It is unstable to heat, however, and is destroyed in canning and overcooking. Americans have been found to obtain 3 to 5 milligrams per day, although the daily requirement appears to be 50 milligrams or more.

At the State University of Iowa College of Medicine, pantothenic-acid deficiencies have been produced in volunteers from a state prison. These young men developed fatigue, headaches, dizziness, weakness, rapid heartbeat, muscle cramps, and continuous colds and upper-respiratory infections. They became easily upset, discontented, irritable, depressed, and quarrelsome. Continuous low blood sugar, or hypoglycemia, caused tremors of their outstretched hands and many other symptoms. Their blood gamma globulin decreased and sedimentation rate increased, indicating susceptibility to infections; and they were unable to produce antibodies even when given immunization shots.

All of the symptoms became worse as the diet continued. The men, though sleepy, suffered from insomnia; some had painful, burning feet. Their adrenal glands became exhausted. Blood pressures dropped below normal. There was such a decrease in stomach acid, digestive enzymes, and movement in the intestinal tract that indigestion, distress from gas, and constipation occurred. After six weeks these men, whose diets were adequate in all nutrients except pantothenic acid, became severely ill; cortisone and 4,000 milligrams of pantothenic acid daily was then given, but recovery was slow.

Pantothenic acid is necessary for every cell in the body. Neither sugar nor fat can be changed into energy without it, nor can PABA or cholin be used. A lack especially harms the adrenal glands, which become enlarged, hemorrhagic, and unable to produce cortisone and other hormones. During any type of stress—illness, injury, effects of drugs, burns, surgery, emotional upsets, or any other—when larger amounts of these hormones are needed, the requirement for pantothenic acid increases proportionately. In fact, if a person has lacked pantothenic acid, taking it is often as effective as being given cortisone.

When rats were deficient in pantothenic acid for varying lengths of time and then injected with bacteria, the severity of the resulting infections was in proportion to the duration of the deprivation. Susceptibility to infections occurs before any other signs of a pantothenic-acid deficiency can be detected. When one is under the stress of a threatening infection and the adrenals are healthy, tonsils, adenoids, and other lymph glands *decrease in size*. Only when the lack of pantothenic acid and/or other nutrients causes the adrenals to be exhausted do the tonsils and other lymph glands enlarge and become infected.

A lack of pantothenic acid appears to be a principal cause of allergies, now being produced in 60 per cent of all bottle-fed babies. Breast milk is rich in this vitamin, but the pantothenic acid in cows' milk is largely lost in pasteurization and none remains in canned milk, prepared formulas, and canned baby foods. Such allergies often last a lifetime. When an adequate diet especially rich in pantothenic acid and vitamin C is carefully followed, however, they readily disappear.

Another common abnormality resulting largely from a pantothenic-acid deficiency is low blood sugar, or hypoglycemia, marked by constant exhaustion, dizziness, nervousness, headaches, and even blackouts. In a healthy person, the blood sugar decreases as energy is produced, but stored body starch, or glycogen, is instantly converted into sugar, thus increasing the supply in the blood. If the glycogen stores have been used up and no food has been eaten to replenish them, adrenal hormones immediately cause body proteins, mostly lymph tissues, to be broken into fat and sugar. Some of this sugar increases the quantity in the blood to normal and a portion is stored as glycogen for future use. When animals given ample pantothenic acid are subjected to stress, the blood sugar remains high and the amount of body starch (glycogen) stored in the liver quickly increases as much as 700 per cent, ready to supply energy for any emergency. In animals and humans alike lacking pantothenic acid, blood sugar stays abnormally low because the adrenal hormones necessary to convert protein to sugar (and fat) cannot be produced. Asthma attacks, temper tantrums, stomach ulcers, and dozens of life's more unpleasant features occur when the adrenals are exhausted and/or the blood sugar is low.

Probably every person suffering from an illness helped by cortisone—arthritis, Addison's disease, lupus erythematosus, and dozens of others—is actually deficient in pantothenic acid. Overweight persons, fasting without pantothenic acid, have actually produced both arthritis and gout in themselves. Because cortisone medication can be highly toxic, the greatest emphasis in overcoming any illness should be to help one's own adrenals produce adequate cortisone by obtaining ample pantothenic acid, vitamin C, the antistress vitamins, and other essential nutrients.

In addition to cortisone, approximately thirty adrenal hormones cannot be synthesized without this vitamin. For example, the adrenals produce a large per cent of a man's sex hormones. If a woman has healthy adrenals, they supply her sex hormones after the menopause, though she can expect difficulty at this time if these glands are exhausted. Male animals deficient in pantothenic acid become sterile whereas females miscarry or give birth to malformed young whose eyes and brains are often damaged.

The amount of pantothenic acid needed daily varies constantly with the severity and number of stresses one is under. This vitamin, however, is never toxic. Dr. E. P. Ralli of New York University College of Medicine studied young men under the stress of swimming in icy water when given no pantothenic acid and again after they had received 10,000 milligrams of the vitamin daily. Her tests showed that the vitamin gave protection in dozens of ways, such as preventing body proteins from being destroyed, blood sugar and blood pressure from dropping, and calcium from being stolen from the bones.

Investigators suggest that 30 to 50 milligrams daily is adequate for a healthy adult. Persons usually recover more rapidly from arthritis, infections, allergies, and other severe stress when they receive 50 to 100 milligrams of pantothenic acid after each meal, between meals, and before bed, always with an otherwise adequate diet. As soon as improvement has occurred, 50 milligrams of pantothenic acid at each mealtime is often sufficient. When stresses decrease, 100 milligrams or less once daily may be adequate, especially if yeast, liver, or wheat germ is eaten. Excessive pantothenic acid taken alone over a prolonged period may increase the need for vitamin B_1 and thus cause neuritis.

Another B vitamin, known as pyridoxin, pyridoxin hydrochloride, or vitamin B_6, is found in descending order in yeast, blackstrap molasses, wheat bran and germ, liver, heart, and kidney. Much vitamin B_6 is lost in cooking, canning, exposure to light, and long storage.

The same Iowa physicians who produced pantothenic-acid deficiencies in prisoners also studied young men lacking vitamin B_6. Though the diet was adequate in all other respects, after only one week these volunteers developed headaches, severe halitosis, irritability, dizziness, extreme nervousness, lethargy, and inability to concentrate. They suffered from burning pain and cramps in the abdomen, and passed much foul-smelling gas. Later an itching, red rash appeared around the genital organs. Some of the men suffered from diarrhea, others from painful hemorrhoids. All became anemic, experienced nausea and vomiting, lost "showers of dandruff," and developed sore lips, mouths, and tongues. Their white blood cells became excessive, as they do when the body must fight an infection, and their lymphocytes, which also help to fight infection, dropped abnormally low. Blood levels of urea and uric acid became elevated and much nitrogen was lost in the urine, showing that proteins were not being utilized normally in the body. In time a seborrheic dermatitis appeared in their eyebrows and hair, and their hands became dry, cracked, and sore. They were unable to sleep, yet were continuously drowsy. All symptoms persisted and became increasingly worse. Even when 600 milligrams of vitamin B_6 was given them daily, nervousness and headaches did not clear up until 4 to 6 weeks later.

Vitamin-B_6 deficiencies have also been produced in hospital patients[1] given a diet considered to be adequate except for this vitamin. They developed mental depression, sore mouths, lips, and tongues and, in time, insomnia, extreme weakness, nervousness, dizziness, nausea, and vomiting. The most striking abnormality, however, was eczema (seborrheic dermatitis), which appeared first in the scalp and the eyebrows, around the nose, and behind the ears, though in the Iowa volunteers eczema had been most severe around the genitalia. One patient, already suffering from eczema, rapidly grew worse. When vitamin B_6 was given these patients, their condition quickly became normal. The investigators then discovered that similar eczemas had appeared in other patients during their hospitalization and while they were eating the "adequate" hospital diet.

[1] A. W. Schreiner, W. Slinger, V. R. Hawkins, and R. W. Vilter, "Pyridoxin Deficiencies in Human Beings Induced with Desoxypyridoxin," *Journal of Clinical Investigation*, XXIX (1950), 193.

Persons only slightly deficient in vitamin B_6 usually suffer from one or two symptoms rather than many. For example, individuals often endure the fatigue of anemia for years, and sometimes even require transfusions, though their physicians overload them with iron; their anemia is quickly corrected when vitamin B_6 is given but recurs if the vitamin is stopped. Similarly, migraine headaches of long duration often clear up when vitamin B_6 is generously added to an otherwise adequate diet. At least fifty persons have told me that they have avoided painful hemorrhoid surgery by increasing their intake of vitamin B_6. For people who suffer from nervousness and insomnia, this vitamin often acts as a tranquilizer. It has also been used successfully in preventing or correcting the nausea of pregnancy, sea and air sickness, and the irradiation sickness resulting from cobalt therapy.

Vitamin B_6 is necessary for the normal functioning of the brain. For example, when diets lacking this vitamin have been given in an attempt to starve cancer cells, convulsions which appear to be identical to epilepsy have been produced in children and adults alike. Some years ago pediatricians recommended a prepared infant formula so deficient in vitamin B_6 that it caused hundreds of babies in America to suffer epileptic-like seizures. The convulsions stopped and the brain waves became normal within minutes after an injection of 100 milligrams of vitamin B_6.

This vitamin is essential in maintaining a normal level of magnesium in the blood and tissues. At the same time magnesium helps to activate dozens of enzymes which contain vitamin B_6; hence these two nutrients work together in the body and neither can function without the other. If health is to be maintained, both vitamin B_6 and magnesium must be adequately supplied at the same time. For example, when either vitamin B_6 or magnesium alone has been given to persons suffering from epilepsy, recovery has not always occurred, but when both magnesium and vitamin B_6 have been generously furnished, recovery has usually been prompt (p. 173).

Vitamin B_6 is essential before the unsaturated fatty acid, linoleic acid, and the many amino acids from protein can be utilized in the body. Without it tissues cannot be built, lecithin cannot be synthesized, and blood cholesterol cannot be kept at a normal level. When this vitamin is undersupplied, the amino acid tryptophane is not used normally; a substance known as xanthurenic acid forms from it and is excreted in the urine. Xanthurenic acid appears in the urine long before any outward deficiency symptoms can be recognized. The test for a vitamin-B_6 deficiency, therefore, is to examine the urine for xanthurenic acid; and the more serious the deficiency, the larger is the amount of xanthurenic acid excreted. Pregnant women, individuals taking oral contraceptives, and persons suffering from epilepsy, diabetes, anemia, and oxalic-acid kidney stones have all been found to excrete abnormally large amounts of xanthurenic acid. Such urine studies indicate that families in which several members suffer from diabetes or epilepsy appear to have an unusually high hereditary requirement for vitamin B_6.

The need for vitamin B_6 increases tremendously during pregnancy; and the abnormalities common during pregnancy, such as nausea, vomiting, anemia, headaches, nervousness, foot and leg cramps, hemorrhoids, retention of water, or edema, and even the convulsions of eclampsia have each been corrected by vitamin B_6. Dr. John Ellis of Mt. Pleasant, Texas, finds this vitamin to be especially effective as a diuretic. When he gave women with severe water retention 25 milligrams of vitamin B_6 with each meal and before bed, one lost 13 pounds in a week and another 8 pounds in 12 days. Since oral contraceptives mimic pregnancy, they too increase the vitamin-B_6 requirement and frequently produce such deficiency symptoms as headaches, hemorrhoids, nausea, water retention, and painful eczema in and around the vagina. Even *grand mal* epilepsy and diabetes have been reported in women taking oral contraceptives.

Many types of nervous disorders such as tics, tremors, twitching, and leg and foot cramps have been relieved when 25 or more milligrams of vitamin B_6 have been taken daily. Muscle weakness has also been corrected even after being so severe that walking has been difficult. Better bladder control and less bed-wetting has been repeatedly reported, especially among persons suffering from multiple sclerosis. Apparently because of faulty absorption, however, seborrheic dermatitis, or eczema, has not always cleared up, even when 600 to 1,000 milligrams of vitamin B_6 were given daily; yet when a salve containing 50 milligrams of vitamin B_6 per teaspoon has been applied, the skin has become normal and xanthurenic acid has quickly disappeared from the urine. The absorption of this vitamin can be markedly increased when the diet contains all the B group, especially vitamin B_2, and generous amounts of magnesium.

Vitamin B_6 protects the body in a surprising variety of

ways. For example, it appears to be particularly effective in preventing tooth decay. Often it stops kidney-stone formation provided magnesium is also adequate. If vitamin B₆ alone is deficient, kidney stones of oxalic acid are produced. Calcium-phosphate kidney stones appear to form when the diet is inadequate in both vitamin B₆ and magnesium. In animals, an undersupply of vitamin B₆ allows so much xanthurenic acid to irritate the lining of the urinary bladder that they develop bladder cancer; whether humans are similarly affected is not yet known.

The amount of vitamin B₆ needed daily to maintain health varies with the intake of protein, fat, and especially of unsaturated fatty acids. The National Research Council has recommended 2 milligrams daily for adults, but when this amount in army rations was tested on conscientious objectors, they showed large amounts of xanthurenic acid in the urine, indicating a severe deficiency. As little as 10 milligrams daily has been found to prevent the nausea of pregnancy, but 250 milligrams were needed to correct it. Similarly, 10 milligrams given daily to one-week-old infants dramatically stopped convulsions although 8 milligrams did not; when the vitamin was discontinued, the convulsions recurred in 5 days.

There is no doubt that certain individuals and even entire families sometimes have unusually high requirements of this vitamin. In general, however, if a recognized deficiency exists, 50 milligrams at each meal, taken preferably with the same quantity of vitamin B₂, is sufficient to rebuild health in a few weeks; then the quantity can usually be reduced to perhaps 10 milligrams daily, taken with yeast and other natural sources. Physicians have given as much as 3,000 milligrams daily without recognized toxicity, but such an amount seems both unnecessary and costly.

Not one of the vitamins discussed in this chapter has ever been added to so-called "enriched" bread. Our sickness statistics indicate that our diets are appallingly inadequate in most of them, yet our Food and Drug Administration claims that we get enough of all of these B vitamins from ordinary foods. I, for one, am afraid to take the chance.

CHAPTER 11

ARE BLUE MONDAYS NECESSARY?

IT MAY NOT BE MERE HAPPENSTANCE THAT ONE PERSON is gay and another grumpy. The grumpy one may have far more to be happy about but may be unable to enjoy his potential happiness because of a niacin deficiency. This B vitamin is variously known as niacin, niacin amide, nicotinic acid, nicotinic acid amide, and vitamin B_3. Pellagra, which has caused the death of thousands of Americans, results predominantly from a lack of this vitamin; hence deficiencies have been thoroughly studied.

The richest sources of niacin amide are yeast, liver, wheat germ, and kidneys. Some is supplied by fish, muscle meats, eggs, and nuts. Aside from these foods, niacin is difficult to obtain. If the adrenals are healthy and the diet high in protein and vitamins B_2 and B_6, a little niacin amide can be made in the body from the amino acid tryptophane, but this supply is limited. There is almost no niacin in milk. For this reason, niacin deficiencies are extremely common in babies and often cause severe diarrhea. Such diarrhea usually stops within a day if a 100-milligram tablet of niacin amide is crushed and placed directly on the tongue of an infant or added to water or formula. Motherhood can be more enjoyable when yeast is included daily in the formula or added to drinking water, not only as a source of niacin amide but of all the B vitamins. My adopted children never received a bottle which did not contain brewers' yeast.

When volunteers have stayed on a diet adequate in all respects except in niacin, the first symptoms noticeable are psychological. The entire personality changes. Persons who were formerly strong, courageous, forward-looking, and unafraid of life become cowardly, apprehensive, suspicious, and mentally confused. They worry excessively and are emotionally unstable, moody, forgetful, and uncooperative. Such persons become depressed; their depression may range from "blue Mondays" to the point where it is impossible to carry on. They lose their ability to keep going when the going is tough. Fortunately, their depression can be eliminated in a few hours by giving niacin amide.

In a person suffering mild niacin deficiency, the tongue is usually so coated with bacterial growth that mouth odor is unpleasant. Canker sores and small ulcers may appear. Such a person frequently contracts Vincent's disease, or trench mouth. He feels tense, nervous, and irritable and often suffers from dizziness, insomnia, recurring headaches, and impaired memory. If skin symptoms appear, they first resemble sunburn and are aggravated by sunlight; later the skin may darken and become dry and scaly. Simultaneously, anemia and digestive disturbances occur; the stomach can no longer produce sufficient enzymes, digestive juices, and acid to allow normal digestion. Constipation may alternate with diarrhea at first, but soon diarrhea becomes persistent. Through the years I have worked with dozens of persons whose diarrhea had been so severe that they had been repeatedly hospitalized because of it; yet within a few days after their diet was improved and 100 milligrams of niacin amide was taken at each meal, their elimination became normal.

If the deficiency is allowed to become more severe, mental dullness, depression, hostility, or suspicion may grow in intensity. In pellagra sufferers, these symptoms gradually give way to actual violence, disorientation, and delusions, such persons often becoming hopelessly insane. Mental hospitals in the South used to be filled with these patients.

Dr. Abram Hoffer, of Saskatchewan, Canada, was the first to discover that massive amounts of niacin amide could help persons suffering from schizophrenia.[1] He gave 1,000 to 3,000 milligrams of niacin or niacin amide at each meal, together with an equal amount of vitamin C and a high-protein diet to maintain normal blood sugar. From 75 to 85 per cent of the schizophrenics adhering to this regime regain their health, but the illness quickly returns if niacin is discontinued. Many mental clinics using the improved diet and vitamins have now had similar results: 75 per cent or more

---

[1] A. Hoffer, *Niacin Therapy in Psychiatry* (Springfield, Illinois: Charles C. Thomas, 1962); A. Hoffer and H. Osmond, *How to Live with Schizophrenia* (New Hyde Park, New York: University Books, 1966).

of their schizophrenic patients have recovered. Psychiatrists, however, are often bitterly opposed to this treatment, arguing that it delays psychotherapy.

No one who has talked to many of Dr. Hoffer's patients or their parents could fail to bless him. Recently a charming woman, obviously of superior intelligence, told me of her recovery under his care. Her illness had set in when she was only six, and for 25 years she had been in and out of mental hospitals. She spoke of her constant fears and depressions; of her desire to take her own life; of her terror that she might murder her own beloved young daughter; of the deep shame she had realized her family felt because of her; and of her awareness each morning on awaking that her mind could not be depended upon. "That," she added, "is the ultimate insecurity." Her years of intense suffering could scarcely be imagined; yet Dr. Hoffer had given her a new life.

You would scarcely have held back tears had you listened to a mother telling me about her only son, a handsome college athlete with the highest scholastic rating in his class. After grueling examinations and inhuman stress, he lay in a stupor, seemingly unable to hear or talk, tearing off his clothes, and urinating and defecating where he lay. After months of despair, they learned of Dr. Hoffer's research, and the boy's health was restored. Later I talked with this delightful young man, now launched on a successful career. He told me how he had relapsed when he had grown tired of taking pills, and of his devastating lethargy, bewilderment, depression, and confusion. He quickly assured me that he expected to adhere to an excellent diet and the high niacin intake as long as he lived.

Schizophrenics who have been ill only a short time more often recover than persons whose illness is already of long standing. Dr. Hoffer tells of one patient, however, who had been ill for 19 years and was well 5 days after massive amounts of niacin and vitamin C were given him. Individuals susceptible to schizophrenia may have an unusually high requirement for niacin. Several investigators believe, however, that they may be unable to utilize this vitamin normally, possibly because of adrenal exhaustion. Such mental breakdowns usually occur immediately following extremely severe stress, often during adolescence when the requirements of all nutrients are high because of rapid growth.

Dr. Hoffer and his associate, Dr. Osmond, have devised an HOD test—Hoffer-Osmond-diagnostic test—for schizophrenia consisting of a long list of questions. It is considered to be a remarkably accurate method of diagnosing the illness. When this test was given to high school students, 15 per cent showed a tendency toward schizophrenia; that is, they revealed mental symptoms characteristic of a niacin deficiency. When given to delinquent boys and convicted prisoners, as many as 80 per cent showed definite schizophrenic tendencies. Alcoholics also have unusually high scores on this test; and an excellent diet together with massive amounts of niacin and vitamin C have been helpful to persons trying to stay sober.

Most of the murders and vicious crimes in this country are being committed by schizophrenics. Suicide, a major cause of death among college students, is extremely high among schizophrenics, yet has dropped to zero in groups given large amounts of niacin amide. It will someday be recognized that our disgraceful crime rate, our tremendous loss from suicides, and our millions of alcoholics are in part brought on by food industries which, ignoring health, flood the market with overrefined and overprocessed products designed merely to make money.

Niacin amide appears not to be toxic in any quantity. Dr. Hoffer even tells of giving one mentally ill person 1,000 milligrams of this vitamin every hour for 48 hours, after which time she was well and remained so. Niacin alone or nicotinic acid alone, however, usually causes the skin to become red, flushed, and prickly for perhaps an hour after it is taken. This reaction can be frightening indeed. Unless it is prescribed by a physician, I feel that anyone wishing to take this vitamin should first make sure it is labeled niacin *amide* or nicotinic acid *amide*.

The amount of niacin amide needed by different individuals obviously varies widely. For years I have obtained excellent results, even with persons who have been mentally ill, with only 100 milligrams taken after each meal, always with yeast, liver, or other natural sources. Since learning more about schizophrenia, I would now recommend 100 milligrams of niacin amide daily for all adolescents and college students under severe stress. If large amounts of this vitamin were given delinquents and prisoners before parole, repeated offenses might be greatly decreased.

Sound nutrition affects the brain as much as it does any other part of the body. Persons whose diets are excellent not only are more mentally alert but usually find that blue Mondays can be largely avoided.

CHAPTER 12

STUDY YOURSELF IN
THE MIRROR

VITAMINS B_1, B_2, AND NIACIN HAVE LONG BEEN MADE
synthetically and are the cheap B vitamins. Liver is the
richest natural source of vitamin B_2, or riboflavin; yeast
runs a close second. Since these foods are rarely eaten, for
all practical purposes milk is the most reliable source. This
vitamin is found in leafy vegetables but can be absorbed
only after they are cooked; it is not available from salads.

According to many authorities, a lack of vitamin B_2 is
the most widespread deficiency in America. Dr. Henry
Borsook, studying workers in defense plants during World
War II, found approximately 60 per cent showing advanced
deficiency symptoms. It has been my experience that symptoms of this deficiency are to be found in almost every person who drinks less than one quart of milk a day.

The symptoms of vitamin-B_2 deficiency are fairly well
understood; studies have been made of human volunteers
living on diets adequate in all nutrients except this vitamin.
The most universal sign is a magenta or purplish tongue,
caused by stagnant blood held in the taste buds. Changes
in the lips, however, usually occur earlier, the lower lip
apparently being affected first. Perpendicular lines or tiny
wrinkles may be seen; later these disappear, and the lip
becomes crinkled and rough, often feeling as if it were
chapped; tiny flakes of skin may peel from it. All too often
these symptoms can be seen merely by studying yourself
in the mirror.

When the deficiency becomes acute, the corners of the
mouth split or crack. These cracks do not heal readily and
repeatedly break open; although they do not bleed, they
become quite sore. They may extend half an inch into the

outer cheek and an equal length or more on the inside of the mouth. These cracks appear or disappear depending upon the vitamin-B_2 intake.

In case the deficiency continues, wrinkles appear radiating from the mouth in much the same direction as is seen when the mouth is puckered for whistling. These wrinkles, which I call whistle marks, may extend halfway to the nose. Lipstick gradually creeps up these whistle marks, giving an irregular and ridiculous appearance. Since most of us are vain enough to smile pleasantly at ourselves in the mirror, whistle marks are rarely noticed by the individual who has them; they are visible only when the face is relaxed.

If the deficiency is slight but of long standing, cracks may never appear; instead, the upper lip becomes progressively smaller. In many cases, the upper lip practically disappears. Women with this symptom usually wear their lipstick far above their upper-lip line. The disappearance of the upper lip is common among elderly persons, who invariably blame their false teeth; persons having their own teeth, however, show the same symptoms. I see whistle marks and atrophied upper lips daily, often in persons thirty years of age or even younger.

An early symptom of vitamin-B_2 deficiency is that the eyes become sensitive to light; like persons deficient in vitamin A, such people usually feel more comfortable wearing dark glasses. If the nutrition is adequate in vitamins A and E, a person's night vision will be normal, but his vision in dim light or twilight is faulty; he feels confused in dim light. If he comes into a room where others are enjoying the twilight, he usually demands irritably, "Why are you sitting in the dark?" and quickly snaps on the lights. Even though his eyes are sensitive to bright light, he cannot work or write with ease unless the lights are bright. As the deficiency becomes more severe, his eyes may water, the lids may itch and burn, and he occasionally feels as if grains of sand are under the lids or particles of dirt are in his eyes. You can notice such a person frequently rubbing or wiping his eyes.

If the eyes are severely strained, they become bloodshot. Enzymes containing vitamin B_2 normally combine with oxygen from the air to supply the cells in the cornea, or tissue covering the eye; when this vitamin is inadequate, the body forms tiny blood vessels in this tissue, thus supplying it with oxygen. After these blood vessels are formed, the blood will drain from them when vitamin B_2 is adequate and they are not needed, but the blood vessels remain; hence blood can quickly enter them again whenever a deficiency recurs. The person whose eyes have once been bloodshot, therefore, often suffers quick recurrences whenever his diet becomes deficient.

A condition similar to bloodshot eyes frequently occurs in the skin of the cheeks. Tiny blood vessels are formed in the outer layers of skin which normally would not contain blood vessels. Such blood vessels can be seen on close examination with the naked eye, and even at a distance they give the cheeks a high color. This abnormal coloring, called acne rosacea, may occur high in the cheeks under the eyes, over the lower jaw, or far back on the face in the lateral line near the ears. In severe cases, most often seen in alcoholics, these blood vessels form in the skin over the nose and sometimes the entire face.

These symptoms disappear when the nutrition is completely adequate, the length of time depending upon the severity of the condition, the amount of vitamins given, and the completeness of absorption. I have seen severely bloodshot eyes appear normal again in 24 hours. The tiny blood vessels in the cheeks usually become invisible within two to four weeks after dietary improvement, but they are sometimes maddeningly persistent.

When volunteers have stayed on diets lacking vitamin B_2, the skin of the nose, chin, and forehead has taken on an oily appearance; tiny fatty deposits, like whiteheads, have accumulated under the skin. Cracks and fissures, like those formed at the corners of the mouth, have sometimes appeared in the corners of the eyelids; the lashes may stick together with an oily secretion, particularly on waking in the morning. Cracks and oily scabs may form at the base of the nose. I have rarely seen these symptoms or perhaps have failed to recognize them.

Such widely different animals as dogs, ducks, rats, chickens, monkeys, geese, and even fish, when put on diets lacking vitamin B_2, develop cataracts. If the vitamin is given early enough, the cataracts disappear. When the deficiency is allowed to progress until it becomes severe, however, the damage can be arrested but not repaired. Blindness results if no vitamin is given. Whether or not an undersupply of vitamin B_2 causes cataracts in humans is controversial. Dr. Sydenstricker of the University of Alabama Medical School studied cataracts and opacities in the eyes of persons showing symptoms of multiple vitamin-B deficiency. When vitamin B_2 was given in generous amounts together with an adequate diet, the eyes became normal, usually in about two weeks.

Bloodshot eyes and lip and tongue abnormalities, characteristic of vitamin-B_2 deficiency, have been produced in persons deficient in any one of several amino acids (ref. 3, p. 37) or in vitamin B_6 (ref. 1, p. 82). Animals lacking any one of these nutrients develop cataracts. These conditions can be corrected by supplying, not vitamin B_2, but the missing nutrient. At first these facts were puzzling indeed. It must be remembered, however, that vitamin B_2 in itself is of no importance; it is merely part of the structure of a number of enzymes. These same enzymes are largely protein made of essential amino acids, the lack of any one of which can limit their production. It is now known that vitamin B_6 is necessary to help combine the amino acids into the protein part of these enzymes. The reason symptoms usually disappear when vitamin B_2 is given is that this vitamin is more often lacking than is adequate protein; vitamin B_6 is usually given with the vitamin B_2. Conversely, if the symptoms do not disappear after vitamin B_2 is made adequate, deficiencies of protein and/or vitamin B_6 should be suspected. The deficiency symptoms are caused by a lack of enzymes rather than of any single nutrient. Such is the intricate relationship of many nutrients in the body and of multiple overlapping deficiencies. Milk or yogurt, supplying vitamin B_2, also furnishes vitamin B_6 and essential amino acids; the yogurt offers protein in predigested form and a "factory" of hard-working bacteria willing to produce B vitamins for future needs.

I have had many persons report that, after their nutrition was improved, their glasses seemed no longer suited to their needs. On going to an oculist, they have been told that their eyes were much stronger than formerly. Such an improvement can be brought about only by a completely adequate diet, although vitamin B_2 undoubtedly plays an important role. Good nutrition, however, cannot correct most conditions for which glasses are needed.

Among elderly persons visual difficulties caused by multiple nutritional deficiencies are almost the rule rather than the exception. In all probability, such deficiencies are often responsible for failing vision so frequently accepted as an inevitable part of growing older. I gave a series of lectures at a women's club where most of the audience consisted of women sixty to eighty years old. On several occasions I tried without success to find one person in the audience who did not show symptoms of vitamin-B_2 deficiency. In this group was a sweet old lady of eighty whom I shall remember; her lower eyelids were so swollen that there appeared to be a half teaspoon of tears poised on each. She had given up reading, sewing, movies, and even television. Only two days after she improved her diet, she could read the newspaper. Later her delight at being able to sew for her grandchildren was touching.

It is important to realize that eyes can be improved during the later years when many activities are denied elderly persons. Under no circumstances should dim vision be accepted without making every effort to keep the nutrition adequate. Years ago Dr. Spies made a study of children whose families were too poor to buy milk. He found marked "old-age" symptoms, including watery and burning eyes and failing vision, which cleared quickly when the nutrition was made adequate and milk was supplied. The worst case I have seen was that of a three-year-old who had been given only soy milk. These visual symptoms are usually corrected in young and old alike by an increased intake of yogurt and/or milk, yeast, and liver. In cases of severely bloodshot eyes, it is wise to take vitamin B_2 temporarily. Milk sugar, or lactose, appears to increase the need for vitamin B_2 unless fat is adequate in the diet (p. 51). If a fat-free diet must be adhered to, the use of powdered milk and especially powdered whey should be restricted, particularly when symptoms of a vitamin-B_2 deficiency occur.

The signs of multiple nutritional deficiencies, perhaps most often caused by lack of vitamin B_2, should not be taken lightly. The woman who may be proud of such high color that she need not wear rouge would be wise to inspect herself carefully in the mirror. Probably she should improve her diet with all possible speed.

CHAPTER 13

IT IS NO MORE IMPORTANT
THAN THE OTHERS

I AM AFRAID TO WRITE ABOUT VITAMIN B$_1$. THE SYNTHETIC form of this cheap vitamin is tossed promiscuously into many of our foods to "enrich" them. Thousands of people take tablets of vitamin B$_1$ or of a few mixed B vitamins, believing that they receive far more than they do. *The action of all the B vitamins is synergistic.* One alone or several together increase the need for the B vitamins not supplied. Deficiencies of the unsupplied vitamins may produce abnormalities which can do more harm than the vitamins obtained can do good.

It is impossible to write about vitamin B$_1$ without saying that an adequate intake aids in producing energy. What is to prevent a tired reader from taking tablets of this vitamin because "Adelle says it will help"? My readers have done that before. Yet the most exhausted woman I have ever seen still walking around had been taking massive doses of vitamin B$_1$ daily for two years.

She was a seamstress, thirty-eight years old, although she appeared to be fifty-five or sixty. Her eyes were bloodshot; she believed they were strained by her work. Her upper lip had completely disappeared; small open cracks cut downward from the corners of her mouth. Such fatigue showed in every line of her face that I wanted to tuck her into bed saying, "There. Don't move a muscle for six months." Most of her hair had fallen out during the past year, she told me; the thin, scraggly remainder was white. She had other abnormalities: her nerves were taut and jumpy; she suffered from insomnia; she worried excessively and felt depressed; the back of her lap was so covered with eczema that she could scarcely sit down; yet she was too exhausted to stand up.

It was only after much questioning that I found the cause of her trouble. She used to be so tired, she said. She had heard that vitamin B_1 prevented fatigue and had found on taking it that at first she did feel better. When the effect "wore off," she asked the druggist for the highest-potency B_1 tablet he had, and when this tablet had not helped, she had gradually increased the amount to four tablets daily. I had difficulty in convincing her that the vitamin B_1 was at fault. She was afraid to give it up. I have seen dozens of cases in which the multiple deficiencies of other B vitamins had been caused by taking vitamin B_1. Fortunately no other cases have been as severe as this one. A little knowledge can indeed be a dangerous thing. If a vitamin has been insufficiently supplied, a pickup is experienced when it is added to the diet; increasing the amount over that needed by the cells cannot produce a further pickup. It can only produce deficiencies of other B vitamins still undersupplied, as it did in this case.

The richest sources of vitamin B_1 (thiamin) are wheat germ and rice polish; liver is not particularly rich. This vitamin is necessary before seeds can sprout; therefore it is found in all cereal grains, nuts, dry beans, peas, soybeans, and lentils, and in unrefined foods prepared from seeds, such as peanut butter, breads, and cereals. Among animal sources, kidneys, heart, and pork rank highest.

A "bird's-eye view" of the difficulties you may avoid by keeping your diet adequate in this vitamin is shown by experiments in which vitamin-B_1 deficiency has been produced in volunteers. Dr. Norman Jolliffe, of the New York University School of Medicine, studied men living on a diet adequate except for vitamin B_1. After only four days they noticed pain around their hearts, palpitation, and shortness of breath on exertion. They became constipated, unusually fatigued and mentally depressed, the symptoms becoming progressively more severe as they continued the diet. Dr. Jolliffe, studying the hearts by fluoroscope and electrocardiograms, found them to be enlarged and sufficiently abnormal as to be diagnosed as heart disease. When adequate vitamin B_1 was given, the symptoms disappeared in three to six days.

In a similar experiment at the Mayo Foundation, volunteers were given a diet containing the amount of vitamin B_1 found in surveys to be that consumed by the general population of our country (0.22 mg. per 1,000 calories). Their report states,[1] "The foods were exclusively those which commonly appear on the American table." The diet consisted of white bread, beef, corn flakes, potatoes, polished rice, sugar, skim milk, cheese, butter, gelatin, egg white, canned fruits and vegetables, cocoa, and coffee. To make sure the diet was otherwise adequate, these persons were given brewers' yeast to supply the vitamins of the B group but with the vitamin B_1 destroyed by heat. The diet was supplemented with iron, calcium, and phosphorus and with cod-liver oil to furnish vitamins A and D. Such a diet, therefore, was superior to that eaten by millions of Americans.

All of the volunteers showed personality changes. They became irritable, quarrelsome, uncooperative, inefficient, forgetful, mentally sluggish, and depressed. (Do they sound like anybody you know?) These symptoms gradually became more exaggerated. In time, the volunteers developed extreme fatigue, sleeplessness, constipation, and sensitiveness to noise; their hands and feet frequently became numb. They developed low blood pressure, anemia of moderate severity, and low basal metabolic rate (p. 23). They suffered from heart palpitation and shortness of breath; electrocardiograms showed that their hearts were abnormal and, in several cases, enlarged. Their capacity to work, measured by an exercising machine, fell progressively as the diet continued; all symptoms were made more severe both by exercising and by cold weather. In time, they became unable to work because of exhaustion. Pain (neuritis) developed in the calves of their legs. It was found that they had little hydrochloric acid in their stomachs, and in some cases this valuable acid was completely absent. By the twenty-first week, they experienced such severe headaches, nausea, and vomiting that the experiment had to be stopped.

Vitamin B_1 was then given; within a few hours the volunteers became cheerful, the fatigue left them, and they reported a feeling of mental alertness and unusual well-being associated with marked stamina and enterprise. Other symptoms disappeared more slowly. The flow of hydrochloric acid became normal in 12 days; their hearts in 15 days.

Despite the fact that these abnormalities are numerous and varied, vitamin B_1 appears to have only one function. As part of an enzyme, it helps to change glucose into energy or fat. During the breakdown of sugar to produce energy, pyruvic and lactic acids are formed. By the help of enzymes

[1] R. D. Williams, H. L. Mason, B. F. Smith, and R. M. Wilder, "Induced Thiamin (Vitamin B_1) Deficiency in Man," *Archives of Internal Medicine*, LXIX (1942), 721.

containing vitamin B_1, pyruvic acid is quickly broken down
still further into carbon dioxide and water; lactic acid is
rebuilt into glycogen. If the vitamin is undersupplied, these
changes cannot take place, and the acids remain in the tissues; they accumulate, especially in the brain, nerves, heart,
and blood; eventually they are thrown off in the urine. The
production of energy from sugar slows down, coming only
from half-burned sugar or from fat; the acids irritate the
tissues. Since energy cannot be produced efficiently from
fat alone, the result is fatigue, lassitude, and a general lazi-
ness throughout the body.

When people deficient in vitamin B_1 are supplied with it,
the relief of fatigue is often dramatic. Frequently they exclaim in amazement, "I can work twice as hard without getting tired!" In an experiment, subjects were given a minimum amount of vitamin B_1 daily; then that amount was
doubled and tripled, and their work capacity was tested by
weight lifting; it was found they could work twice and then
three times as long without tiring. The first thing I do when
I employ help to work in the garden or house is to feed
them B vitamins; they not only work three times as hard for
the same amount of money but work three times as cheer-
fully.

The reason for personality changes and such symptoms
as mental depression, confused thinking, and forgetfulness
which occur when vitamin B_1 is undersupplied is twofold:
first, brain cells derive their energy only from sugar, and
glucose cannot be converted into energy without this vitamin; second, the accumulation of pyruvic and lactic acids in
the brain cells is somewhat toxic. At a Philadelphia hospital
persons who had eaten foods inadequate in the B vitamins
were given a battery of psychological tests before dietary
improvement, after vitamin B_1 was given, and again after all
the B vitamins were supplied. When vitamin B_1 was injected,
clarity and quickness of thinking, ability to remember, fore-
sight, and judgment somewhat improved. The improvement
was far more marked when all the B vitamins were supplied
by natural foods. Unfortunately, intelligence as such remained the same under all three conditions.

A deficiency of vitamin B_1 causes digestive disturbances
in a number of ways. Energy production is so faulty that
muscular contractions of the stomach and intestinal walls
slow down; food can no longer be well mixed with digestive
juices and enzymes; and the already digested food cannot be
brought into frequent contact with the absorbing surface
where it can pass into the blood. A partial or complete lack

of hydrochloric acid allows several vitamins to be destroyed, proteins to be incompletely digested, and many minerals to stay insoluble. Gas pain and flatulence are inevitable. If the nutrition is not improved, more serious deviations from health can be expected.

Interference with energy production so limits the contractions of the walls of the large intestine that waste material remains in the large bowel longer than it should. The purpose of the large intestine is to conserve water by absorbing it back into the blood; the longer the wastes remain, therefore, the harder and drier the stools become. This condition is constipation. Poor elimination can be corrected by a diet adequate in the B vitamins. Except in cases of diarrhea or severe psychological disturbances, your elimination is a fair index of your energy production. Whenever energy is not produced as it should be, constipation occurs; when energy is readily produced, elimination is usually normal.

Heart abnormalities are also caused by the body's inability to burn sugar efficiently without vitamin B_1. Since the heart must work from birth until death, it must be continuously supplied with energy. In a mild deficiency a resting pulse may drop to 50 or even 40 beats per minute instead of the normal 72. As the vitamin deficiency becomes progressively more severe, the pulse alternates between slow during relaxation and rapid during exertion. Eventually it remains rapid, sometimes reaching 180 beats per minute or more. Irritation of the heart muscles by the accumulated lactic and pyruvic acids is believed to cause both the rapid beat and the enlarged waterlogged heart. I recall a sixteen-year-old girl, suffering from exophthalmic goiter, whose resting pulse dropped from 180 to 80 beats per minute during the first week after she added yeast to her diet. If adequate B vitamins are not given, the condition can increase in severity; the almost complete lack of vitamin B_1 can quickly result in death.

Neuritis frequently develops when vitamin B_1 is inadequately supplied. Like the brain cells, the nerves are particularly affected by this deficiency because they are exclusive sugar burners. Neuritis, which may take the form of trifacial neuralgia, shingles, sciatica, or lumbago, is characterized by a sliding scale varying from a dull ache to excruciating pain following the nerve channels. Such pain is thought to result first from the accumulation of acids and later from actual damage to the nerve cells. Headache and nerve irritation which bring about nausea and vomiting may likewise be caused by these acids.

Neither persons nor experimental animals undersupplied with vitamin B$_1$ show all the symptoms of the deficiency. Symptoms of any deficiency vary in endless degrees among individuals and even in the same person from day to day. These same symptoms, however, occur again and again in both people and animals.

Any woman who reads about the experiments conducted at the Mayo Foundation must surely come to the conclusion that it is selfish wisdom to see that her family is given daily foods rich in the B vitamins.

CHAPTER 14

FOODS TASTE SO MUCH BETTER

YOU MEN CAN SKIP THIS CHAPTER UNLESS YOU HAPPEN TO be one of those creatures who enjoy fooling around a kitchen.

At first it may seem complicated to get your B vitamins from natural foods. Perhaps I can help you most by telling you how I have solved the problem in my family. I have had no white flour in the house for perhaps 20 years. All my flour is stone-ground whole wheat; usually it is "organically grown," that is, grown on soil rich in humus, without commercial fertilizers. Such flour has a flavor infinitely more delicious than that of ordinary varieties. The machinery which grinds ordinary flour creates such heat of friction that the flour is precooked; its flavor is comparable to last night's chops reheated. So-called "enriched" flour is my idea of outright dishonesty; at least 25 nutrients are largely removed during refining, and one-third the original amount of iron, vitamin B_1, and niacin may be replaced. Such flour is "enriched" just as you would be enriched by someone stealing 25 dollars from you and returning 99 cents.

I frequently make my own bread, always with wheat germ added. Bread-making, I believe, is a creative art which will give satisfaction to the soul of any woman who masters it. To my way of thinking, the smell of bread baking is one of the joys of home life. The only argument against making it is that such bread is so delicious that one can easily eat too much. I get the flour from a health-food store or have the miller send it to me the day it is ground; then I make many loaves of bread the next day. Any bread not needed immediately and any flour left over I keep in the freezer; if either is left at room temperature, vitamin E and flavor may be destroyed. Flour, I believe, should be treated as a perishable commodity; I see no more reason for buying a quantity of flour now to be used next month than to buy milk today to be drunk 30 days hence.

The only other bread we have in the house is a wheat-germ bread made by a baker. I buy many loaves of this bread at a time and keep it in the freezer. Children, given genuinely good bread, eat tremendous quantities of it.

I use stone-ground, whole-wheat pastry flour for thickening gravies and making wheat-germ waffles, hotcakes, muffins, cookies, etc. I hold that no one has ever tasted delicious waffles until he eats them made with wheat germ and bakers' yeast (ref. 7, p. 41). I serve them frequently for suppers with creamed tuna, ham, or chicken.

All wheat germ should be refrigerated. If a fresh, sweet-smelling wheat germ cannot be obtained, the toasted kind is preferable. You can toast your own by spreading it on cookie sheets and putting it in the oven at 250°F. until slightly brown.

Wheat germ I use in dozens of ways. Brownies made entirely of wheat germ are delicious. My favorite dessert for guest dinners is walnut torte made by using wheat germ and no flour. Recently a friend's husband wired me, "Loved your party loved your guests especially loved your dessert." I suspect that persons who think delicious foods cannot be prepared with whole-grain flours have never tasted genuinely good food. A friend who serves only health-building foods told me of entertaining guests intolerant of nutrition. One guest remarked on leaving, "Such delicious food could be prepared only by loving hands."

I rarely serve cereals because they contain so much starch. If used, they should be the whole-grain cereals. When I do use them, I cook them in milk and add generous amounts of powdered milk and wheat germ. I buy prepared cereals at health-food stores. My youngsters also enjoy toasted wheat germ mixed with powdered milk and fresh cream.

Rice polish (the bran removed when rice is polished) is about half as potent in most B vitamins as is wheat germ. Except in making cookies, I find it difficult to use. Brown rice is preferable to white. "Converted" rice is now available, so treated that the vitamins are carried into the center of the rice before milling; I use it almost entirely. I purchase whole-wheat macaroni, spaghetti, and noodles from health-food stores and keep them under refrigeration; or I buy these same foods prepared for diabetics from the wheat protein (gluten) after the starch has been removed. The flavor in both cases I find superior to that of the usual varieties. Soy flour, which supplies protein, cholin, inositol, and some antistress vitamins, I sometimes use in fortified milk and the best hotcakes I have ever tasted. It is good in breads, if you do not object to a heavy texture, and in cookies. Every effort should be made to see that your supplies are fresh. Nothing is so revolting as rancid wheat germ, weevily flour, or lumpy powdered milk.

Any of these supplies can be purchased from a health-food store. One cannot recommend such stores without qualification. A few of these stores are run by persons who have gained an amazing knowledge of sound nutrition and are doing tremendous good. Other owners make claims for products such as lecithin capsules, linoleic acid in capsules, and yeast tablets, which in my opinion have little or no value. Health-food stores, however, are usually the only out- let for stone-ground whole-grain breads, cereals, and flours which are free from preservatives and are kept refrigerated; cold-pressed, unrefined oils; unsalted nuts; nut butters to which no hydrogen, sugar, or saturated fat has been added; yogurt and acidophilus cultures; non-instant powdered milk having almost twice the nutritive value per cup of any puffed-up instant variety; and perhaps fertile eggs, safe raw milk, and fruits and vegetables grown on rebuilt soil rich in humus. All labels should be carefully read in health-food stores and ordinary markets alike.

The yogurt I make is far less expensive and we think more delicious than the commercial varieties. My favorite recipe is to blend, using a liquefier, 6 cups of water, 1½ cups of non-instant powdered milk, a large can of evapo- rated whole milk, and yogurt culture or 3 tablespoons of commercial yogurt or of the last yogurt made. This mixture is then poured into jars and set in an electric yogurt-maker or in a large pan of warm water coming to the brim of the glasses, and kept at 105° to 120°F. for approximately four hours, or until it becomes the texture of pudding.

We most often eat yogurt plain or made into a sundae with frozen, undiluted orange juice. I also serve it with fresh or canned fruits, blended into applesauce, and as a salad dressing. When the children were small, I made thousands of popsicles by stirring together a quart of homemade yo- gurt, vanilla, and a large can of frozen, undiluted orange juice; this mixture was frozen in paper cups with small wooden tongue depressors for handles. Often we discov- ered children we had never seen before getting into our freezer for these popsicles.

Unfortunately, too much highly sweetened fruit has been added to most commercial yogurt. Although yogurt is an excellent source of calcium, this mineral can be absorbed only in acid medium. Sugar stimulates the flow of alkaline digestive juices in the intestine so quickly that calcium absorption is largely prevented. Furthermore, yogurt made by the foregoing recipe has twice the calcium, protein, and vitamin-B_2 content of commercial yogurt. Families who make their own inexpensive yogurt usually eat far more of it, and hence achieve a higher degree of health than if they had to purchase each jar of it. If a glass yogurt-maker is used, however, it should be covered with a towel during the culturing process; vitamin B_2 in milk is destroyed by light. Making yogurt with fresh milk is often unsuccessful; cows are frequently given penicillin, some of which is excreted in milk and kills the yogurt bacteria, whereas in canned and powdered milks the antibiotic has been destroyed.

Many excellent foods can contribute B vitamins which cumulatively are worthwhile indeed. Kidney creole (ref. 7, p. 41) is hard to beat. Brains, rich in cholin and inositol, I bake in bacon rings or cream with ham, tuna, or sweetbreads. Some people enjoy lecithin stirred into natural peanut butter. A "candy" can be made by mixing equal parts of honey and peanut butter, then adding enough wheat germ and/or non-instant powdered milk to give the desired texture. All nut butters are nutritious provided they have nothing added except salt. Read the labels carefully, however, and avoid all brands with hydrogen added, usually spoken of as "homogenized"; hydrogenation destroys vitamin E and linoleic acid, increases the need for cholin, and raises blood cholesterol. Nuts and nut butter, lecithin, and all oils should be refrigerated after they have been opened.

When I am working under pressure, I eat liver daily for breakfast, searing it lightly on both sides with a little vegetable oil, then letting it cook slowly, uncovered. Both raw and rare liver are nutritionally superior to well done. Every type of liver, however, whether lamb, pork, beef, rabbit, or any other, supplies excellent protein, iron, copper, trace minerals, and all the B vitamins including those especially needed during stress. Pork liver, usually the least expensive, furnishes the most iron.

If you are one of those people who hate liver yet truly desire the best health you can obtain, desiccated liver, dried under vacuum below body temperature, is available; not by the farthest stretch of the imagination, however, could one call it palatable; 2 heaping tablespoons are equivalent to one serving, or ¼ pound, of fresh liver. I often tell people about it, saying they might try it if they want to. I have been surprised at the number of people who not only take it daily but claim it makes them feel so much better that nothing could make them give it up. I use it, stirred into water or tomato juice, when I cannot get fresh liver. Tablets of dried liver are expensive; 30 tablets are usually equivalent to a serving, or ¼ pound, of fresh liver.

For all practical purposes, brewers' yeast is the cheapest and best source of the B vitamins for a person not under stress. In fact, more nutrients are more concentrated in yeast than in any other known food. The use of yeast alone could correct the majority of the world's nutritional problems: the proteinless meals of China and India; the B-vitamin needs in the Orient and the tropics; the iron starvation of women the world over; and the trace-mineral deficiencies of both sexes of all ages of every nationality. Yeast can be grown in a few hours without acres of land or sweat of a laborer's brow, its nutritive value increased by the touch of a chemist's hand. It is said that three hundred years have been required to introduce most new foods, for example, potatoes and tomatoes. Perhaps by the year 2275, yeast will save our overpopulated planet from famine.

Yeast contains almost no fat, starch, or sugar; its excellent protein sticks to your ribs, satisfies the appetite, increases your basal metabolism, and gives you pep to work off unwanted pounds. If any food could be said to be "reducing," yeast is that food. Powdered yeast is preferable to flaked yeast, which usually has a lower vitamin content, weight for weight. Moreover, 1 tablespoon of powdered yeast is the equivalent of 5 to 9 tablespoons of the light flakes. Yeast tablets are quite all right; 90 tablets are equivalent in mineral, protein, and vitamin content to 1 heaping tablespoon of powdered yeast.

As to flavor, I find torula yeast more palatable than any other. Most health-food stores carry many varieties; you might try several to see which you dislike least. The taste of some yeast is unforgivably bad. I recently met a young man who had been climbing mountains in Alaska. He had carried yeast with him, knowing that it would increase his energy output, but had found it so unpalatable that he could not swallow it. Yet he declared that he actually enjoyed a yeast I suggested he use. Uncooked bakers' yeast grows in the intestine and absorbs the B vitamins supplied by foods or supplements, using them for its own needs; the body may thus be so deprived that multiple B-vitamin deficiencies can result.

Just as you may not have enjoyed your first taste of coffee, you may not enjoy your introduction to yeast. The best way for a beginner to take it is to add no more than 1 teaspoon to a large glass of fruit juice; increase the amount very gradually as you become accustomed to it. If you dislike the yeast you have, feed it to the cat and/or dog, and buy a different brand. A few varieties, to one who is used to yeast at least, are quite palatable. The flavor is, of course, a matter of personal preference.

One reason for taking yeast in small amounts at first is that, in case your digestion is below par, yeast may blow you up like a zeppelin. Since faulty digestion is usually the result of inadequate B vitamins, the more gas you get from yeast, the more deficient you can know that you are in B vitamins, and the more you need the yeast. You might eat sugar by the cup and get no gas because it cannot support the growth of bacteria. Yeast is an excellent food, however; hence bacteria thrive on it. If you lack hydrochloric acid in your stomach or produce too few digestive enzymes, much of the yeast remains undigested, and your intestinal bacteria have a feast; they form the gas. The healthy person digests the yeast completely and has no gas or feeling of fullness from taking it.

A method of taking yeast which will give you many times the quick energy of yeast mixed in juice is taking it in a drink I call pep-up or fortified milk. If you once acquire a taste for yeast and make your pep-up properly, it can be quite palatable. Because all nutrients are used together in the body, health can be rebuilt faster when as many nutrients as possible are furnished together and thus made available at one time. Except for vitamins A, D, and E, this fortified milk supplies most of the essentials: the amino acids from complete proteins; linoleic acid; all B vitamins; some vitamin C if orange juice is used; and calcium, magnesium, and trace minerals. For years every member of our family has had a small glass of some such fortified milk for breakfast. When the children used to be in a hurry to get off to school, they often drank a large glass which served as their entire breakfast menu. The ingredients of pep-up are as follows:

1 quart skim, low fat, or whole milk, preferably medically certified raw
1 teaspoon to ½ cup yeast, depending on whether you are a beginner or a veteran
¼ to ½ cup non-instant powdered milk
1 tablespoon soy, peanut, or safflower oil or mixed vegetable oils

½ teaspoon magnesium oxide (p. 176)

1 tablespoon granular lecithin; more if blood cholesterol is above 180 milligrams per 100 cc. (p. 47)

1 or 2 eggs as desired

½ cup frozen, undiluted orange juice or ½ cup apricot nectar or grape juice or ½ banana or 3 or 4 tablespoons chunk pineapple or frozen berries or any strong-flavored fruit

A number of other health-building ingredients can be added to pep-up: ½ teaspoon of bone meal; 1 teaspoon of calcium lactate or powdered mixed minerals or 2 rounded teaspoons of calcium gluconate (p. 167); and several tablespoons of wheat germ and/or yogurt. When gas is a problem, digestion is more complete if ¼ cup of lemon juice or more is added slowly after other ingredients are blended. Much gas is simply air unconsciously swallowed when one drinks rapidly; as it heats to body temperature, it expands, often causing much distress. This type of gas can be prevented if you sip your pep-up slowly through a straw.

A great many of our most nutritious foods—liver, yeast, wheat germ, lecithin, and most meats—are extremely rich in phosphorus yet are low in calcium and all but lacking in magnesium. Much of the phosphorus in the body can be used only with calcium. When phosphorus is much in excess of calcium, it is excreted in the urine, unfortunately as a calcium salt; thus the body is robbed of already undersupplied and badly needed calcium. Even though milk is our richest source of calcium, bottle-fed infants often develop calcium-deficiency convulsions known as tetany; the excretion of excess phosphorus in cows' milk causes calcium to be lost in the urine. It is to be hoped that, to obtain some calcium, wheat germ is eaten with milk and that milk is drunk at the same meal with liver. Yeast and lecithin, however, should not be used liberally unless ¼ cup of calcium lactate and 1 tablespoon of magnesium oxide are stirred or sifted into each pound. Manufacturers add these minerals to some yeasts before they are marketed.

In case working adequate B vitamins into your diet seems complicated and you have difficulty in getting started, perhaps you would find comfort in knowing that others have had rough going too. A young man once consulted me because of extreme fatigue; he was finishing his doctorate at the University of California, but his fatigue was such that he feared he could neither face nor pass his comprehensive examinations. I suggested that temporarily he eat a half-pound of liver daily for breakfast. Apparently the ink did not take; he believed that I intended him to eat two pounds of liver each morning. He did his best but sent me the following complaint:

> My dear Adelle it is plain hell to follow your directions;
> But I do try hard, avoid all lard and all the fine confections.
>
> There is much to encourage and much to intrigue,
> So much to be grateful for this lack of fatigue.
>
> With devotion to you and in spite of my pride . . .
> One thing that I can hardly abide
>
>> Is rising each morning at the clang of clocks
>>   and facing the white vastness of the icebox.
>> I withdraw with fright and begin to shiver
>>   on seeing that mountain of slippery liver.
>
> But once it is down, I lift high my cup,
> And I can drink deep of the milk and pep-up.

CHAPTER 15

I WISH I KNEW

PERHAPS A HUNDRED TIMES EACH YEAR I AM ASKED, "IS IT all right to take tablets of B vitamins indefinitely?" I simply do not know the answer. I wish I did.

Such tablets are often of value; I have recommended their use for short periods and have taken them myself. No one knows the harm they may do, however, when some B vitamins are omitted and others are disproportionately high, especially if continued over a long period. When they are taken together with liver, yeast, wheat germ, yogurt, and the most carefully selected diet possible, they probably do little or no harm. In this case they may not be needed unless your requirements are unusually high.

These tablets generally contain a day's requirement of vitamins B_1, B_2, and niacin, a small amount of pantothenic acid, and just enough vitamin B_6 to permit a statement of its content on the label. A few other B vitamins may be included but usually are not. Misleading labels often state that such tablets contain 200 to 500 milligrams of liver or yeast; one serving of liver, or less than ¼ pound, is 100,000 milligrams; a heaping tablespoon of yeast is approximately 45,000 milligrams. What earthly value could 500 milligrams, or $\frac{1}{50}$ ounce, of either be?

The proportions of each vitamin found in animal and human tissues and the amounts of each excreted daily in the urine of healthy persons on adequate diets have been carefully studied. These proportions should apparently be maintained if health is to result. In case you take a tablet of mixed B vitamins, examine the label for the following: if your tablet supplies 2 milligrams of vitamin B_1, it should also contain equal amounts, or 2 milligrams, of vitamins B_2, B_6, and folic acid; approximately 20 times more niacin amide, pantothenic acid, and PABA than B_1, or 40 milligrams of each; 500 times more inositol and cholin, or 1,000 milligrams of each of these two. I know of no studies of the amount of biotin required. Only 1 to 3 micrograms of vitamin B_{12} appear to be needed daily.

Unfortunately, most B-complex tablets supply dangerously little vitamin B_6 and pantothenic acid and often no cholin and inositol. Many contain a great excess of vitamin B_1, thereby claiming to be "high potency." Our Food and Drug Administration limits over-the-counter sales of PABA to 30 milligrams and of folic acid to 0.1 milligrams; therefore no supplement having the proportions of vitamins found in healthy human tissues can be obtained unless purchased on prescription or in Canada or Europe.

It is now known that many individuals have unusually high requirements for certain nutrients. Examples are the schizophrenics' great need for niacin amide and the pregnant woman's high requirement for vitamin B_6. If health is to be protected during times of stress, the intake of all B vitamins must be increased, particularly pantothenic acid. Furthermore, a deficiency of a single B vitamin often predominates, such as a lack of vitamin B_2 when the eyes are bloodshot; at such times, individual B vitamins may be of great value, but in my opinion they should be taken only with natural sources of these vitamins, such as yeast, liver, or wheat germ. If you continue taking one or more B vitamins over a long period, you increase your need for all the other vitamins in the B group. The increased need for the ones you do not take may cause you to develop deficiencies of them.

During World War II, when defense plants were selling tablets which supplied only three or four of the B vitamins, dozens of persons with eczema consulted me. Invariably these persons had figured that if one tablet daily was good, several would be better. I told them to discontinue the tablets immediately. Usually it took a few days before they purchased the foods I recommended, and in this interval the eczema often cleared up. I became convinced that the B vitamins they were taking had increased their need for pantothenic acid, vitamin B_6, PABA, and/or biotin, a lack of any one of which could have caused the eczema. These people not only suffered from eczema but also from fatigue, constipation, and multiple symptoms which these very tablets are supposed to prevent.

The problem of obtaining adequate amounts of all the B vitamins largely from natural sources when living in a hotel or traveling is a challenging one. I travel a fair amount and often must live in hotels. At such times my requirements for these vitamins are unusually high because I am lecturing or rushing from one engagement to the next or interviewing people. For me, fatigue prevention at such times is paramount. I carry tablets of mixed B vitamins, plastic spoons, and yeast and/or desiccated liver or liver tablets. At most hotels, fresh liver and yogurt are available; if not, I ask the *maître d'hôtel* to order them for me. Wonderful people from coast to coast simplify my travel problems by inviting me to their homes. I doubt that there is another person in this entire United States who is served such marvelous meals of nutritious and delicious foods, although one hostess told me recently that the thought of my coming made her as nervous as if she were entertaining Socrates. Had she known that I washed my face in a granite wash pan until I was nearly old enough to vote, she might have relaxed.

The question of the quantity of B vitamins which should be taken daily is impossible to answer. The foods themselves vary widely. No two people have the same requirement, and every individual's requirement changes from day to day. For these reasons, the daily allowances suggested by the National Research Council (p. 275) have little value.

Since all the B vitamins appear to be needed by every cell in your body, the amount required depends on how many cells you have. If you are small-boned and short, you have relatively few cells, and your B-vitamin needs are probably moderate. Stored fat, of course, has no nutritional requirements. Your need for these vitamins, therefore, is in proportion to your ideal weight rather than to your actual weight. The larger your body structure and especially the more pounds of actual muscle you have, the larger the quantity of these vitamins you need.

Vitamin B_1 is used in changing sugar into energy or fat; hence the more starches and sugar you eat, the more of this vitamin you need. Similarly, if your diet is high in fat, you need more inositol and cholin. In one way or another, all B vitamins appear to be concerned with the utilization of foods. The person who eats large amounts of food, therefore, needs far greater quantities of these vitamins than do persons with small food intakes.

Since these vitamins are concerned with the production of energy, the more exercise you take and/or the harder you work, the more of these vitamins you need. Obviously, your requirement will be higher on the days you work hard than when you are vacationing. Also the less sleep you get, the more of these vitamins you need.

The requirement of all vitamins appears to be greatly increased by stress. Your need, therefore, will depend upon the number and severity of stresses you are under. A person might be upset over a pending divorce (stress 1), working long hours under pressure (stress 2), getting too little sleep (stress 3), taking thyroid tablets and benzedrine to keep going (stresses 4 and 5) and sleeping tablets to relax (stress 6), worrying over a sick child (stress 7), and suffering from a sinus infection (stress 8); his requirements for these vitamins are tremendous indeed. I frequently find persons harassed by as many as 15 or 20 different stressor agents at one time. If you are such a person, it seems to me you have three possibilities: live on yeast, liver, yogurt, wheat germ, and even B-vitamin tablets; or remove the stresses; or look forward to ill health.

Your need for these vitamins also appears to be in proportion to the amount of liquid you drink. Years ago, Dr. George R. Cowgill, of Yale University, produced B-vitamin deficiencies in animals by force-feeding them water. Alcoholic drinks of all varieties increase the need for the B vitamins; these vitamins are needed in utilizing the alcohol in the body and are washed through the body by the liquid. Recently—I am sincerely sorry to write this—scientists at the University of Wisconsin have produced multiple B-vitamin deficiencies merely by feeding animals coffee. Animals thrived when given caffeine without water. It would appear that caffeine, by stimulating the heartbeat, increases the flow of blood plasma through the kidneys and thus causes more of the B vitamins to be lost in the urine. So far no one seems to have investigated tea, but it is a fairly safe bet that the effect will be the same as that of coffee.

Heavy coffee drinkers almost invariably show symptoms of B-vitamin deficiencies even when their diets are excellent. I strongly suspect drinking large amounts of coffee is one factor contributing to the graying of hair and perhaps to baldness. Even drinking too much water may be unwise. This problem of liquid intake is probably more important than is appreciated.

Through the years I have been consulted by many persons who make a fetish of building health. For example, a woman recently told me that her breakfast was whole-grain cereal, hand-ground immediately before it was cooked, on which she put powdered whey, bone meal, sunflower seeds, powdered milk, yeast, rice polish, cream, and "raw" sugar. Her husband commented that it was like compiling a compost heap; he was (understandably) intolerant of her ideas (an understatement). Even with such carefully selected foods, this woman and others not unlike her showed symptoms of severe B-vitamin deficiencies. Invariably I find these people not only believe that one should drink eight glasses of water daily but actually do it. Large amounts of water, coffee, beer, soft drinks, or any liquid wash these vitamins out of your body. On very hot days when B vitamins are lost in perspiration and you drink large amounts of liquids, your need for these vitamins is tremendously increased.

It seems to me there is only one way to determine the quantity of these vitamins which will make you feel your best: find your own dosage. Learn how to vary the amounts from day to day depending upon your own body structure, the quantity and type of food you eat, the strain of your work and exercise, the stresses you are under, and the amount of liquid you drink. For example, during the summer when I vacation in the mountains, I eat yogurt occasionally and take only a tablespoon of yeast daily, usually in juice. When working moderately hard, I drink 1 or 2 glasses of pep-up made with ¼ cup of yeast and have some yogurt daily. If under stress, I eat a cup of yogurt and ¼ pound of fresh liver or take 2 tablespoons of desiccated liver in addition to the fortified milk; on the days when the going is really tough, I have liver and yogurt and drink a quart of pep-up containing ½ cup of yeast.

The one day when I experienced the most exuberant feeling of well-being and felt that my mind was clearest was a time when I was under considerable strain. I was asked to give an intensive post-graduate course in nutrition to physicians and dentists. The procedure was to lecture from 9 A.M. until 5 P.M. with a five-minute break every hour. I was told that the last lecturer to give such a course had blacked out from exhaustion at the end of the day. I realized that if I were to sell nutrition, I had to stay rested, with my mind alert. Frankly, I was frightened. I therefore had fruit with yogurt, liver, and pep-up at breakfast; milk and a huge serving of lobster for lunch, chosen because lobster is rich in glycogen, which would be changed slowly to sugar as the protein digested and would thus give a sustained pickup; and perhaps ¼ cup of the fortified milk at each hourly break. Although I stood except during lunch and spoke without a microphone, I did not experience one second of fatigue throughout the day or evening or even the next day, when I kept expecting a letdown. This experience convinced me that, for the relatively healthy person, fatigue can be completely prevented.

The real test, I believe, is this: if you are never tired, the chances are that your intake of B vitamins is adequate or that your intestinal bacteria are pretty efficient. If you experience fatigue, your intake is probably too low. A man said to me recently, "You never realize how terribly tired you were until you've found out you don't need to be tired at all."

CHAPTER 16

REDUCING BLOOD CHOLESTEROL

AN IMPORTANT FUNCTION OF AT LEAST THREE OF THE B vitamins—cholin, inositol, and vitamin B_6—is to help maintain normal blood cholesterol (p. 116), which becomes excessive when any one of these vitamins is undersupplied. Cholesterol deposited in the arteries has become a national problem in the United States, and many investigators believe it to be the major cause of death from heart disease. Problems of cholesterol deposition arose only after 1910, when machinery first came into use which removed most of the minerals and vitamins from breads and cereals. Since then, these three B vitamins (and vitamin E) have been largely discarded and have never been added to so-called "enriched" flour.

If the diet is adequate, cholesterol stays in small particles and passes readily into the tissues to be used. Only when nutrients are lacking does cholesterol remain in such large particles that it cannot pass through the arterial walls. Amounts in the blood increase. The quantity deposited in the walls of the arteries produces a condition spoken of as atherosclerosis. The arteries throughout the body thus become constricted, leaving less space through which the blood can flow. Circulation is impaired, often seriously. Oxygen and food less readily reach the tissues. Gradually the tissues are harmed, the degree of damage varying with the severity of the atherosclerosis and the length of time the blood cholesterol has been excessive.

Atherosclerosis to some degree now seems to affect almost every American. Autopsies of infants dying under a year of age have revealed cholesterol in their tiny arteries. Baby monkeys, fed commercially prepared formulas recommended by thousands of pediatricians, were found to have arteries completely plugged with cholesterol by the time they were a year old. The few studies made of growing children indicate that many have atherosclerosis, which markedly increases during the late teens. Autopsies of 300 boys killed in the Korean War—young men at the height of their physical development—showed that 72 per cent had cholesterol deposits in their coronary arteries, some with advanced atherosclerosis. The arteries of boys dying in Vietnam were found to be in even worse condition.

Scientists believe that any blood cholesterol above 180 milligrams in approximately ½ cup of blood (100 cc.) is excessive and incompatible with health. Persons whose blood cholesterol exceeds 260 milligrams per 100 cc. are known to be susceptible to heart attacks, though it has not been proved that the cholesterol deposits actually cause the attack. They do, however, drastically impair circulation to the heart muscles as well as to all parts of the body.

Fortunately, if the diet is made adequate, the cholesterol in the blood can again be broken into the smallest of microscopic particles, which pass quickly into the tissues. Experiments have shown that cholesterol already deposited can again be broken up, pass back into the blood, and eventually go into the tissues, leaving the arteries open. At times this process can be observed, especially when yellow fatty accumulations of cholesterol can be seen around the eyes; after the diet has been made adequate, these gradually disappear, often in a few months.

Because of our high death rate from coronary disease, the effect of cholesterol on the heart has held the limelight. Many studies indicate, however, that if cholesterol is being deposited in any one artery in the body, it is likewise being laid down in all arteries. Apparently none escape. For example, persons who have been hard of hearing have improved significantly after their excessive blood cholesterol was held at a normal level for several months. The onset of cataract and other visual problems is said to be complicated by cholesterol narrowing the blood vessels to the eyes, and vision has gradually improved when it has been reduced. Smokers with high blood cholesterol have been found to die of lung cancer earlier than do smokers whose blood cholesterol is low. Similarly, the plugging of the arteries with cholesterol causes literally millions of Americans to suffer from leg cramps, especially at night, when inactivity further reduces circulation. Not infrequently the oxygen supply is cut off so completely that toes or a foot become gangrenous and amputation is sometimes necessary. Millions of persons, often formerly brilliant individuals, become confused, forgetful, slow-witted, and absent-minded, especially during their later years, because cholesterol deposits interfere with the oxygen supply to the brain. Still more millions exist whose circulation to the heart muscles is decreased by narrowed arteries; and regardless of the cause of a heart attack, lowering the blood cholesterol gradually increases the oxygen supply and speeds recovery. The individual whose blood cholesterol is high, therefore, appears to be much like the famous one-hoss shay: he is falling to pieces at all the seams at the same time.

Though thousands of studies have dealt with the effect of diet on blood cholesterol, relatively few concern B vitamins alone. When animals, however, are put on a diet lacking cholin, which plays an essential role in utilizing cholesterol and solid (saturated) fats in the body, large amounts of cholesterol are held in the walls of the arteries, causing a condition analogous to human atherosclerosis. Such experimental atherosclerosis can be prevented or corrected by giving either cholin or lecithin,[1] which supplies cholin, inositol, and essential fatty acids.

Dr. Lester M. Morrison, working at the Los Angeles County Hospital, studied 600 patients who had survived heart attacks.[2] Alternate ones were given cholin but no medication. Their diets were inadequate in many respects; and they ate as much cream, butter, eggs, liver, and other foods high in cholesterol as they wished. Yet they quickly reported a feeling of well-being and general improvement in health; and many returned to work. The amount of cholesterol in their blood decreased. They had fewer recurring heart attacks and fewer deaths than in the alternate group, which was given standard medical treatment, such as phenobarbital, digitalis, and nitroglycerin.

When Dr. Morrison gave similar groups cholin, inositol, and a liver concentrate supplying all the B vitamins, his results were even better.[3] Patients reported having less shortness of breath and pain around the heart, and an increase in sex interest, morale, and general well-being. Many de-

[1] H. D. Kesten and R. Silbowitz, "Experimental Atherosclerosis and Soya Lecithin," *Proceedings, Society for Experimental Biology and Medicine,* XLIX (1942), 71.

[2] Lester M. Morrison and W. F. Gonzales, "Results of Treatment of Coronary Arteriosclerosis with Cholin," *American Heart Journal,* XXXIX (1950), 729.

[3] Lester M. Morrison, "Results of Betaine Treatment of Atherosclerosis," *American Journal of Digestive Diseases,* XIX (1952), 381; "The Therapeutic Action of Betaine-Lipotropic Combinations in Clinical Practice," *Geriatrics,* VIII (1953), 649.

clared they had "never felt better in their lives." Blood cholesterols dropped despite the generous use of eggs, liver, and butter. No deaths occurred during a year's observation, whereas death took 25 per cent of the group which Dr. Morrison describes as receiving "treatment by neglect."

When the diet is adequate, the liver produces daily wax-like substances collectively known as lecithin (p. 47) but spoken of scientifically as phospholipids. Lecithin breaks cholesterol into tiny particles which can pass readily into the tissues. It is only when too little lecithin can be produced that the particles of cholesterol become large and thus get trapped in the blood and the arterial walls.

Lecithin is made of fat, cholin, inositol, and essential unsaturated fatty acids; and it cannot be produced without the help of co-enzymes containing vitamin B_6 and magnesium. An undersupply of any one of the last five of these nutrients prevents the synthesis of lecithin and allows blood cholesterol to become excessive. Even given separately, each of these five usually reduces an excessive blood cholesterol. It has become well known that vegetable oils, as sources of linoleic acid, are needed to decrease blood cholesterol, yet the equally essential cholin, inositol, vitamin B_6, and magnesium are still largely ignored. If a person's diet is adequate, especially in these nutrients, he can produce all the lecithin his body needs.

When 2 tablespoons of granular lecithin were given at each meal to patients whose blood cholesterol had long been excessive and who had suffered heart attacks, their blood cholesterols fell remarkably within three months, although no other change had been made. Many of these patients had been resistant to cholesterol-lowering medications for as long as ten years. Even as little as a tablespoon of lecithin daily has sometimes decreased the cholesterol level. Lecithin capsules, however, contain too little to be of any value.

Every physician is aware that experimental atherosclerosis is produced merely by giving animals pure cholesterol and an inadequate diet extremely high in saturated fat. He is usually unaware that such a diet must also be deficient in magnesium, and that the need for cholin is proportional to the intake of solid fats; hence the animals' cholin requirement immediately skyrockets, but the amount of this vitamin in the diet is not increased. Without adequate cholin, lecithin production is limited. Moreover, few physicians are aware that experimental high blood cholesterol cannot be produced by feeding cholesterol and saturated fats if even a small amount of lecithin is included in the diet. When lecithin is generously supplied, no amount of cholesterol and saturated-fat feeding can cause atherosclerosis.

Unawareness of the importance of lecithin has resulted in appalling confusion. Medical treatment for atherosclerosis has now run the gamut of diets containing no eggs, no liver, almost no fat, and no cholesterol to diets supplying all the calories from vegetable oils[4] (the latter so unappetizing that they had to be given by stomach tube), or high in liver, eggs, and even cholesterol. The late Dr. Laurance Kinsell gave groups of patients whose cholesterol was excessive 10 eggs daily or 16 egg yolks, or the fat from 32 egg yolks, or even 60 grams—about 4 tablespoons—of pure cholesterol; in no case did the blood cholesterol increase provided all the nutrients essential for lecithin production were supplied in the diet. Dr. Kinsell also found that lecithin itself "lowered cholesterol profoundly." Only when given with an inadequate diet could butterfat, eggs, or any other cholesterol-bearing foods increase the cholesterol in the blood.

Physicians wisely advise patients whose blood cholesterol is excessive to increase vegetable oils, avoid all hydrogenated fats, and decrease their intake of solid animal fats by avoiding pork and rich gravies. Many ask that beef and/or lamb be eaten no more than three times a week. Broiled or roasted fish and fowl, however, can be on the daily menu; fish oils are unsaturated, the fat of fowl only partially saturated. Unfortunately, adding oil to the diet without simultaneously increasing the vitamin-E intake (p. 161) may actually cause a heart attack. Furthermore, patients are often asked to avoid such excellent foods as eggs, liver, kidneys, brains, shell fish, cream, butter, and whole milk. These foods, especially liver, supply the very nutrients needed to reduce cholesterol. Furthermore, when no cholesterol is obtained from the diet, the body produces cholesterol far more rapidly than when the intake is high.

Although no cholesterol is found in foods of vegetable origin, many vegetable fats are more saturated either by nature or by hydrogenation than are solid animal fats. These saturated vegetable fats increase the blood cholesterol by increasing the need for cholin. Coconut "oil," used in "filled" milk, in imitation milk, and in both powdered and liquid imitation sweet and sour creams, is the worst possible offender. Palm oil is also a saturated fat. Solid fats, regard-

---

[4] Laurance W. Kinsell, "Effect upon Serum Cholesterol and Phospholipids of Diets Containing Large Amounts of Vegetable Fat," *Journal of Clinical Nutrition*, I (1953), 224.

less of origin, increase blood cholesterols, whereas liquid fats, such as fish oils, do not. Even fat formed in the body from unneeded calories is saturated and can increase the cholin requirement, again causing the blood cholesterol to become excessive. Most people who have been overweight long have definite atherosclerosis.

Persons in Switzerland, Finland, and Denmark, whose intake of dairy products is very high, have few deaths from heart disease. Certain dairying tribes in Kenya who drink 9 to 14 quarts of whole milk daily were found to have "remarkably low" blood cholesterol; 60 per cent of their caloric intake was butterfat. The diets of these peoples are adequate in nutrients needed to produce lecithin. The late Dr. Francis M. Pottenger, Jr., then professor of medicine at the University of Southern California, told me that no patients ran a high blood cholesterol in his tubercular sanitarium, although they consumed huge amounts of eggs, liver, butter, and whole milk. Their diets were adequate in other respects.

As I see it, cholesterol deposition and its many related problems can be expected to get worse each year. People frequently try to control weight, for example, by missing meals; the body uses a little food continuously and is overwhelmed by a day's supply coming at one time. In both animals and humans, the blood cholesterol soars when only one or two meals are eaten daily; it decreases when small, frequent meals are obtained. Furthermore, many new foods containing coconut oil are reaching the market, though the label states only that the product contains a vegetable fat. Coconut butter is a highly saturated fat which increases blood cholesterol as quickly as the most saturated animal fat. Unfortunately, even pediatricians, tragically untrained in nutrition, recommend formulas containing coconut oil. Others give infants skim milk, completely lacking linoleic acid necessary for lecithin production.

Even when the blood cholesterol remains at 180 milligrams or below for a prolonged period, there is no guarantee that all the cholesterol deposits laid down over perhaps a half century have been picked up. The removal of cholesterol, once deposited, can be slow indeed. An adequate, cholesterol-lowering diet should therefore be maintained year after year.

Here again is an instance where the refining of foods, particularly the milling of grains, has affected the health of our entire nation. In Denmark during World War I and in England during World War II, when the B-vitamin intake greatly increased because wheat germ remained in all the breadstuffs, health improved in many ways and the incidence of deaths from heart disease dropped markedly.

How much longer are we going to allow the greed of the few to impose ill health on the many?

CHAPTER 17

THE TWO-HUNDRED-YEAR-OLD VITAMIN C

ALTHOUGH THE WORD VITAMIN WAS NOT COINED UNTIL THIS century, vitamin C has been known for over 200 years; its deficiency disease, scurvy, has played a major role in history. In 1754 James Lind wrote a treatise on scurvy recommending lemon juice for its prevention or cure. Despite the fact that we live in a land of plenty and our need for this vitamin can scarcely be called news, surveys show that three-fourths of our population receive less than the minimum daily allowance recommended by the National Research Council.

All fresh, growing foods contain vitamin C, or ascorbic acid. The richest sources are citrus fruits, guavas, ripe bell peppers and pimientos, and the seed pods of wild roses, known as rose hips. During World World II, the English extracted quantities of vitamin C from rose hips, simultaneously using hops from beer for the B vitamins; a wit remarked that England's magnificent strength was maintained by "her hips and her hops." Tomato juice, cabbage, and fresh strawberries are fair sources. Scurvy has resulted whenever people have been unable to get fresh foods.

One function of vitamin C is to help form and maintain a strong cement-like material, known as collagen, which holds together all the cells in your body. The amount of collagen required uses about a third of all the body protein. The collagen serves much the same purpose as cement does in a brick building except that the "concrete" in a healthy body is in the form of a stiff jelly, like gristle or a tough gelatin, known as connective tissue; thus every cell in your body "reposes" in a protective bed of jelly. This connective tissue is concentrated in the cartilage, the ligaments, the walls of all the blood vessels, the base of the bones and of the developing teeth, and gives all of these structures both great strength and elasticity. Although vitamin C is necessary for the formation of this tough jelly, adequate calcium must be present before the "jel" can set.[1] Calcium is not part of the structure; it merely has a stiffening effect much as pectin does. In fact, pectin is to the plant world what connective tissue is to the animal body; neither can be formed without vitamin C or be strong in the absence of adequate calcium.

Strong connective tissue plays a role of far greater importance than has heretofore been appreciated. Cell walls are only a few molecules thick; almost any harmful substance can penetrate them, whether it be virus, poisons, toxins, dangerous drugs, allergens, or other foreign materials which often gain access to the body. Strong connective tissue is not easily penetrated; thus the cells are protected. An undersupply of vitamin C, however, allows this tissue to break down; a lack of calcium allows it to weaken; protective doors are flung open, and pirates are invited in.

The walls of blood vessels must be able to expand or contract, depending on the amount of blood needed at a certain place and time; hence elasticity and strength are of paramount importance. Normal blood vessels are amazingly elastic, like rubber bands. Although a partial lack of vitamin C causes changes in all blood-vessel walls, those of the capillaries, made of single cells cemented with minute quantities of connective tissues, are affected most. When a deficiency exists, therefore, the capillary walls readily break down, and blood is freed into the tissues. These tiny hemorrhages occur first in the intestinal walls, the bone marrow, and joints, sometimes causing pain spoken of as "rheumatism." When the walls break near the surface of the skin, the freed blood discolors to produce a bruise. Regardless of the severity of a blow, a bruise shows brittleness and loss of elasticity in the blood-vessel walls; it is usually the first visual evidence of a vitamin-C deficiency, especially in women and children. "Pink toothbrush" may be the first symptom in men, who bruise infrequently because their muscles are generally harder than women's. Bruises and bleeding gums are both important danger signals. When adequate vitamin C is added to the diet, however, the capillary walls become strong within 24 hours.

A subtle lack of this vitamin causes profound changes in

[1] Mary E. Reid, "Interrelation of Calcium and Ascorbic Acid," *Physiological Review*, XXIII (1943), 76.

growing teeth. A deficiency in childhood causes slow dental growth or temporary cessation of growth. The dentin formed during a deficiency is porous and soft; if decay later penetrates the enamel, it meets little resistance; the pulp quickly becomes infected; the tooth dies and is probably lost. Experiments with labeled minerals show that when vitamin C is added to the diet of a child lacking it, normal dentin formation is resumed within a few hours.

If vitamin C is inadequate, the foundation of the bones partially breaks down, minerals are lost, the bones become rarefied and brittle and lack elasticity and strength; such bones break easily. Even when generous amounts of calcium and phosphorus are available, they cannot be deposited in the bones because the collagen base is too weak to hold them.

When a deficiency has existed and vitamin C is generously added to a diet otherwise adequate, dramatic changes take place in the bones whether during childhood or advanced age. New bone foundation forms within 24 hours, and minerals, if available, are quickly laid down. Bones thus continually change; a deficiency of vitamin C during the winter, followed by generous amounts from summer fruits and vegetables, produces alternate softening and strengthening of the bones, causing them to break easily at one time and to resist fractures at another.

Gum tissue fits tightly around the base of each tooth in a healthy mouth; it does not bleed even when brushed vigorously with a stiff-bristled brush. If vitamin C is undersupplied, the gums become puffy and spongy and bleed easily. Ever-present bacteria live on the dead cells of the gum tissue, and infections such as pyorrhea pockets often develop. When such patients have the pockets cleaned out and an adequate diet is eaten, soreness and inflammation often show marked improvement in a few days. A lack of vitamin A or niacin, however, also causes susceptibility to gum infections.

In pyorrhea the gums not only bleed easily and become infected, but much bone surrounding the teeth is destroyed, causing them to become loose. When guinea pigs (used experimentally because most animals produce their own vitamin C) are kept only mildly deficient in this nutrient, a condition strikingly similar to pyorrhea develops in nine months, which is equivalent to 40 years of human life, the age when pyorrhea most frequently appears. It seems probable that a subtle undersupply of vitamin C over a period of years plays a causative role in the onset of pyorrhea.

Typical pyorrhea, however, is not uncommon among malnourished children and adolescents. If the infection is not too far advanced, an entirely adequate diet unusually high in vitamin C can restore oral health.

Scar tissue formed in healing wounds and injuries is a connective tissue made of collagen which depends on both vitamin C and calcium for strength. During World War I it was noticed that wounds healed slowly or failed to heal unless fresh foods were eaten. Experiments prove that speed of healing and strength of the scar tissue are directly proportional to the vitamin-C intake. Operative patients deficient in this vitamin not only heal slowly, but their wounds frequently break open. When 4,000 milligrams or more of vitamin C have been given daily to such patients, the speed of healing is often dramatic. Medical journals have urged all physicians to recommend large amounts of this vitamin before and after surgery.

Vitamin C is especially important in the healing of broken bones. When it is lacking, a collagen bone base fails to form; hence the ends of the broken parts are unable to knit. Such abnormal healing occurs frequently in older persons whose diets are notoriously deficient in multiple nutrients. Bones heal readily at any age when an adequate diet is given and steps are taken to assure normal absorption. Protein, calcium, vitamin D and other nutrients, however, are equally as important as are large amounts of vitamin C.

Although not yet understood, vitamin C apparently plays a role in maintaining normal vision. In healthy eyes, the vitamin is concentrated in the lens; the vitamin is lacking or reduced in the lenses of persons having certain types of cataract. Experimental cataracts have been produced by a restricted vitamin-C intake. Marked improvement in eye infections and inflammation of the eyes often follows when large amounts of vitamin C are taken.

This vitamin cannot be stored in the body. The tissues, however, can be saturated as a sponge might be saturated with water. The state of saturation, in which every cell has all of this vitamin it can use, is considered to be most compatible with health. After saturation occurs, any excess vitamin C obtained is promptly thrown off in the urine. The amount of vitamin C found in foods, blood, or urine can easily be measured. The tissues of seemingly healthy persons whose diets have been inadequate frequently soak up as much as 4,000 milligrams of this vitamin before any is excreted; this amount is equivalent to 40 glasses of fresh citrus juice. After saturation, the amount of vitamin obtained minus that lost in the urine gives the requirement for a particular day. By this method requirements of different people under various circumstances have been studied.

About 50 milligrams of vitamin C appear to be needed daily by the genuinely healthy adult to prevent scurvy, provided his tissues are already saturated; 60 to 80 milligrams are recommended by the National Research Council as the minimum intake. This amount can be supplied by a glass of fresh orange or grapefruit juice. The scurvy-preventing requirements of vitamin C appear to increase with advancing years, probably because absorption is often faulty and much of this vitamin is destroyed in the intestine when the stomach fails to produce normal amounts of hydrochloric acid. Studies show that the aged are appallingly deficient in this vitamin. Dr. Walter H. Eddy when at Columbia University pointed out years ago that many signs considered typical of old age are actually symptoms of scurvy: wrinkles, or loss of elasticity of the skin; loss of teeth; brittleness of bones. Certainly the person who wishes to retain his youthfulness should see that his ascorbic-acid intake is ample.

The vitamin C in all plants is produced, by the aid of enzymes, under conditions of warmth and moisture at which the plant grows best. Unfortunately, the action of the enzymes is reversible; they can quickly destroy what they have made. After a food is harvested, the destruction of the vitamin occurs most rapidly under the same conditions as those at which the plant grew best, that is, in a heated market or a warm room. Furthermore, the enzymes destroy the vitamin by combining it with oxygen; hence, if a fruit or vegetable is peeled or chopped, the destruction is unusually rapid. The enzymes are kept inactive by refrigeration or are destroyed by heat at about 140°F. Since the vitamin dissolves in water, much or all of it is lost when foods are washed slowly, soaked, or boiled. The average housewife, untrained in nutrition, extravagantly destroys vitamin C before the food can be swallowed.

For practical purposes, the best source of this vitamin is citrus fruits and juices. Fresh orange juice averages 130 milligrams for an eight-ounce glass; grapefruit and lemon and canned orange juice, about 100 milligrams. Frozen orange juice may be as rich as fresh or may contain little, depending on the type of oranges from which the juice came, the method of extraction, and the length of time it has been stored. Often culls, containing little vitamin C, are used for juice. In general, the sweeter oranges, to which no sugar need be added, have the highest vitamin-C content. Other juices, such as apple, pineapple, or grape, are not good sources, whether canned, frozen, or fresh. Tomato juice may supply 30 milligrams of vitamin C per glass or may contain none. A ripe pimiento or bell pepper or one California persimmon often contains 300 milligrams of vitamin C, whereas ½ cup of guavas may supply 1,000 milligrams.

Tomatoes, both fresh and canned, all salad greens, fresh strawberries, and raw cabbage average 30 to 50 milligrams per serving. Green vegetables, such as spinach, Brussels sprouts, and broccoli, may be good sources, but 50 to 90 per cent is often lost in the water in which these foods are cooked. Apples, bananas, lettuce, potatoes, and peas may supply only 20 to 30 milligrams per serving but are important sources because of the quantities eaten. Foods such as butter, cheese, eggs, all breadstuffs, and dry beans lack ascorbic acid. Milk and cooked meat other than liver contain almost none.

Climate, soil, the degree of ripeness, storage, temperatures and methods of handling, cooking, canning, or freezing all affect the vitamin-C content of foods. Little ascorbic acid is destroyed when foods are quickly frozen, but losses of 90 per cent may occur within an hour after the food has thawed. Much vitamin C is lost if foods are stored at room temperature or are soaked or boiled and the water discarded.

Since citrus fruits are the most dependable sources of vitamin C, one or more grapefruit and/or oranges or a glass of fresh unstrained juice should be taken daily by every child and adult. It is wise to serve a fresh salad at each lunch and dinner and to have appetizers of fresh fruit on the menu frequently. Even today when frozen foods are widely used, fewer vitamin-C deficiencies occur in summer and fall when more fresh foods are available than in winter and spring. This deficiency is especially common among the poor of all ages and the aged of all economic groups. If care is given to the purchase and preparation of food and the planning of menus, much vitamin C can be obtained even when little money is available.

A group of substances known as the bioflavonoids occur in the pulp—but not the juice—of citrus fruits and especially in the white of the rind. Experiments indicate that these bioflavonoids reduce the need for vitamin C and make it more effective, thereby increasing the strength of capillary walls, reducing inflammation, and decreasing the seepage of blood cells and proteins into the tissues. When given to athletes, the bioflavonoids speeded the healing of muscle strains, skin abrasions, and joint injuries. Some investigators believe it is not the bioflavonoids responsible for such improvement but a yet unidentified nutrient associated with them. Until more is known, it seems wise to include them in the diet.

Because the changes in collagen breakdown can be swift, harmful, and hidden, a bruise should be interpreted as a danger signal, indicating that more vitamin C should immediately be added to your diet.

CHAPTER 18

A FINGER IN EVERY PIE

ALTHOUGH IT HAS BEEN KNOWN FOR CENTURIES THAT A person dying of scurvy could make a startling and dramatic recovery if fresh foods were given him, vitamin C can bring about other startling and dramatic recoveries only recently discovered. Much of the research being done is still unpublished.

Aside from helping to build collagen, this vitamin appears to be a busybody with its finger in every pie. When toxic or poisonous substances gain access to the body, adequate vitamin C, if available, often detoxifies them, making them harmless. The toxic substance apparently combines with the vitamin, and the two are excreted together in the urine; this combination is now given the name of ascorbigen.

It has long been known that during infections and diseases, vitamin C disappears from the blood and urine; that the more vitamin C given, the less ill the person usually is, and the more quickly he recovers; and that 20 to 40 times more of the vitamin has to be given during illnesses to keep the tissues saturated than during periods of health. Furthermore, antibodies are unable to render bacteria harmless unless vitamin C is adequately supplied. Antibodies must be helped by a complement; if there is no vitamin C, there is no complement. Vitamin C seems equally helpful whether the disease is caused by virus or bacteria or is non-infectious, as is gout, arthritis, or a stomach or duodenal ulcer. Almost countless infections and diseases have been studied: colds, pneumonia, meningitis, rheumatic fever, tuberculosis, diphtheria, infections of the prostate, ears, eyes, sinuses, and tonsils, the childhood diseases, and many others. In every case, vitamin C appears to be the good Christian ready to soothe the aching brow.

It has been found that vitamin C can often prevent or cure chemical poisoning. This vitamin has been valuable in correcting the toxic effects of lead, bromide, arsenic, benzene, and many other substances which sometimes gain access to the body, especially of persons doing industrial work.

Studies have proved that vitamin C helps to prevent allergies; if enough is given, it can detoxify the harmful effects of allergens which have entered the blood, whether they be pollens, dusts, dandruff, or foods. This vitamin seems to be equally effective in treating all varieties of allergies, whether rhinitis (stuffy nose and/or postnasal drip), hay fever, asthma, eczema, or hives; spectacular relief often results from massive doses of vitamin C. Even the effects of poison oak, poison ivy, snake bite, black widow spider bite, and carbon monoxide poisoning have been overcome when massive amounts of vitamin C have been taken.

Any foreign substance reaching the blood appears to be more or less toxic; the harm is prevented by vitamin C, but the vitamin itself is destroyed in the process. For example, every drug apparently destroys vitamin C in the body. When a drug promises to save your life, the vitamin destruction is unimportant; if it is being taken promiscuously without a physician's prescription, both the drug and the vitamin loss may be unnecessary. It has been found that a single tablet of any one of several drugs widely used and considered harmless can continue to destroy vitamin C in the body for three weeks or longer after the drug is taken. The *Journal of the American Medical Association* carried an editorial entitled "Is Aspirin a Dangerous Drug?"[1] pointing out that aspirin, which frequently causes internal hemorrhages, can be dangerous unless our diets contain enough vitamin C to detoxify it.

This vitamin appears to play no major role in producing energy; yet it helps to prevent fatigue. For example, a group of soldiers was given vitamin C until the tissues were saturated. Their performance was compared with that of a similar group not given the vitamin. After maneuvers involving carrying heavy equipment, walking miles, and climbing mountains, the soldiers given vitamin C experienced little fatigue, recovered quickly, and had no leg cramps, whereas the other soldiers suffered severely from cramps and fatigue and did not completely recover for days. The harmful "ashes" left from incompletely burned fats, known as acetone bodies, which accumulate in the

[1] CXXIV (1944), 777.

tissues when the blood sugar falls below normal, is a major cause of fatigue; these acetone bodies are detoxified by vitamin C.

Vitamin C seems to help everything by being destroyed by everything. For a nutrition consultant, the situation as regards vitamin C becomes progressively more embarrassing. No one seems to be in danger of coming down with scurvy; yet almost every person has abnormalities which vitamin C has been proved to help. In order to do good work, a nutritionist seems to have to accept the fact that people think him a crackpot hipped on liver, yeast, orange juice, and vitamin-C tablets. But all people do require the same 40 nutrients.

The quantity of vitamin C needed to detoxify a foreign substance depends upon the amount of that substance gaining access to the body. Relatively small quantities are required by the healthy person to prevent harm, particularly when adequate calcium is absorbed. Many toxic substances, however, might enter the body simultaneously. For example, a person suffering from allergies and doing industrial work where toxic chemicals have reached his blood might suffer from a serious infection which prevents him from eating and for which he is given various drugs; his temporary need for vitamin C would be tremendous indeed. Fortunately, even massive doses of this vitamin seem to be completely harmless; any excess not needed in the body is quickly lost in the urine.

Dr. Fred R. Klenner, chief of staff at the Memorial Hospital in Reidsville, North Carolina, appears to have given the largest quantities of this vitamin to date, administered by injection when his patients are too ill to swallow.[2] Some years ago it was my good fortune to visit with Dr. Klenner and hear him lecture. He showed slides of hospital records and fever charts and told of case after case of meningitis, encephalitis, virus pneumonia, and serious complications following scarlet fever and other diseases treated with massive amounts of vitamin C. Many patients had not been expected to live; often huge amounts of antibiotics had been given without success; in most instances, fevers ranged from 103° to 105°F. Within a few minutes after

[2] Fred R. Klenner, "The Use of Vitamin C as an Antibiotic," *Journal of Applied Nutrition*, VI (1953), 274; "Massive Doses of Vitamin C and the Virus Diseases," *Southern Medicine and Surgery*, CXIII (1951), 101; "The Vitamin Treatment for Acute Poliomyelitis," *ibid.*, CXIV (1952), 194; "Virus Pneumonia and Its Treatment with Vitamin C," *ibid.*, CX (1948), 36.

the vitamin was injected, fevers started to drop and temperatures frequently reached normal within a few hours. Usually the patient enjoyed the next meal and was ready to be discharged from the hospital in two or three days. The amount of vitamin given varied with the severity of the illness. The initial dose was usually 2,000 to 6,000 milligrams (2 to 6 grams), followed four and eight hours later by a second and a third injection of 2,000 to 4,000 milligrams if the temperature did not remain normal; injections were continued around the clock when needed.

Dr. Klenner told of an eighteen-month-old girl suffering from polio. The mother reported that the child had become paralyzed following a convulsion, after which she soon lost consciousness. When Dr. Klenner first saw the child, her little body was blue, stiff, and cold to the touch; he could neither hear heart sounds nor feel her pulse; her rectal temperature was 100°F. The only sign of life he could detect was a suggestion of moisture condensed on a mirror held to her mouth. The mother was convinced that the child was already dead. Dr. Klenner injected 6,000 milligrams of vitamin C into her blood; four hours later the child was cheerful and alert, holding a bottle with her right hand, though her left side was paralyzed. A second injection was given; soon the child was laughing and holding her bottle with both hands, all signs of paralysis gone. Dr. Klenner quite understandably speaks of vitamin C as "the antibiotic par excellence." A physician who later obtained striking results at the Los Angeles County Hospital by treating severe infections with vitamin C matched Dr. Klenner's enthusiasm with the remark, "If anything should be called a miracle drug, it is vitamin C."

With his extremely ill patients, Dr. Klenner found that no vitamin C whatsoever could be detected in the blood only a few minutes after massive doses were injected; nor was any vitamin C found in the urine. It is his belief that this vitamin combines immediately with toxins and/or virus, thus causing the fever to drop. In cases where the fever rises again later, he believes that too little vitamin C has been given in the initial dose; that virus not destroyed multiplies and again causes the temperature to increase. For this reason, he emphasizes that if the original dose is sufficiently large, no further massive amounts need be given.

Many other investigators have obtained remarkable results with massive doses of vitamin C in treating mononucleosis, phlebitis, slipped discs, bursitis, and a wide variety of other abnormalities. In an attempt to saturate the tissues, physicians have recommended as much as 1,000 milligrams every hour during the day from 1 to 3 days to persons suffering from arthritis, gout, and almost any infectious disease, infection, or allergy, the same amount being repeated during subsequent acute attacks. They have also recommended that this quantity be taken immediately at the onset of a cold or any infection and that the amount be decreased only after all symptoms have disappeared. On the other hand, satisfactory results have been reported when a mild allergy or lead poisoning has been treated with as little as 300 milligrams daily. These problems, however, are medical ones; our problem is prevention.

Physicians have pointed out that patients with hepatitis or mononucleosis, for example, have often been sick several days before a doctor is called in and a diagnosis made. By the time such cases are checked into a hospital they are in what has been described as "a sorry state." Vitamin C has proved to be most effective when taken at the onset of an infection, at which time a patient rarely sees his physician. Relatively smaller amounts are needed than those required after an illness becomes serious. If sufficient quantities of the vitamin are obtained, especially when taken every 2 or 3 hours around the clock with pantothenic acid (p. 79) and fortified milk, serious illness may often be prevented. It appears desirable, therefore, for persons to learn when large amounts of vitamin C are needed and how much should be taken. Such information has great comfort value.

I asked several nutritionally oriented physicians if they felt it wise to recommend that families keep vitamin-C tablets in the medicine chest and use them at the onset of any illness. The most frequent reply was, "They are certainly safer than aspirin." Several physicians remarked, "Tell people to take them when they need to, but the rest of the time to stick to orange juice and natural sources." Others pointed out the importance of advising large initial doses rather than smaller frequent ones, the total of which might be larger than would be needed if the original dose were sufficient.

When persons are too ill to eat or retain food, as were many of Dr. Klenner's patients, injections of vitamin C are obviously advantageous. If the vitamin is taken immediately at the onset of an illness, however, such difficulties rarely arise. Occasionally undissolved tablets can be seen in the stools, particularly if diarrhea occurs. In this case and when a child is too young to swallow tablets, I tell people to put one cup of hot water in a liquefier, add 50 tablets of vitamin C, 500 milligrams each, blend well, sweeten to taste with honey, pour into a glass jar, and keep refrigerated. If one does not have a liquefier, the 50 tablets can be pulverized and dissolved in a cup of hot water. Each teaspoon of such a solution contains 500 milligrams. If 100 tablets (500 milligrams each) are dissolved in a cup of water, each teaspoon of solution would supply 1 gram, or 1,000 milligrams, of the vitamin; similarly 200 tablets per cup of water would give a solution having 2,000 milligrams of vitamin C per teaspoon and so on. These solutions are quite palatable. There is available chewable vitamin C, which most youngsters enjoy, and powdered vitamin C which can be stirred into any cooked or canned fruit or juice. Since the synthetic vitamin does not contain enzymes found in natural foods, it is quite stable to heat and storage, but if stirred into uncooked fruit or juice, enzymes can readily destroy it.

Although I have never been up a night with a sick child, I know that giving a tablespoon or more of vitamin-C solution every hour or two to a sick, feverish infant can be a godsend when a physician cannot be reached. The knowledge that this vitamin could help in emergencies brought me great comfort as a mother and I am sure other mothers have felt much the same. For example, a friend's little boy, then the only child, died of meningitis. Three children were born later. The mother's fear that something would happen to one of these children was ruining her life and theirs. They were not allowed to go to a public pool or mingle in crowds. The mother gathered articles concerning diseases from newspapers and magazines; she became overcautious about sanitation and still lived in fear and dread. I saw her recently for the first time in years; the children were at a park, swimming. I commented on her change of attitude. "I never worry about them any more," she answered. "At the first sniffle I give extra vitamin C. The kids haven't been sick a day in years."

My first personal experience wtih massive doses of vitamin C came when our son, then five years old, had the mumps. One morning when we awoke, the evidence was unmistakable. Starting at 7 A.M., I gave him 1,000 milligrams of "melted" vitamin C directly from the spoon every hour except when he slept, making a total of 10,000 milligrams during the day. By that evening, all swelling was gone, and there was no further sign of illness. Within the next two months every member of our family had the one-day mumps. The children weathered all of the childhood "diseases" in the same delightful fashion. There was no irritability, nausea, or vomiting; no meals were missed; and after vitamin C had been given, there was no fever.

The quantity of vitamin C to take depends on the type and severity of the illness and whether it is of short duration or chronic. Large amounts are usually needed at first to saturate the tissues; the quantities can later be reduced. Persons suffering from arthritis, asthma, or other chronic diseases have often taken drugs for months or even years; these drugs must apparently be detoxified before vitamin C is available to the tissues. It is difficult to realize what large amounts of vitamin C can be destroyed by drugs. It has long been known that if more of the vitamin is taken than is needed, the excess is quickly lost in the urine; and that none is lost until the tissues throughout the body are saturated, or contain all the vitamin C they need. A healthy person's tissues may be saturated with as little as 200 milligrams or less of the vitamin daily. Yet I found one study of the quantity of this vitamin needed by a number of persons taking tranquilizers; no vitamin C whatsoever appeared in the urine of several until 15 grams—15,000 milligrams—were given daily. In planning diets, I usually suggest that 500 milligrams of vitamin C be taken with each dose of medication, and that if bruises appear, this amount be increased until the physician decreases the drug. It is known, however, that vitamin C increases the value of every type of drug and at the same time decreases its toxicity.

The quantity of vitamin C most advantageous under all circumstances for all persons can probably never be known. Our requirements vary daily. Almost every person is exposed to chemicals from water purifiers, smog, smoke, or smoking; from arsenic, DDT, and other pesticides, traces of which are found in fruits, vegetables, meats, and milk; many people take drugs occasionally; and most of us are threatened by one or more infections per year. Each individual must find his own dosage, depending upon his symptoms and the number of toxic substances he is exposed to. If you are going to use massive doses over a prolonged period, however, first make sure that your diet is adequate in every respect. During normal times, use natural sources first: 1 or 2 oranges daily; a glass of orange juice; salads; and fresh fruits for desserts and mid-meals. Watch for bruises; if they occur, know that your intake of vitamin C is not meeting your needs; then supplement your natural sources with vitamin-C tablets, solution, or powder.

Massive doses of vitamin C seem never to be toxic. Occasionally a person taking large quantities will develop a skin rash which appears to be caused by the filler holding the tablets together; this problem can generally be solved by changing brands or using powdered vitamin C. If the quantity taken greatly exceeds the amount which can be absorbed, diarrhea may occur; the vitamin should then be decreased or temporarily discontinued. Large amounts of vitamin C can act as a diuretic, causing excessive urination, which is advantageous in case the tissues have been water-logged. Any dehydration is usually accompanied by a corresponding thirst and is easily corrected.

In a recent phone conversation, Dr. Klenner told me that he is now giving his severely ill patients intravenous injections of 50 to 100 grams of vitamin C—50,000 to 100,000 milligrams—in 5-per-cent dextrose solution; and as soon as they are able, he also has them take as much vitamin C by mouth as they can tolerate without having diarrhea, a problem which never arises when the vitamin is given by injection. He said that geriatric patients, especially those who appeared to be hopelessly ill with pneumonia, have often recovered after a single injection of vitamin C, though he has sometimes given a second 30 grams the following day.

Dr. Klenner felt that his results in treating severely burned persons with massive amounts of this vitamin had been particularly rewarding. He remarked that the pain disappeared so quickly that pain killers often were not needed, that the wounds healed readily and cleanly, and that no skin grafts were necessary. He told me that he even sprayed open burns every few hours with a 3-per-cent solution of vitamin C or laid cloths moistened with this solution over the burn and that patients found it especially soothing. Such a solution could be prepared by blending 12 tablets of vitamin C, 500 milligrams each, with a cup of water.

"We take arthritic cripples and put them back to work," Dr. Klenner exclaimed. "Even the worst cases are rehabilitated in six months." He added that each takes by mouth 10 grams—10,000 milligrams—of vitamin C daily. He explained that when his patients started by taking only one 500-milligram tablet with each meal and before bed for a day or two, then increased the amount by 1,000 milligrams daily until they were taking 5 tablets, or 2,500 milligrams, four times each day, the huge amounts were well tolerated and no diarrhea occurred. This quantity, or 10 grams daily, they continued indefinitely, even after they recovered. When I asked about the amount of vitamin C lost in the urine, he told me that he had found it to be surprisingly little. He again stressed that vitamin C enhances the value of any drug, even though much of the vitamin is destroyed by the drug.

Dr. Klenner is still enthusiastic about the use of massive amounts of vitamin C in treating every variety of infection, allergies, snake and insect bites, and myriads of conditions resulting from excessive stress. After 25 years of clinical research, this wonderful physician has found vitamin C to be far safer than drugs and far more valuable than most. He considers it to be the antibiotic of choice.

I am convinced, however, that the greatest value of massive doses of vitamin C will never be shown by research or found in a laboratory. It lies in the hearts and prayers of the parents of the nation. They will render silent tribute to the wonderful scientists and physicians who have brought them peace of mind.

CHAPTER 19

THE NICEST PEOPLE I KNOW

IT IS UNDISPUTED THAT VITAMIN D AIDS THE ABSORPTION OF calcium, favors its retention, and improves its utilization. Certainly it is a fact that calcium is needed by adults; this mineral helps to relax nerves, induce sound sleep, and decrease sensitivity to pain. The National Research Council concedes that small amounts of vitamin D are desirable for people working at night, for elderly persons, and for nuns and others whose clothing shields them from the sunlight. According to this Council, however, "vigorous persons leading normal lives" appear not to need vitamin D. What about the almost vigorous person leading an almost normal life? It seems to me the scientific scientists are indulging in unscientific double talk here.

Vitamin D is scantily distributed in foods. There is some in egg yolks provided the hens sat in the sunshine and preened their feathers well; 50 to 200 eggs daily might supply your needs quite adequately if modern hens were not forced to live in shaded cages. Caviar contains some vitamin D; there is a little in the milk from cows pastured on high mountain slopes. Artificially produced vitamin-D milk is excellent, but compared to a few years ago relatively little of it is now sold. Fish-liver oils are the only natural foods containing sufficient quantities of this vitamin to promote health.

This vitamin D can be produced in foods or oils by exposure to ultraviolet light; the commercial concentrate, viosterol, is made by such a method. Vitamin D is formed by ultraviolet light from sunshine in the oils *on* the skin, provided you have oils on your skin and the shortest rays from the sun reach the earth. In winter, these rays do not penetrate our atmospheric blanket; during the summer they reach the top of the Empire State Building but usually not the street below it. Sunshine would be an excellent source of this vitamin if it were not for the facts that people are surrounded by smog, wear clothes, live in houses, and have bathtubs and hot-water heaters.

Most medical textbooks say that vitamin D is formed by sunlight on the oils *in* the skin although it was proved years ago[1] that the oils must first be *on* the skin, then exposed to ultraviolet light, and later absorbed back into the body. If persons take a bath before going into the sunshine, the oils are washed off, and no vitamin D is formed; if they do not bathe before exposure to sunshine but bathe immediately afterward, the oils are removed before the vitamin can be absorbed into the body. Most of the oils appear to be washed off by cold water, and still larger quantities by warm water; warm soapy water does the job thoroughly. Time was when wood was hard to split, water hard to carry, and soap hard to make (and smelled too bad to use anyway); the Saturday-night bath was then a family institution. During the remainder of the week the oils stayed on the skin and absorbed any ultraviolet rays which reached them. The early settlers described the Indians as being great of stature with teeth "as even as piano keys," both the advantages of having no hot-water heaters and no soap. Now as a nation we are bath-happy and soap-happy; I, for one, call it progress.

There are to be found in any medical library many books and thousands of articles concerning the need of vitamin D by children. Except for a few articles and short paragraphs on diseases known as osteomalacia, meaning literally bad bones, and osteoporosis, meaning porous bones, the need of adults for vitamin D is rarely mentioned. These diseases are identical except in degree; bad bones are worse than porous ones. In both, so few minerals are available that the bones become porous and honeycombed; the persons so afflicted may become shorter and may suffer from muscle cramps, twitches, and even convulsions, or tetany. Osteoporosis is usually painless, but in osteomalacia pain is experienced, especially in the hips; such pain is customarily spoken of as rheumatism; spontaneous fractures and breaks may occur. This disease is common in China and India, particularly when the need for minerals is increased by pregnancy and "becomes more piteous" (p. 684 of ref.

[1] A. C. Helmer and C. H. Jansen, "The Absorption of Vitamin D Through the Skin" and "Vitamin D Precursors Removed from Human Skin by Washing," *Studies of the Institutum Divi Thomae,* I (1937), 83, 207.

2, p. 43) with each child, especially when the mother "suckles her infant in the vain hope of thus warding off her tragic fertility." Skeletal remains indicate that the Norse colony founded by Eric the Red in Greenland gradually became extinct because the pelvic deformities of women suffering from osteomalacia hindered childbirth; it is thought that the colonists did not eat the local diet of fish and fish-liver oils; too little vitamin D could be obtained from the Arctic sun. Osteomalacia results from famines and food shortages during and after wars. It occurs in American and English cities "where solitary old people live in proud self-respecting poverty rather than apply for charity" (p. 684 of ref. 2, p. 43). This disease can be cured by vitamin D alone, but to speed recovery calcium and phosphorus are customarily given with the vitamin.

Sir Robert McCarrison, the great English physician, wrote of osteomalacia in India among the Mohammedan women observing the custom of purdah. These women veil their faces at adolescence and rarely go outside their homes. No milk or other food rich in calcium is eaten. Vitamin D, however, either from sunshine or cod-liver oil, so increases the absorption and utilization of the meager dietary calcium that health is restored. Here, at last, is proof that vitamin D alone, without any increase in calcium or phosphorus, can help adults as well as rapidly growing children.

Most Americans have no more cause to worry about osteomalacia than about scurvy; 60 per cent or more of our population, however, obtain too little calcium in their diets. Much of this supply fails to reach the blood. Calcium is tricky in that it does not dissolve easily; your teeth and bones, even though washed by saliva or tissue fluid, do not dissolve. Unless calcium from food is dissolved, it remains in the intestine and is lost in the feces. The calcium supply to the tissues can be increased by eating more foods containing calcium or by obtaining ample vitamin D; both should be adequate.

Excessive amounts of vitamin D can be toxic, causing such symptoms as weakness, fatigue, weight loss, nausea, vomiting, diarrhea, abdominal cramps, headaches, dizziness, and demineralization of bones. Blood calcium becomes excessive, the blood pressure increases, and calcium is laid down in soft tissues. As little as 1,800 units of vitamin D given daily can be toxic to infants and 25,000 units daily, if taken over a prolonged period, to adults. For a time, the British added vitamin D to so many baby foods that infants often received 4,000 units or more daily; a number of these children died of vitamin-D toxicity. Follow-up studies of survivors showed that the symptoms disappeared in a few weeks after the vitamin was withdrawn and no permanent damage was done. Vitamin D toxicity can be largely prevented by generous amounts of vitamins C, E, or cholin. It is made far worse by a deficiency of vitamin E or magnesium; either deficiency causes large amounts of calcium to be laid down in soft tissues.[2] Unfortunately, the diets of infants and children are severely lacking in both vitamin E and magnesium.

Almost all toxicity has resulted from vitamin D artificially produced by irradiation (viosterol) and not from that in natural fish-liver oils or fish-liver-oil concentrates. Yet fear of toxicity has caused the National Research Council to recommend only 400 units daily for persons of all ages, regardless of the source of the vitamin or individual variations in requirements. A few years ago I saw a two-year-old boy with the classical symptoms of the vitamin-D-deficiency disease, rickets: his forehead was huge and bulging; his chest caved in at the top while the lower ribs flared outward; his knees rubbed together; and his legs were severely bowed. Yet this child, whose mother is extremely conscientious, had been given 400 units of vitamin D daily. The youngster, however, was growing unusually rapidly and was obviously going to be like his father, who is a huge man; his need for vitamin D was probably two or three times greater than that of a slow-growing child. This child was then given 2 teaspoons of cod-liver oil daily for a year and a teaspoon daily since and has now become a beautifully formed, handsome boy.

The symptom of rickets, or of too little vitamin D, I see most frequently in babies 3 to 15 months old is a bulging forehead. If the bones are developing normally, the forehead, viewed in profile, forms a straight line above the eyes. The bulging forehead characteristic of rickets is largely thick cartilage laid down only when normal, brain-protecting bone cannot be formed. A partial lack of vitamin D also results in many varieties of homeliness: narrow, underdeveloped faces and chests; buck teeth, irregular teeth, and crooked teeth; sloping or protruding chins and/or foreheads; eyes so deep set as to give a thug appearance; and dozens of other abnormalities. People often argue that these abnormalities are hereditary, and indeed they frequently

[2] Hans Selye, *Calciphylaxis* (Chicago: University of Chicago Press, 1962); Eörs Bajusz, *Nutritional Aspects of Cardiovascular Disease* (Philadelphia: J. B. Lippincott Company, 1965).

appear to be; parents whose faces are deformed because of poor nutrition may give their children such inadequate diets that their faces are also deformed. The tiny full or rounded chest and round face of a healthy newborn infant reveals its heredity; when the diet meets the child's needs, these contours remain throughout life. If by the time the youngster is ten his face is shaped like a pear or a banana, you may be sure he received too little vitamin D and calcium.

Vitamin D can be absorbed into the blood only in the presence of fat. A great increase in rickets has been reported in both the United States and Canada because physicians, untrained in nutrition, recommend that infants and children be given skim milk. Even vitamin D given in capsules is poorly absorbed by growing children up to approximately twelve years of age. Such capsules contain too little oil to insure absorption. Because of frequent bathing and too little time spent in the open, one cannot rely on sunshine as a source of this vitamin; a high incidence of rickets has been reported in such sunny lands as Greece and Israel.

Personally I feel that nothing produces such beautiful children as old-fashioned cod-liver oil, provided it is always refrigerated, given only after a meal and with vitamin E, and continued throughout the entire growth period. Unless the child is growing particularly fast, a half teaspoon or less is usually adequate for a baby up to a year of age, especially one receiving vitamin-D milk; read the label and allow a total of no more than 1,000 units of vitamin D daily. The amount should gradually be increased to 1,500 units, or about a teaspoon of oil daily for a child up to eight years old, and then two teaspoons or more as long as it can be accepted graciously. My children were given cod-liver oil daily until they were twelve, after which they were allowed to take capsules of vitamins A and D.

Many youngsters find mint-flavored cod-liver oil quite palatable. When cod-liver oil is not tolerated, the drops of vitamins A, D, and E in oil now available at health-food stores should be given directly on the tongue and after a meal which contains the most fat. It should never be put into a bottle because it adheres to the sides. I have rarely seen good bone structure in children who have been given water-dispersed vitamins A and D added to the formula. If the child is to grow up to be physically attractive, he must be given a dependable source of vitamin D daily throughout the entire growth period.

Almost nothing is known of the amount of vitamin D which can be taken advantageously by an adult. Dr.

Johnston[3] of the Henry Ford Hospital in Detroit studied the needs of adolescent girls, some of whom had ceased growing. He found that even though a generous amount of calcium was supplied by the diet, if no vitamin D was taken, more calcium was excreted than was eaten. When the vitamin was supplied, the amount of calcium absorbed into the blood paralleled the vitamin-D intake. For example, when 650 units of vitamin D were given daily for a time, and later 3,900 units were given, the quantity of calcium absorbed was increased tenfold. In some cases 1,950 units of vitamin D were given with more calcium than could be obtained from an average quart of milk (1,343 milligrams); still no calcium whatsoever was retained in the body; this amount of calcium was well absorbed when vitamin D was increased to 3,900 units daily.

Dr. Johnston's study indicates that adolescents and probably adults may profit by taking approximately 4,000 units of vitamin D daily. The assumption has been that everyone except infants gets all the vitamin D he needs from sunshine; yet Michigan nurses working indoors throughout the summer were found to have no vitamin D whatsoever in their blood. As much as 5,000 units daily had to be given them before the quantity in their blood was comparable to that found in the blood of healthy women living in the subtropics, receiving ample vitamin D from the sun. I am convinced, therefore, that 4,000 or 5,000 units of vitamin D should be taken daily by all adults, especially during pregnancy, lactation, and menopause.

This vitamin is particularly needed during the menopause, when the calcium intake is usually low. Hot flashes, night sweats, leg cramps, irritability, nervousness, and mental depression, so frequently experienced at this time, can be overcome in a single day by giving calcium and vitamin D; when the calcium intake is already adequate, vitamin D alone relieves these symptoms. The positive results gained by any adult in taking adequate vitamin D throughout life are identical with the advantages of having ample calcium, to be discussed in Chapter 21.

Vitamin D helps to prevent tooth decay. All decay is apparently caused by sugar being broken down by bacteria-produced enzymes into lactic and pyruvic acids; any acid can combine with calcium. If the saliva can reach the area where the acids are being formed, and if it contains ample

[3] J. A. Johnston, "The Calcium and Vitamin D Requirements of the Older Child," *American Journal of Diseases of Children,* LXVII (1944), 265.

amounts of dissolved calcium, these acids are neutralized by the salivary calcium, and no decay results. Dental erosion appears to be prevented in the same manner. Although the subject is still controversial, an increasing amount of evidence indicates that both the enamel and dentin of mature teeth can be built up provided the nutrition is adequate, especially in calcium and vitamin D.[4]

Ample vitamin D undoubtedly plays an important role in the prevention of pyorrhea. If the diet is markedly improved and all infection is removed, even severe pyorrhea can usually be arrested. Although pyorrhea is a disease involving infection and resulting from multiple nutritional deficiencies, the loss of teeth is caused by decalcification of the bones. When too little calcium or protein is supplied the tissues, minerals are withdrawn from the jaw bones; the bones themselves become smaller and recede, and the gums can no longer fit tightly around the base of each tooth. Eventually, so little bone structure remains that it cannot hold the teeth firmly in place; the teeth, though they may be free from decay, become loose and must be removed.

Even when the teeth and all infection are removed, the destruction of jawbones does not cease, nor does this destruction cease to be a problem. Dentures can fit well only when sufficient jawbone remains on which to anchor them. If the nutrition is poor, so much bone tissue can be lost even six months or less after perfectly fitting dentures are made that the dentures shift, wobble, or refuse to stay in place. One of the delightful memories of my childhood is an occasion when a malnourished Methodist minister, apparently believing that the gospel was more effective when thundered, shouted his upper dentures into the congregation. An innocent dentist was probably blamed even by this good Christian; at least a dentist usually is. It is not a dentist's fault that a person's diet cannot maintain normal bone structure. Often set after set of dentures has to be made as the destruction continues. Furthermore, persons whose bones are undergoing rapid destruction are so deficient in calcium that they are nervous wrecks; often they cannot stand to wear dentures no matter how well they fit. For a time a dentist referred to me many patients who complained that new dentures did not fit. As soon as the patients' diet was made adequate and their nerves relaxed, there were no more complaints.

[4] "Isotope Studies in Dental Tissues," *Nutrition Reviews,* XI (1953), 89.

The calcification of the jawbones, shown by dental X rays, is probably a good index of the density of bones throughout the body. Fragile bones break easily. When bones are so poorly calcified that teeth are lost from pyorrhea, the condition of the bones throughout the body can degenerate but little more before they may crumble or break at any minor twist or fall. Millions of Americans, including thousands of relatively young persons and almost every person sixty years old and older, have porous bones. An estimated six million elderly persons in our country are said to have aching backs because of the severe demineralization of their bones. Formerly it was believed that bones naturally became porous with age. When experimental animals are kept on adequate diets, however, the longer they live, the stronger their bones become. Such evidence indicates that poorly calcified bones are the result of nutritional deficiencies; elderly persons have eaten faulty diets more years than has the younger person; hence the condition is more universal among them.

If you think bones do well without care, you should go through an orthopedic hospital and talk with patients; you would soon be convinced that anything which helps to build strong bones and prevents such misery as you would find is worthwhile. Let me tell you about a few cases I have known personally.

A woman in her late thirties hobbled in to see me not long ago and, after putting her crutches aside, told me the following story. Several years ago she had somehow twisted her leg while walking across a lawn; the femur, or thighbone, had broken near the pelvic joint. She lay in the hospital month after month before healing was sufficient for her to walk with crutches; in time they were discarded. Then one day, without warning, she simply fell in a heap. This time the bone had crumbled at the spot where it had been broken before. A plastic head was put on the femur, which involved deep, drastic, and expensive surgery; the gold pin which held it in place showed clearly in the X rays. Again months were passed in hospital beds before she graduated to crutches, but pain in that joint remained acute. She had been told that the pain was probably caused by calcium forming in rough deposits over the plastic head of the femur; she came to me requesting a *calcium-free diet*. She left with a nutrition program which included generous amounts of both calcium and vitamin D and was as adequate in all respects as I could make it. Only three days later she phoned to say the pain had completely disappeared. A month later she came to see me, carrying a cane; she walked, however, without using it and without a limp.

A plasterer, forty-two years of age, who had fallen from scaffolding, used to come on crutches to hear me lecture. He too had broken his femur; months had passed without healing. The jagged ends of the bone kept breaking apart. Apparently in desperation, his physicians put a steel plate around the bone to hold the ends together, but X rays cannot be taken through such a plate to see whether healing has occurred. Eventually the plate had been removed, but the bone still had not knitted. Infection, called osteomyelitis, set in, and operation after operation followed. Great deep scars about two inches apart and each a foot long went round his entire thigh. The wound from the last operation was still draining, the bone was badly infected, and amputation had been recommended. During all these tragic years, he had never once been given vitamin D; certainly he had not been in the sunshine. No diet had been recommended rich in calcium, in protein necessary to form bone base, or in the B vitamins needed to insure that adequate hydrochloric acid could be produced to help the absorption of what little calcium he chanced to obtain. No extra vitamin C or pantothenic acid had been given to help prevent or fight the infection. When his nutrition was made adequate, improvement was rapid. He now walks to work but with a limp he will have throughout life. Do you suppose he thinks that vitamin D is a nutrient only for babies?

I have seen perhaps three dozen similar cases, most not so severe but many equally tragic. The elderly persons whose hipbones crumble after a minor fall, usually in a bathtub, seem to me most pathetic. Yet they themselves have unknowingly produced these abnormal bones. Not long ago I visited a friend whose mother had broken her hip in just such a fall. This woman told me that she had always hated milk and had never taken calcium or vitamin D. Her pain was so acute when she sat still or lay down that she moved slowly about the room with a walker, yet she groaned with every step. Such is the price paid for indifference to nutrition.

Because I do not wish my twilight years to become a nightmare, I take 5,000 units of vitamin D daily, a quart of milk, and enough tablets to supply an additional gram of calcium. In fact I would be terrified not to obtain these nutrients.

Once when I mentioned something about saving teeth by taking vitamin D, a friend remarked, "Some of the nicest people I know wear dentures." He is right of course. There are some 32,000,000 nice people in these United States wearing dentures. I myself would gamble that all of these 32,000,000 nice people wish they had 32 nice teeth stuck firmly in their own jaw bones.

CHAPTER 20

NEEDED BY EVERY CELL

MEDICAL LIBRARIES HAVE THOUSANDS OF SCIENTIFIC REPORTS showing the tremendous value of vitamin E, or d-alpha tocopherol acetate; few physicians, however, have read as many as half a dozen of them. They rarely recognize vitamin-E deficiencies; and repeatedly persons have told me their doctors advised them not to allow children vitamin E for fear of making them oversexed.

Fifty years ago, when rats were given food in which iron salts had caused the total destruction of the then unknown vitamin E, sterility was produced in the males. Females conceived normally, but the embryos died early or the young, born prematurely, often had congenital malformations such as retarded heart development; severe brain, lung, and kidney damage; and small, abnormal eyes. Older animals lacking vitamin E develop a wide variety of symptoms: anemia; enlarged prostate; liver and kidney damage; and early onset of old age. Muscle degeneration occurs in all species, many developing fatal muscular dystrophy. These same symptoms occur in humans whose blood vitamin E is low or absent.

Vitamin E is measured in both units and milligrams having equal value; hence the terms are used interchangeably. Our intake of this vitamin has been estimated to have been 150 units daily before wheat germ was discarded during the milling of flour, but now it averages 7.4 units. Vitamin E occurs in several forms known as mixed tocopherols, abundant in food. It is found in the oils of all grains, nuts, and seeds. Except for alpha tocopherol, however, the vitamin is lost during exposure to air, heating, freezing, and storage. Frying in oil, for example, destroys 98 per cent of the mixed tocopherols. Not one unit of vitamin E remains in oils extracted chemically or in refined flour and packaged cereals; none is added to "enriched" products. Nuts, fresh wheat germ, cold-pressed oils, and recently stone-ground whole-grain breads and cereals are almost our only sources. Even when ample vitamin E is obtained, it cannot be absorbed unless the vitamin, fat, and bile are all simultaneously present in the intestine. If babies, for instance, are given skim-milk formulas, none of the vitamin reaches the blood; and twice as much is absorbed when taken with whole milk as with milk containing only half as much cream.

Despite the wide variety of symptoms produced by vitamin-E deficiencies, this vitamin appears to have only one function: to prevent unsaturated fatty acids and fat-like substances from being destroyed in the body by oxygen.[1] These substances include vitamin A, carotene, the essential unsaturated fatty acids, and the pituitary, adrenal, and sex hormones. The vitamin itself is used up, or destroyed, however, in preventing this damage by oxygen.

Vitamin E is necessary for the formation of the nucleus of each body cell, including RNA and DNA. Furthermore, the essential fatty acids are now known to form not only part of the internal structure and wall of every cell in the body but also the connective tissue between all cells. When a lack of vitamin E allows these acids to combine with oxygen, they break down and cause the cell to disintegrate. The more oxygen present, the more rapidly the cells break down. As somewhat of a by-product, vitamin E tremendously reduces the body's need for oxygen by preventing vitamins, hormones, and fatty acids from wastefully combining with it.

A vitamin-E deficiency reveals itself by "clinkers" in the form of brown ceroid pigment which remains whenever unsaturated fatty acids are destroyed by oxygen. In humans and animals alike this pigment is found in the uterus, lymph nodes, spleen, liver, kidneys, brain, muscles, body fat, walls of blood vessels, and the sex, adrenal, and pituitary glands. No such pigmentation occurs in animals given ample vitamin E. Ceroid pigmentation—the remains of oxidized unsaturated fatty acids—is an "early and constant" finding in autopsies of persons dying of heart disease and/or of those having heavy cholesterol deposits in their arteries. The large amount of this pigment in blood clots is said to prevent enzymes from dissolving the clot readily, a problem in varicose veins, phlebitis, strokes, and many heart attacks. Au-

[1] O. A. Roels, *Present Knowledge of Nutrition* (New York, New York: The Nutrition Foundation, Inc., 1967), p. 87.

topsies of 151 children revealed heavy ceroid pigmentation in the tissues of those dying of diseases in which fat could not be absorbed, such as pancreatic fibrosis. I suspect the ugly brown spots on the backs of hands of persons middle-aged or older result from a vitamin-E deficiency; they usually appear at the menopause, when the vitamin requirement skyrockets, especially when female hormones are taken which increase the vitamin-E need tenfold. A lack of vitamin E in children can also cause depigmentation of their teeth, leaving them ugly and chalky-appearing for life.

Scientists have found that if less than 0.5 milligram of vitamin E is in a half cup of blood (100 cc.), a deficiency exists. This state can also be determined by analyzing the urine for creatine, a substance from the breakdown of muscle cells, the amount of which parallels the severity of the vitamin-E deficiency. The method most often used to determine this vitamin deficiency is to observe the number of red blood cells destroyed in the presence of oxygen, though the breakdown of cells from the eye, liver, kidney, muscle, or any part of the body could be used instead. This method has revealed that premature infants are particularly deficient in vitamin E.

All babies are born low in the vitamins which dissolve in fat, A, D, E, and K, but a lack of vitamin E in mothers is a major cause of premature births. Before birth an infant's environment is low in oxygen. The larger the amount of oxygen available after birth, the more quickly essential fatty acids are destroyed in the absence of vitamin E, and the more rapidly cells break down. For example, hundreds of premature infants have become blind after being put in oxygen tents, where high oxygen pressure caused an eye condition known as retrolental fibroplasia. Dr. W. C. Owens, of the Johns Hopkins Medical School, observed 23 premature infants given 150 milligrams of vitamin E daily, started immediately after birth. None of these children became blind, whereas 21.8 per cent of those not given the vitamin lost their sight. Dr. Owens found that when the vitamin was first started at 6 weeks of age, the babies might retain their vision but become permanently myopic, or nearsighted. I suspect one cause of the near-sightedness now so common among children is that pediatricians rarely allow babies any vitamin E. Retrolental fibroplasia is still said to cause more blindness in babies than all other causes combined.

When no vitamin E has been given a mother, the exposure to atmospheric oxygen immediately after birth may cause so many of the baby's red blood cells to be broken down that jaundice occurs. The yellow color characteristic of this abnormality comes from disintegrating red blood cells. As soon as vitamin E has been given such babies, the destruction of red blood cells stops and the jaundice clears up.[2]

A lack of vitamin E is a major cause of anemia in infants; the body is unable to replace quickly enough the many blood cells continuously breaking down. Such anemia can be prevented if the mother obtains vitamin E during pregnancy or even takes 600 units just before delivery. Dr. Dick-Bushnell of the University of Wyoming found infants' formulas and baby foods to be grossly deficient in vitamin E; hence anemia in bottle-fed infants continues for months. The fortunate breast-fed baby has no such problem.

Vitamin-E deficiency anemia occurs at any age and has been produced in volunteers by a diet undersupplied in this vitamin. When the vitamin E in the blood of 233 persons was determined, it was found that anemia occurred whenever the quantity was less than 0.5 milligram per 100 cc. Such anemia appears to be widespread during adolescence and the menopause as well as during pregnancy and infancy. Anemia caused by a lack of vitamin E is impossible to distinguish from iron-deficiency anemia unless tests for vitamin-E adequacy are made. Since physicians make no such tests and are usually unaware of the value of vitamin E, they merely recommend larger and larger amounts of iron. Unfortunately, most iron salts, if not all, destroy vitamin E. Anemic children often recover rapidly after being given vitamin E, whereas they have frequently remained persistently anemic despite supplements of iron, protein, and vitamin B_6. If iron must be given for anemia, it should be taken 8 to 12 hours before or after vitamin E is given; iron might follow breakfast and the entire day's quota of vitamin E be taken after dinner.

During space flights of more than eight days, or up to the flight of Apollo 10, astronauts lost 20 to 30 per cent of their red blood cells and returned to earth anemic and exhausted, their hearts so weakened as to puzzle their physicians.[3] They breathed an atmosphere rich in oxygen which, in the absence of vitamin E, rapidly destroyed the unsaturated fatty acids in their cells. Dr. David Turner of Toronto,

[2] J. B. MacKenzie, *Pediatrics,* XIII (1954), 346.
[3] W. E. Shute and H. J. Taub, *Vitamin E for Ailing and Healthy Hearts* (Pyramid House, 1969).

Canada, who formerly worked with the Shute brothers, recognized the problem as a vitamin-E deficiency. Since that time the food for the astronauts has been "substantially enriched" with vitamin E and no anemia has occurred.

The muscle cells of a vitamin-E-deficient person break down as readily as do the red blood cells, causing creatine and amino acids from these destroyed cells to be lost in the urine. When pregnant women are not given vitamin E, the babies are born with such weak muscles that their heads wobble. Usually they are slow in sitting up, crawling, standing, and walking. Repeatedly mothers have told me that their children, who could not sit up alone at six months of age, could sit well within a single week after 100 units of vitamin E were given daily. On three occasions, pediatricians have convinced these mothers that vitamin E was dangerous; within two weeks after the vitamin was withdrawn, the child could no longer sit alone. The muscles of animals deficient in vitamin E split easily, or develop hernias; the hernias so common in the muscles of infants may also be related to the lack of this vitamin.

When 400 units of vitamin E were given daily to 112 patients with muscular weakness, stiffness, pain, and spasms, improvement was prompt and elderly persons were benefited as much as younger ones. Cross eyes in children have sometimes been corrected by giving vitamin E because weak muscles behind the eyes have been strengthened. Protruding eyes occur in animals deficient in vitamin E. I once planned a diet including 600 units of vitamin E daily for an invalid suffering from severe myositis; her eyes protruded so much that they seemed ready to pop out of her head. In a surprisingly short time, she had completely recovered and her eyes became normal. Improvement of such muscle abnormalities as myitis and myositis have been frequently reported in medical journals. One reason for the abominable posture in persons of all ages in the United States is undoubtedly their weak muscles caused by a lack of vitamin E.

Studies of vitamin-E-deficient animals show that wherever cells break down, a tiny quantity of calcium is deposited; thus the calcium content of soft tissues often increases 500 per cent or more. By producing such experimental calcium deposits, Dr. Hans Selye (ref. 2, p. 141) has induced all appearances and characteristics of advanced old age even in young animals. This damage could be prevented only by huge amounts of vitamin E. Dr. Selye points out that similar calcium deposition occurs in arteriosclerosis, arthritis, scleroderma, and many diseases; and that the shift of calcium from bones to soft tissues, formerly considered to be the result of aging, is probably the actual cause of aging. In one study of 320 infants with "fatal" scleroderma, 75 per cent fully recovered after being given vitamin E.

Muscular dystrophy, produced in every type of animal severely deficient in vitamin E, is said to have doubled in the past 10 years. In this disease, muscle cells break down and are replaced by useless scar tissue. If vitamin E is given before the disease becomes advanced, recovery occurs quickly. It is usually advanced before being diagnosed, however, and no amount of vitamin E can then reverse it. Diets unusually high in all nutrients appear to retard the disease.

For a number of years I planned a diet high in vitamin E for a charming youngster who has had muscular dystrophy since he was three. He was then unable to walk, and doctors assured his parents he could not live. His courageous mother tied both his hands and his feet to a tricycle and taught him to ride; thereafter he used it as a wheelchair, taking himself to the bathroom, dining table, and play areas. At the age of 11, he now attends school, is an excellent scholar, and appears to be a happy, outgoing youngster although he must use a wheelchair and a small motor-driven car to get around.

In September, 1965, I planned a diet for a youngster who was then in Johns Hopkins Hospital with muscular dystrophy. Fortunately his illness was not advanced. Today's mail brought the following report from his mother: "My son is miraculously and happily functioning as a normal, healthy boy in junior high school. His doctors are amazed but I know why he is well."

Vitamin E given to men frequently increases the number, quality, and motility of sperm. In a study of families who had had one or more defective children, after the fathers had taken vitamin E several months prior to a later conception, all had normal infants. One physician states that out of thousands of infants he has delivered, as long as both parents had adequate vitamin E before conception and the mother continued the vitamin during pregnancy, not one baby has been malformed or mentally defective.

Dozens of studies show that women who had miscarried two or more times or had given birth prematurely have delivered healthy, full-term infants after taking vitamin E. In one study of several hundred who had repeatedly miscarried, 97.5 per cent had given birth to healthy babies after taking the vitamin; without the vitamin, a third miscarried again. Because muscles become weak, women deficient in vitamin E may have delayed deliveries with prolonged and difficult labor, often causing the child to die or suffer brain damage from a lack of oxygen; some such women have been found to have no vitamin E whatsoever in their blood. Because vitamin E decreases the body's need for oxygen, it can prevent brain damage in infants both in early embryonic development and during delivery.

If vitamin E is not supplied, oxygen is continuously wasted; hence the body's need for oxygen is tremendously increased. When animals have been given less and less oxygen until they died, those generously supplied with the vitamin lived far longer on "remarkably little oxygen." Volunteers have breathed "rarefied air" until they became unconscious, then repeated the experiment after taking 300 units of vitamin E daily. The vitamin allowed them to remain conscious much longer and to have greater comfort, fewer palpitations, and far less exhaustion. Similarly, athletes, especially persons climbing mountains in rarefied air, have more and far greater endurance when taking vitamin E. An engineer who had worked high in the Peruvian Andes told me that his company purchased vitamin-E capsules for their employees, who then reported a marked improvement in health and well-being; and that when they later considered discontinuing this practice, every employee threatened to resign.

Scar tissue appears to require less oxygen to form than does normal tissue; hence it occurs in areas of oxygen deprivation. Surgery, accidents, and burns damage blood vessels and thus reduce the oxygen supply. Drs. E. V. and W. E. Shute of London, Ontario, Canada, show slides of patients piteously burned, mangled in accidents, or with gangrenous skin grafts, massive varicose ulcers, or ulcerated amputation stumps. After being given 600 units or more of vitamin E daily, all miraculously healed not only with scarcely a scar but without the contraction and the itching, drawing pain so often characteristic of healing. Even old disfiguring scars sometimes disappeared. I have repeatedly seen near-miracles occur after vitamin E was given: horrible burns, even radiation burns, healed without a scar; a young girl's face was so cut in an accident that years of plastic surgery were said to be required, yet became lovely in a few weeks, no surgery needed; a toddler whose esophagus was so constricted by scar tissue from drinking lye that she could be fed only with a tube—after receiving hundreds of units of vitamin E daily, her throat is now normal. I have seen persons whose flesh was literally cooked, yet with the contents of vitamin-E capsules dropped twice daily over the burned area and 200 units of the vitamin taken after each meal, they have suffered almost no pain and healed without a blemish.

Though the fact that vitamin E could prevent pain and scarring from burns has been known for 20 years, I have heard of no hospital in the United States where burned patients are allowed this vitamin. The suffering imposed on these burned patients is heartbreaking. The mother of a ten-year-old girl caught in a gasoline explosion told me she had pleaded with physicians to allow her to give the child vitamin E but that they had refused. Now after three years of hospitalization, uncountable hours of pain, and thousands upon thousands of dollars spent on skin grafts, the child is hopelessly scarred. Her face is distorted, her mouth and smile crooked, her ears partly missing; scars on her arms and chest have caused her to give up swimming and to wear high-necked, long-sleeved dresses the year round. Eight more surgeries on her face are recommended, but the child now refuses, and the family is at last ready "to try" vitamin E without the doctors' blessing. The pain already endured by this little girl and the lifelong psychological suffering ahead of her, multiplied by hundreds of thousands, gives some concept of the cruelty resulting when persons are forbidden an essential nutrient.

Scarring inside the body often causes severe problems. Adhesions are scar tissue. In pancreatic fibrosis, muscular dystrophy, and cirrhosis of the liver, useless scars replace large areas of normal tissue yet can never perform its function. After infections of the bladder, scars may contract so severely that almost no urine can be retained. In rheumatic fever, the scarring of heart valves can cause lifelong murmurs, but if the vitamin is given during the acute stage and continued, no scarring occurs. Arthritis, bursitis, myositis, arteriosclerosis, constriction of the urethra or ureters, and dozens of other abnormalities are complicated by scarring, probably all preventable were vitamin E adequate.

Vitamin E has been used successfully in treating Dupuytren's contracture, where scar tissue pulls the fingers into fixed claws; Peyronie's disease, in which scar tissue, forming on the penis, causes pain and often impotence; and keloids, the painful, itching tumor-like growths of excessive scar tissue so often torturing to colored people. The more recent the scar, the more easily it is replaced. Some old scars never disappear, largely, I believe, because the diet is not adequate enough to rebuild normal tissues.

One is said to be less sensitive to pain when the vitamin-E intake is adequate. The excruciating agony of severe burns usually stops within minutes if capsules of vitamin E are pierced with a sterile needle and their contents squeezed over the burned areas. Similarly, the pain of frostbite is said to disappear if the frosted area is covered with vitamin E. The pain of angina pectoris, caused by insufficient oxygen, usually disappears after an adequate diet is supplemented with this vitamin. An obstetrician tells me that suffering is decreased when women take 600 units of vitamin E at the onset of labor. Certainly the vitamin prevents the itching, pulling, and drawing pains of a healing wound. Recently when I was stung by bees, I quickly applied vitamin E; the surprisingly severe pain disappeared immediately. The pain of sunburn can be relieved by vitamin E squeezed from capsules or by ointment containing either vitamin E or PABA (p. 71).

Clots readily form in the blood vessels of animals deficient in vitamin E, though they cannot be produced by a lack of any other nutrient. As we have seen, cells break down whenever vitamin E is undersupplied; and if blood vessels are cut or broken, clots form to prevent hemorrhage. In the absence of vitamin E, therefore, the breakdown of cells in blood-vessel walls causes clots to form. Varicose veins, for example, are caused by clots and have been repeatedly produced in animals lacking vitamin E.

I recently talked to a young woman, an avid tennis player, who had developed huge, ugly varicose veins during pregnancy, when the vitamin-E needs skyrocket. Her physician assured her that she could never again play tennis. At the seventh month a marble-sized purple clot appeared near the skin, causing her entire leg to become inflamed and continuously painful. Her doctor kept her in bed, urged her to allow labor to be induced, and told her that surgery would be necessary. At this point she started taking 300 units of vitamin E after each meal; and because of the inflammation, she also took 1,000 milligrams of vitamin C six times daily. This girl and her mother both declared that not only the clot but also the varicose veins disappeared before their eyes. A week after her delivery, she was again playing tennis, her legs having become completely normal.

In varicose veins, the clot usually attaches itself to the blood-vessel wall, causing inflammation and swelling. The combination of swollen walls and clot throws up a "road block," plugging the vein so completely that no blood can flow through it. The large vein near the center of the leg normally carries 90 per cent of the blood returning from the feet to the heart. When this vein is blocked, the huge amount of blood must return by the only means available: through the small surface veins, which quickly become distended, ugly, blue, and unsightly. If vitamin E is increased immediately and the diet kept adequate, varicose veins usually disappear in a few days or weeks, though they can quickly recur unless the vitamin is continued. A few persons have told me their varicose veins of twenty years' standing disappeared after they added vitamin E to the diet. When no vitamin E is taken and varicose veins are repeatedly stripped, circulation is interfered with so much that painful ulcers often appear. In time the discolored legs are permanently encased in elastic stockings and become so painful that even walking is constantly difficult.

In attaching itself to the blood-vessel wall, a clot can cause inflammation, tenderness, pain, and redness along the entire vein, a condition spoken of as phlebitis or thrombophlebitis. Phlebitis has been produced in vitamin-E-deficient rabbits and dogs. If the vitamin is then given, many new blood vessels quickly form parallel to the obstructed vein, allowing blood to return efficiently to the heart; clots soon dissolve and inflammation clears, none of which occurs when the vitamin is withheld. Similarly, after 327 persons with phlebitis were given 300 to 800 units of vitamin E daily, clots "melted away," pain quickly left, and the results were said to be "gratifying and dramatic"; improvement often occurred in 12 hours after the vitamin was started. Other patients were completely healed in 4 days. "Clearance tests" in which dye is injected into the blood vessels of persons with varicose veins or phlebitis, allowing them to show in X rays, have also revealed that clots have disappeared and normal circulation has been resumed.

Because phlebitis often occurs following operations, a study was made of a hundred persons given 200 units of vitamin E immediately before surgery; a few had small clots but none developed phlebitis. Of a similar number not given vitamin E, 15 developed phlebitis, 30 suffered from clots, and 2 had pulmonary embolism, or clots which formed elsewhere, lodging in the lungs.

Recently a letter reached me saying: "I am afraid my sister is dying. She is only 46 years old but she has phlebitis with blood clots all over her body. It started last spring with a blood clot in her lungs. Now she is swelling more and more. Her legs are terrible. Can you please, please help?" Fortunately a high-protein diet supplemented with large amounts of vitamins C, E, and pantothenic acid brought relief.

Pulmonary embolisms and strokes caused by clots lodging in the lungs or brain can occur when vitamin E is undersupplied. Blood analyses show that 80 per cent of stroke victims are grossly deficient in this vitamin; and giving them vitamin E has resulted in marked improvement even long after the stroke occurred. Because oral contraceptives increase the need for vitamin E, women using them have suffered from varicose veins, phlebitis, pulmonary embolisms, and even strokes.

Heart attacks, which kill ten times more people in the United States than in other civilized countries, are often caused by a clot lodging in a coronary artery, thus cutting off the oxygen supply. The value of vitamin E in preventing coronary thrombosis has been disgracefully little investigated. It is known that this vitamin decreases the need for oxygen; helps to dissolve clots; and stimulates the formation of blood vessels to bypass clots.

When 100 survivors of heart attacks caused by clots were given only 200 units of vitamin E daily and compared with a similar group, four times more individuals not receiving the vitamin suffered recurring attacks. Similarly, when the vitamin was given to another group of 457 patients who had experienced coronary thrombosis, no attack recurred until the vitamin was discontinued. Of 246 controls not receiving vitamin E, 23 experienced heart attacks said to be caused by clots.[4] Survivors of such attacks consistently have both low blood vitamin E and abnormal electrocardiograms. Autopsies show degeneration, massive scarring, and much ceroid pigment in the heart muscles; and tissue analyses reveal marked vitamin-E deficiency.

Patients given 600 to 1,600 units of vitamin E daily soon after heart attacks have shown improved electrocardiograms, more regular pulse, marked relief from pain, and less shortness of breath. Physicians who have worked with this vitamin state that it is far more effective in preventing clots than the dangerous anticoagulant drugs; and that if the vitamin is generously supplied, the need for oxygen is

[4] Medical references for topics discussed in this chapter may be found in Adelle Davis, *Let's Get Well* (Harcourt Brace Jovanovich, Inc., 1965).

so reduced that a patient may survive an attack which otherwise could be fatal.

Congenital heart abnormalities often disappear when vitamin E is given daily from early babyhood. I have planned diets for many children with such congenital defects for whom heart surgery was said to be necessary. Each of these youngsters has received 100 units of vitamin E daily since early babyhood; none has required surgery, and several have even become athletes.

Since animals deficient in vitamin E often develop nephritis, or kidney damage, a few physicians have given this vitamin to children suffering from this disease. Only 300 to 450 units daily caused water retention (edema) to decrease, blood and albumin to disappear from the urine, the blood pressure to fall, and the anemia which accompanies this disease to improve. A kidney specialist angrily told me recently it was not proved that vitamin E would help nephritis; and until it was, he would not give it to his patients. Though kidney damage has many causes, I wanted to say that nothing is proved unless it is tried; and that no human being, even a physician, has the right to keep patients on inadequate diets.

If the vitamin-E intake is generous, the liver can often detoxify such harmful substances as food preservatives, bleaches added to flour, residues from pesticides, nitrites and nitrates from chemical fertilizers, industrial poisons such as carbon tetrachloride, and a wide variety of toxic drugs. Any of these substances can cause liver damage unless vitamin E is adequate. Such liver damage, however, has been found to occur in two-thirds of hospital patients who are also severely deficient in vitamin E.

Vitamin E is particularly helpful to persons with thyroid problems. The thyroid glands of animals deficient in this vitamin become a mass of scars incapable of producing thyroxin or absorbing iodine; their eyes become as prominent as do those of persons with exophthalmic goiter. When 500 units of vitamin E were given daily to 70 adults with abnormal thyroid function, the uptake of iodine doubled and protein-bound iodine in the blood increased; underactive glands markedly improved; and the cases of overactive thyroid became normal. Nodules on the thyroid glands also often disappear after vitamin E is taken.

This vitamin is essential to glandular function. If adequately supplied, the pituitary, or master gland, contains 200 times more vitamin E than any other part of the body.

A vitamin-E deficiency decreases the production of all pituitary hormones: of STH, the pituitary growth hormone; of ACTH, essential to stimulate the adrenals; and the hormones which stimulate the thyroid and sex glands. As soon as vitamin E is given, hormone production rapidly increases. Even when produced normally, the pituitary, adrenal, and sex hormones are destroyed if vitamin E is undersupplied. Years ago the late Dr. Francis M. Pottenger, Jr., predicted that if our inadequate diets continued, the pituitary and sex glands would function so inefficiently that normally developed breasts and narrow masculine hips would disappear, and that one would have difficulty in telling boys from girls. His prophecy could scarcely have been more accurate.

When the unsaturated fatty acids forming part of the connective tissue and cell walls are destroyed by oxygen in the absence of vitamin E, viruses, bacteria, and allergens are allowed free access into the tissues. In cystic fibrosis, for example, where vitamin E is not absorbed, infections become rampant. Furthermore, since vitamin A is destroyed unless protected by vitamin E, children unnecessarily suffer frequent infections because they are not given vitamin E. Similarly, physicians sometimes recommend that adolescents take vitamin A because of acne, but no improvement occurs because vitamin E is inadequate. The more vitamin E in the diet, the less vitamin A needed and the more vitamin A stored. The water-soluble and water-miscible drops of vitamins A and D, often recommended by pediatricians, destroy vitamin E so rapidly that all available vitamin E is used up; without it the vitamin A quickly loses potency. Vitamin A from fish-liver oils is far more stable but still must be protected by vitamin E. The toxicity of excessive vitamin A can be prevented by a liberal supply of vitamin E.

This vitamin appears to be important in cancer prevention. Older animals deficient in it readily develop spontaneous cancer; the number of cancers induced by azo dyes decreases when vitamin E is given; the growth of cancer cells in blood plasma is inhibited if vitamin E is added; and transplanted cancers do not grow if the animals are allowed ample vitamin E. Dr. Otto Warburg[5] has shown that cancer cells grow only when deprived of oxygen, largely by the loss, destruction, or absence of oxygen-carrying enzymes. It is known that vitamin E tremendously reduces the need for oxygen. Early skin cancers sometimes heal when vita-

[5] Otto Warburg, *The Prime Cause and Prevention of Cancer*, trans. by Dr. Dean Burk (Bethesda, Maryland: National Cancer Institute, 1967).

min E is applied daily by squeezing the contents of a capsule onto them.

Vitamin E helps many unrelated diseases. For example, when given this vitamin, hemophiliacs have experienced "constant and quick" improvement. Diabetics have often decreased their insulin dosage. Persons with allergies and/or low resistance to infections have improved; when the fatty acids forming part of the cell structure break down in the absence of vitamin E, cells become porous and viruses and allergens can easily penetrate them. Detached retina, where harm is done by contracting scar tissue, has been helped. This vitamin is especially valuable in illnesses where the oxygen supply is limited: asthma, emphysema, and Buerger's disease. Vitamin E reportedly has corrected diaper rash, adolescent acne, and inflammation of the vagina; it has helped warts to drop off, and improved lupus erythematosus and scleroderma. Physicians have noted greater mental alertness when vitamin E has been given to elderly patients. Because this vitamin increases the utilization of acetyl cholin, it is invaluable to persons with myasthenia gravis.

The amount of vitamin E needed daily varies widely; and some individuals require four times more than others. The need is increased by stress, the intake of oils, long deprivation of this vitamin, rapid growth, the menopause, and the taking of sex hormones. Because a small increase in the intake of oils, or unsaturated fats, can increase the need for vitamin E sixfold, it is extremely dangerous to add oil to the diet without simultaneously obtaining more vitamin E. Yet without mentioning vitamin E, innumerable physicians recommend oil in the hope of preventing heart disease; and pediatricians now give oil-containing formulas to babies already deficient in vitamin E. The tremendous harm thus being done can only be guessed at.

Estimates of the daily requirement run from a bare minimum of 30 units to several hundred units. Careful studies indicate that an adult usually needs 140 to 210 units daily but requires 100 additional units for each tablespoon of oil in the diet. A small excess is stored in the pituitary, adrenal, and sex glands, but is quickly exhausted, especially during illness. The amounts which have produced excellent results have usually been 600 to 1,600 units daily, always taken after meals containing fat. Persons who have uncontrolled high blood pressure or hearts damaged from chronic rheumatic fever, however, should take no more than 100 units of vitamin E daily for the first six weeks (ref. 3, p. 151). The amount can then be increased to 125 units daily and six weeks later to 150 units.

Vitamin E is repeatedly said never to be toxic. Premature infants have been given 1,400 units of alpha tocopherol daily for short periods and children 2,000 units with no signs of toxicity. One 41-year-old man, however, taking 4,000 milligrams of synthetic vitamin E daily for three months, developed diarrhea, abdominal distress, and sore mouth, tongue, and lips. Toxicity has also been produced in animals, causing degeneration of adrenals, thyroid, and sex glands. Amounts of the vitamin larger than 1,600 units daily, therefore, should probably be used only for short periods.

This vitamin is needed in proportion to the amount of oil in the diet. Our oil consumption has tripled since 1946; our intake of vitamin E continues to decrease and now averages only 7.4 units daily. Unless every person's diet is quickly supplemented with vitamin E, we can expect each abnormality discussed in this chapter to become more severe and more frequent. Yet this vitamin is discarded with every pound of flour refined and every quart of oil chemically extracted. Can we afford such an appalling waste?

CHAPTER 21

YOUR DISPOSITION
TELLS THE STORY

NO PERSON AWARE OF THE REWARDS OF ADEQUATE CALCIUM would allow himself to be even slightly deficient in this nutrient. Calcium can be as soothing as a mother, as relaxing as a sedative, and as life-saving as an oxygen tent.

Although 99 percent of the calcium in the body is in the bones and teeth, symptoms resulting from an undersupply to the nerves and soft tissues can make life quite unbearable. For example, calcium aids in the transportation of nerve impulses. When this mineral is undersupplied, nerves become tense, and you become grouchy. The calcium-deficient person wastes energy, and his nervous tension and inability to relax induce fatigue out of all proportion to the work he actually does. He is usually so restless that it is tiring to be around him. His irritability and quick temper add nothing to his popularity. A mother whose seventeen-year-old son had an overdose of these symptoms, relieved by adequate calcium, said to me not long ago, "Thank you for making Johnny into a human being again." If the blood calcium becomes unusually high, as it does when toxic doses of vitamin D are given experimentally, relaxation reaches the point of lethargy or sometimes coma; even the excitability of nerves and muscles to electrical stimulus is greatly reduced.

Often the person undersupplied with calcium becomes an air swallower. Since such a person usually talks rapidly, the air may be forced from the throat into the stomach during conversation, a trick nervous women are particularly good at. Either sex may unconsciously form the habit of vigorously swallowing saliva and air simultaneously. Frequently a man gulps his food and, like a ravenous baby, swallows air as he eats; since no one burps him, he often suffers from "indigestion." The volatile oils from such foods as onions, green peppers, and garlic already in his stomach pass into the air bubbles, are tasted whenever he belches, and are blamed for the "indigestion." In time his can't-eat list usually becomes impressive. Often he is an enthusiastic user of soda or alkalinizing preparations. Besides forming enough carbon dioxide to force open the upper valve of the stomach and thus allowing gas and air alike to escape, these substances neutralize the valuable hydrochloric acid in his stomach; any calcium his food may have contained is made insoluble and cannot be absorbed into the blood. The swallowed air sometimes passes into the intestines, expands as it heats to body temperature, and may cause considerable distention and even pain. He becomes, in short, his own worst enemy. His symptoms, however, are quickly relieved provided adequate calcium reaches the nerves.

A calcium deficiency often shows itself by insomnia, another form of an inability to relax. The harm done by sleeping tablets, to say nothing of the thousands of dollars spent annually on them, could largely be avoided if the calcium intake were adequate. Since milk is our richest source of calcium, warm milk drinks taken before retiring have long been advertised for relief of insomnia; heat quickens digestion, calcium soothes the nerves, and restful sleep may follow. Such advertising has the blessing of both the American Medical Association and the Food and Drug Administration. For the person whose tissues are starved for calcium, however, the amount in a milk drink is a mere drop in a bucket. I usually tell persons whose insomnia is severe to take temporarily two or three calcium tablets with a milk drink before retiring and to keep both milk and the tablets on a bedside table and take more every hour if wakefulness persists. Twenty years ago I discussed this subject with a physician who himself suffered from insomnia; he still calls calcium tablets "lullaby pills" and tells me he continues to recommend them for patients annoyed by wakefulness.

An undersupply of calcium also causes irritability of the muscles which may take the form of cramps or spasms. If the blood calcium drops extremely low, convulsions known as tetany can occur; fortunately the usual muscle symptoms are less severe. Leg or foot cramps are the most common, although either cramps or spasms may occur in almost any muscle. For example, spasms in the intestine, spoken of as spastic colitis or spastic constipation, are usually relieved by adequate calcium.

A lack of calcium (and magnesium) can make adolescent youngsters, whose requirements have skyrocketed with growth, become so irritable that the most tolerant mother sometimes feels her teen-agers should have been put to death at birth. During the year before menstruation begins, a girl's blood calcium drops so abnormally low (ref. 3, p. 143) that she may become nervous, suffer from insomnia and tooth decay, and be so irritable that she is almost impossible to live with. If, in addition to drinking a quart of milk daily, such a youngster will take 2 or 3 calcium tablets—preferably containing also magnesium and mixed minerals—after each meal and before bed her entire personality often improves almost overnight. Vitamin D, however, must be taken to insure calcium absorption (p. 140).

The amount of calcium in a woman's blood parallels the activity of the ovaries; the blood calcium falls to such an extent during the week prior to menstruation that nervous tension, irritability, and perhaps mental depression result. At the onset of menstruation, the blood calcium takes a further drop, often causing cramps of the muscular walls of the uterus. This condition is especially severe during adolescence. In such a case, if calcium tablets are not taken regularly, they should at least be started the week prior to menstruation and continued until menstruation has ceased. If the slightest menstrual cramping occurs, calcium tablets should be taken every hour until cramps are gone; usually such cramps will stop within half an hour.

During the menopause, the lack of ovarian hormones causes severe calcium-deficiency symptoms to occur; at these times unusually large amounts of calcium should be obtained and every step be taken to insure its absorption into the blood and to prevent its loss from the kidneys. When these precautions are taken and the diet is adequate in other respects, the woman at menopause usually loses her irritability, hot flashes, night sweats, leg cramps, and mental depression. Even after the cessation of menstruation, a pseudo-menstrual cycle can usually be observed, and calcium-deficiency symptoms can be particularly noticed during one week of each month. The calcium intake should be increased at such times.

Another reason for an adequate calcium intake and for keeping calcium tablets in the medicine chest at all times is that this mineral is a pain killer par excellence. Old medical textbooks give as the treatment for the sharp stabbing pains of pleurisy—than which there are few worse —injections of calcium. Why calcium has not been used more widely in alleviating other pain remains a mystery. One physician tells me that he uses no opiates but injects one to four grams of calcium gluconate into the veins of patients suffering even excruciating pain and that relief occurs almost immediately. Though the severely ill person or one enduring a blinding headache usually cannot absorb enough calcium taken by mouth to relieve pain, a less ill person can. The migraine sufferer, for example, can be helped most by taking calcium (and vitamin B_6) between headaches. For years I have told people to take calcium tablets before visiting a dentist; the mineral helps them relax and feel less pain, and makes life easier for the dentist. Adequate calcium often relieves the itching of hives and the pain of arthritis. My advice to expectant mothers has long been to take, as soon as labor starts, a capsule containing vitamin D and two or three calcium tablets every hour until they are wheeled into the delivery room. I have been amazed at the number who have written or told me that they experienced no pain during delivery, often adding, "I thought I was having gas pains when the baby was born."

A further reason for obtaining adequate calcium is that it is necessary for the clotting of blood. This need for calcium in blood clotting can be a matter of life or death, especially after an accident. Calcium decreases cell-wall permeability (ref. 1, p. 123) and thus prevents harmful substances such as allergins and viruses from entering the cells. This mineral is also essential in maintaining normal muscle tone, or excellent posture, and strong muscular contraction; it is for this reason so valuable during labor at childbirth. Calcium has been found to delay fatigue and to hasten recovery.

A lack of calcium causes susceptibility to decay of teeth and demineralization of bones which cannot be overcome with any amount of vitamin D alone. Both calcium and vitamin D must be adequately supplied, absorbed, and retained if dental and skeletal health is to be maintained. Although phosphorus is combined with calcium in bones and teeth and is possibly more important than any other mineral in the body, it is usually overabundant in the American diet.

Numerous surveys have shown that the deficiency of calcium is more widespread than that of any other nutrient;

milk is our only dependable source. There is, of course, calcium in sour milk, cultured buttermilk, yogurt, and any food prepared with milk. The calcium is often lost in the making of cheese. Churned buttermilk contains little calcium because cream is a poor source; cultured buttermilk, made from skim milk, is an excellent source.

Appreciable amounts of calcium can be obtained from mustard and turnip greens, soybeans, and blackstrap molasses, but these foods are rarely eaten daily. The quantity needed to meet an adult's calcium requirements per day from the following foods, listed in medical textbooks as good sources of calcium, would be 72 apples, 80 bananas, 42 oranges, 11 cups of carrots, 33 eggs, 77 potatoes, or 214 dates; the quantities of other foods listed are even more ridiculous. Certainly there are healthy peoples who do not drink milk, but each has a source of calcium; the Hawaiians' source is poi; the Orientals', soybean curds. The Eskimos, the African natives, and formerly the American Indians obtained calcium from bones of fish, small game, and birds. The late Dr. Michael Walsh found that Mexican Indians, "starving" by our standards, had a calcium intake equivalent to eight quarts of milk daily; this calcium was obtained from the soft limestone used in grinding corn for tortillas. In America the calcium needs of a person who does not drink milk are not met unless he takes a calcium supplement, a poor substitute indeed for milk.

Many calcium salts are available in tablets or powder which can be taken in milk or juice. Calcium gluconate and calcium lactate, or calcium combined with the sugars glucose and lactose, usually absorb more readily than does dicalcium phosphate or calcium chloride. Fine bone powder or ash is a concentrated source of calcium but unfortunately is high in phosphorus. Although calcium salts are not harmful, only a limited quantity can be absorbed even under ideal conditions.

Before calcium can pass through the intestinal wall into the blood it must first be dissolved by hydrochloric acid in the stomach. Lactose, the sugar obtained by drinking milk, causes a pronounced increase in calcium absorption because it is broken down by intestinal bacteria into lactic acid. If the diet is excessively high in phosphorus, calcium and phosphorus combine in the intestine to make insoluble salts which do not dissolve even in acid. The taking of soda or any alkaline substance, which neutralizes the stomach acid, or eating candy or other concentrated carbohydrate, which stimulates the flow of alkaline digestive juices, decreases or prevents calcium absorption. Because fat increases calcium absorption, children, particularly babies, should be given whole milk rather than skim. If an adult prefers skim milk, it should be drunk at mealtime, perhaps with a salad tossed with oil.

If the diet is too high in phosphorus, large quantities of calcium are lost in the urine. Ideally, no more than twice as much phosphorus as calcium should be obtained; yet persons often ingest 10 times more phosphorus than calcium. Phosphorus is necessary to the life processes of every cell not only in all animals but in all plants. The American diet, poor in calcium, is therefore rich in phosphorus. In the maintenance of bones and teeth, calcium is used in chemical combination with phosphorus. If calcium is undersupplied in proportion to phosphorus, there is nothing for phosphorus to combine with. In this case, phosphorus is excreted. There is, however, always calcium in the blood; if not supplied in the diet, it is withdrawn from the bones. Unfortunately, urinary phosphorus is excreted in the form of calcium-phosphorus salts, and the body is robbed not only of its limited calcium supply but of phosphorus which may also be greatly needed. For these reasons, calcium gluconate and calcium lactate are preferable to calcium salts containing phosphorus.

Liver, yeast, lecithin, and wheat germ are unusually rich in phosphorus and yet poor in calcium; if large quantities of these foods are consumed, calcium lactate or calcium gluconate should be obtained simultaneously. When such a precaution is not taken, the proportion of phosphorus to calcium may become so high that the excretion of the excess phosphorus in the urine can induce a severe calcium deficiency. Sometimes a person who uses little or no milk becomes enthusiastic about obtaining large amounts of the B vitamins; his high intake of phosphorus and lack of calcium can cause him to become a nervous wreck. Phosphorus, calcium, and vitamin D are interdependent. When liberal quantities of milk, cultured buttermilk, yogurt, and foods prepared with fresh and powdered milk are used, calcium is supplied, and no problem arises unless large amounts of liver, yeast, lecithin, and/or wheat germ are eaten temporarily; in this case, a calcium salt can both prevent harm and be of great value.

Excess calcium which is absorbed and retained is stored in the shafts at the ends of the long bones as a lacy network of bony structure known as trabeculae, absent when no excess minerals have been available. You probably have noticed this lacy structure when a soup bone has been cut lengthwise. Calcium thus stored can be used at times of dietary insult; thus health can be protected. When no minerals are stored, calcium and phosphorus, aided by a hormone from the parathyroid glands, are removed from the bones to supply the needs of the soft tissues. The amount of calcium in the blood therefore remains at a normal level even when bones become progressively more porous and fragile, teeth become susceptible to decay or erosion, and multiple symptoms of calcium deficiency become evident. When deficiency symptoms are persistent, the bones are probably in a precarious condition.

Instead of bones being lifeless structures, unchanging after the cessation of growth, a continuous tidal flow of minerals passes in and out of them every hour of life. If sufficient calcium is obtained and absorbed, the tide flows into the bones, building and repairing until all porosity is gone. Unfortunately millions of Americans suffer from aching backs, a price they pay largely because they failed to get adequate calcium and vitamin D. If health is to be obtained, adults should have daily at least one gram of calcium, the amount supplied by four glasses of milk, yogurt, or cultured buttermilk. Still larger amounts may be advantageous. In times of prosperity, the daily calcium intake of the Finns and Swiss averaged six grams; many primitive races obtain even larger amounts of calcium. If a small excess is allowed for daily storage, large amounts of calcium would never be needed nor would calcium deficiencies ever exist.

There are few nutrients which can increase the graciousness of a home as much as can calcium. Without it, tempers flare and irritabilities are constant. With it, serenity can at times prevail.

CHAPTER 22

NATURE'S OWN TRANQUILIZER

ANOTHER NUTRIENT, MAGNESIUM, PROTECTS YOUR NERVES
as much as does calcium. Persons only slightly deficient in
magnesium become irritable, high-strung, sensitive to noise,
hyperexcitable, apprehensive, and belligerent. If the deficiency is more severe, or prolonged, they may develop
twitching, tremors, irregular pulse, insomnia, muscle weakness, jerkiness, and leg and foot cramps; their hands may
shake so badly that their writing becomes illegible. Electro-
encephalograms, electrocardiograms, and electromyograms,
or the records of electrical waves in the brain, heart, and
muscles, all become abnormal. If magnesium is severely
deficient, the brain is particularly affected. Clouded thinking, confusion, disorientation, marked depression, and even
the terrifying hallucinations of delirium tremens are largely
brought on by a lack of this nutrient and remedied when
magnesium is given.

Fortunately, improvement is usually dramatic within
hours after magnesium is taken, as is shown by a medical
report of a 68-year-old man who suffered from a magnesium deficiency brought on by diarrhea. For nine days this
man had been "irrational, disoriented, confused, noisy,
combative, and wildly restless." Only hours after a half teaspoon of Epsom salts, or magnesium sulfate, had been
given him, he was free from all symptoms and "a delightful gentleman." Another example is that of correcting
muscle weakness resulting from a lack of magnesium. Bed-
wetting, produced in volunteers on magnesium-deficient
diets, can be caused by an inability to control the muscles
closing the urinary bladder. This symptom frequently
occurs in persons suffering from multiple sclerosis. One
woman with multiple sclerosis told me she had endured
this embarrassing problem daily for four years, but that

it had ceased completely the very day she had added magnesium to her diet.

Magnesium deficiency is not easy for physicians to detect because this nutrient stays largely inside the cells; the quantity in blood plasma varies little. The magnesium in the cells, however, has been found to be unusually low in persons who have taken diuretics or antibiotics or who suffer from tremors, muscle weakness and/or spasms, epilepsy, diarrhea, diabetes, nephritis, or delirium tremens.

Animals lacking magnesium for only a few days develop convulsions. Later they show kidney damage and pass gravel and kidney stones. They quickly develop "heart trouble," and in addition to abnormal electrocardiograms, they have hemorrhages, areas of dead cells, and calcification of the heart muscles. Calcium is also laid down in many soft tissues: the skeletal muscles, the kidneys, and particularly the walls of the arteries. Potassium (p. 194) cannot be retained by the cells unless magnesium is adequate. All symptoms, particularly the calcification of tissues, are made worse by *an undersupply of calcium*, especially when the diet is high in phosphorus, as is that eaten by most Americans. Death is usually caused by "heart attacks."

If animals are put on an atherosclerosis-producing diet high in saturated fat and containing large amounts of cholesterol, no heart disease will develop as long as magnesium is given them. Similarly, races of people whose diets are rich in magnesium are amazingly free from heart attacks and arteriosclerosis (ref. 4, p. 158). There can no longer be doubt that magnesium deficiency plays a role in our disgracefully high death rate from heart disease. Magnesium is especially effective as a blood-cholesterol-lowering agent; and when a little Epsom salts has been given daily to patients who survived heart attacks, the response has been "truly remarkable." In one study alone, individuals having high blood magnesium (2.06 milligrams per 100 cc.) averaged 170 milligrams of cholesterol; persons with low magnesium (1.71 milligrams per 100 cc.) average 470 milligrams of cholesterol, the danger zone where a heart attack can be expected at any time.

It is extremely important to realize that calcium deposits in soft tissues become worse when the diet is *low in calcium*. Persons suffering from arthritis, bursitis, scleroderma, hardening of the arteries, and any abnormality where calcium deposits or spurs may cause pain are often afraid to eat foods rich in calcium. Actually they can never improve until both their calcium and magnesium intakes are adequate. Not infrequently physicians tell individuals with kidney stones to avoid all milk, thereby causing stones to form even more rapidly. Such calcium deposits can also occur when vitamin E is undersupplied. After open-heart surgery, when both magnesium and vitamin E are drastically needed and could be easily given, the calcification of heart muscles often becomes so severe that it can cause death within a few days (ref. 3, p. 151).

It has been assumed that magnesium was generously supplied in the American diet, as indeed it once was; and deficiency symptoms are still rarely recognized by physicians. Only during the past ten years have thousands of scientific studies made it clear that magnesium deficiencies are extremely widespread. Whenever chemical fertilizers are used, especially if the soil is limed, the moisture in the ground quickly becomes so saturated with the readily soluble fertilizers that magnesium cannot be absorbed into the soil solution or picked up by the plants. Soils east of the Mississippi are also particularly deficient in magnesium. If no chemical fertilizers are used and the soils are enriched with magnesium-containing dolomite or oyster-shell powder, the magnesium content of the food is high. The magnesium in foods, however, is lost if they are soaked or boiled and the water discarded. Even when the magnesium intake is high, losses caused by diarrhea, kidney disease, diabetes, diuretics, or drinking alcohol can induce a deficiency. Social drinkers who have 2 ounces of liquor daily containing 95-proof alcohol excrete three to five times more magnesium in their urine than they do when avoiding alcohol. Any enthusiastic social drinker not supplementing his diet with magnesium is asking for a heart attack.

Because deficient animals so readily develop convulsions, persons with epilepsy have been given magnesium; the blood and cells of such individuals have been found to be markedly deficient in this nutrient. Often the results have been spectacular. One medical report concerned a 38-year-old man with kidney damage (nephritis) which allowed magnesium to be lost in the urine. He developed severe epilepsy, suffering almost continuous seizures not controllable by anticonvulsant drugs. A single hour after a little magnesium was given, all epilepsy stopped and did not recur despite continued urinary losses. Similarly, Dr. L. B. Barnet, a Texas physician, gave 450 milligrams of magnesium daily by mouth to 30 epileptic children, and all anticonvulsant drugs were discontinued. Several had been so seriously ill that their seizures could not be prevented by large amounts of such drugs. Every child except one showed marked improvement. The magnesium corrected *grand mal,* or severe convulsions, as readily as *petit mal,* or minor seizures. One 13-year-old epileptic boy had been thought to be mentally retarded for 10 years, yet as soon as he was given magnesium he showed above-normal intelligence. Consistently good results, however, cannot be expected unless the entire diet is adequate, especially in vitamin B_6 (p. 83). One physician told me that he starts all his epileptic patients on both 25 milligrams of vitamin B_6 and an entire teaspoon of Epsom salts at each meal. Three days later he stops all anticonvulsant drugs. He reports that his results have been consistently excellent. After a week, he advises these people to take the vitamin B_6 and magnesium only after breakfast but to continue this quantity indefinitely, increasing it immediately if another seizure threatens. Magnesium and vitamin B_6 appear to be equally essential in preventing the severe convulsions of pregnancy known as eclampsia.

I am continuously amazed at the number of parents afraid to give magnesium to their epileptic children. When I was a youngster parents had no such timidity. It was then a fundamental rule imposed on children "to keep their mouths shut but their bowels open," and Epsom salts were ladled out by the tablespoon at the first sniffle. Many parents today allow their children to have seizures and stay in a perpetually drugged state rather than add a little harmless magnesium to their diets; they fail to realize that physicians are too overworked to keep up with the thousands of research projects reported each year. Furthermore innumerable brilliant, fine individuals suffering from epilepsy are literally held prisoners in our degrading mental institutions, and are receiving the most inadequate diets imaginable. Many states still have laws forbidding anyone once diagnosed as an epileptic to marry or drive a car. Yet physicians give antibiotics and diuretics which, by destroying vitamin B_6 and increasing the urinary losses of magnesium, actually induce such convulsions. Seizures have also been produced by inadequate baby formulas recommended by pediatricians (p. 174).

Magnesium is needed by every cell in the body including those of the brain. It is essential for the synthesis of proteins, for the utilization of fats and carbohydrates, and for hundreds of enzyme systems, especially ones involved in energy production. Because most of these enzymes also contain vitamin B_6, which is not well absorbed unless magnesium is generously supplied, a lack of either vitamin B_6 or magnesium may result in the same symptoms: convulsions, tremors, insomnia, kidney stones, and many others.

When magnesium is deficient, large amounts of calcium are lost in the urine even though sorely needed by the body. Such a tragedy occurs in infants. Milk, proprietary infant formulas, and baby foods are extremely low in magnesium, the requirement for which is increased by the baby's high calcium intake. Pediatricians, untrained in nutrition, fail to give magnesium supplements or to recognize deficiency symptoms. As a result, marked sensitivity to noise, insomnia, tremors, painful muscle spasms, hyperactivity, and convulsions are not unusual in infants. The continuous loss of calcium contributes to the abominable bone structure so common now even in small children. I have seen parents of magnesium-deficient babies desperate from lack of sleep themselves, kept awake night after night by the child's crying; since a lack of magnesium causes one to become sensitive to noise, the least sound awakens such an infant. Because potassium leaves the cells when magnesium is undersupplied, a lack of this nutrient can even cause infant colic (p. 191). Yet symptoms resulting from an undersupply of magnesium can be prevented or corrected by as little as ¼ teaspoon of magnesium salts added once daily to a bottle of formula. As little as 500 milligrams of Epsom salts have stopped epilepsy in infants.

Because large amounts of calcium are lost in the urine when magnesium is undersupplied, the lack of this nutrient indirectly becomes responsible for much rampant tooth decay, poor bone development, osteoporosis, and slow healing of broken bones and fractures. In case any of these abnormalities become a problem, magnesium should immediately be added to the diet. In areas where magnesium is high in the soil and water, as in Deaf Smith County, Texas, there is remarkable freedom from tooth decay; fractures are rare, even among the extremely elderly.

The same high urinary losses of calcium during a magnesium shortage play a role in forming kidney stones. Such stones occur when the diet is deficient in either magnesium or vitamin B_6. If magnesium alone is undersupplied, the stones are made of calcium combined with phosphorus rather than with oxalic acid, as they are when only vitamin B_6 is missing. Stone formation has been found to stop almost immediately after these nutrients are obtained and well absorbed, but it recurs as quickly if the supplementations are withdrawn.

The best sources of magnesium are nuts, soybeans, and cooked green leafy vegetables such as spinach, chard, kale, and beet tops, provided these foods are grown without chemical fertilizer and no cooking water is discarded. Unfortunately these foods are eaten infrequently by most persons. Sea snails, the richest source, would scarcely whet an appetite.

The amount of magnesium needed daily appears to be about 500 milligrams for infants, children, and most women, and 800 milligrams for adolescents, men, convalescents, and expectant mothers. These quantities give a bare margin over the amounts lost daily in the urine, feces, and perspiration.[1] Deficiencies have been produced in volunteers merely by giving them foods eaten daily by millions of people: white bread, polished rice, macaroni, noodles, tapioca, sugar, candies, jams, bakery goods, and soft drinks. Even when unrefined foods are eaten entirely, only about 100 milligrams of magnesium are obtained per 1,000 calories, half of which may not be absorbed. The adults of races whose diets are rich in magnesium and who have no heart disease or arteriosclerosis have an intake of approximately 5 milligrams per pound of ideal weight daily, or 10 milligrams per kilogram.

The magnesium requirement is in proportion to the calcium intake. The more calcium in a diet, the more magnesium needed. Calcium given alone can induce a magnesium deficiency. In fact, calves given only milk die because in the presence of so much calcium the little magnesium in milk is excreted in the urine. Similarly a mother or physician who gives an infant a milk formula without adding magnesium can produce convulsions in the child as surely as they are produced in animals in the laboratory. Taking excessive amounts of magnesium can also prevent calcium from being absorbed.

The correct proportion appears to be approximately twice as much calcium as magnesium, or 500 milligrams of magnesium for each 1,000 milligrams of calcium. Children, pregnant women, and ill and convalescent persons have especially high magnesium requirements. Men need more than do women. Whenever a calcium supplement is used, magnesium likewise must be increased. Health-food stores carry tablets containing the proper proportions of

[1] M. S. Seelig, "The Requirement of Magnesium by the Normal Adult," *American Journal of Clinical Nutrition*, XIV (1964), 342.

natural magnesium-rich limestone (dolomite), and of magnesium salts added to bone ash or various calcium salts. Magnesium carbonate, magnesium bicarbonate, magnesium oxide, magnesium chloride, and magnesium sulfate have all been successfully used in overcoming deficiencies. A fourth or a half teaspoon of any one of these supplements, furnishing 250 to 500 milligrams of magnesium, can be added to milk or juice with little or no change in flavor provided the drink is not allowed to stand before being taken. Magnesium oxide neutralizes the hydrochloric acid in the stomach so completely that it should not be used by persons having digestive difficulties.

Persons who take magnesium compounds as laxatives or antacids obtain such an excess that they experience muscular weakness, listlessness, lethargy, drowsiness, lack of co-ordination, speech difficulties, slow heartbeat, nausea and vomiting, and even coma, or unconsciousness. Such symptoms can be overcome by taking calcium, but the relationship between the two minerals should always be carefully balanced; both should be adequate and neither excessive.

Because of the tremendous importance of magnesium, it appears that the diet of every man, woman, and child should be supplemented with this nutrient unless he is lucky enough to eat foods grown entirely on magnesium-rich soils without chemical fertilizers. The principal reason physicians write millions of prescriptions for tranquilizers each year is the nervousness, grouchiness, and jitters largely brought on by inadequate diets lacking magnesium. I recently talked to a psychiatrist who told me she had formerly put most of her patients on tranquilizers. She said she had then become interested in nutrition, and after insisting that persons who worked with her follow a good diet especially adequate in magnesium and calcium, she had found not only that tranquilizers were no longer needed, but that psychotherapy progressed more rapidly. It was her conviction, as it has long been mine, that nature supplies her own tranquilizers.

CHAPTER 23

AS I SEE IT, THERE'S NO EXCUSE

I FIND IT DIFFICULT TO UNDERSTAND HOW ANY INTELligent person could let himself be deficient in either iron or iodine. The need for both has been known for decades. Iron is found in almost every natural food, whereas iodized salt has been sold at no extra cost for years. The fact that deficiencies of both iron and iodine are still widespread gives me a depressing you're-butting-your-head-against-a-brick-wall feeling. Then I remind myself, more logically, that people will never apply sound nutrition until convinced it has personal value for them.

Long ago a physician referred to me a man suffering from a fatal disease, siderosis, in which excessive iron is held in the body. This man's identical twin had already died of the disease. My problem, supposedly, was to plan a diet which could maintain maximum health but which supplied no iron, meaning no meat, eggs, fruit, vegetables, yeast, wheat germ, or whole-grain breads or cereals. Such a diet is not possible.

Anemia can result from inadequate protein, iodine, cobalt, copper, vitamin E, or almost any one of the B vitamins, particularly folic acid, niacin, or vitamin B_6. Approximately half of all persons suffering from anemia have abnormal or sore tongues, indicating a lack of B vitamins. Probably every nutrient plays some role in building healthy blood. Much anemia does exist, however, which can be corrected by iron.

Red blood cells, or corpuscles, are made in the bone marrow. It is estimated that approximately one billion per minute are produced by a healthy adult. In a cubic millimeter of blood, an imaginary cube about 0.04 inch on every side, there are normally about 5,000,000 red corpuscles. This number is spoken of as the blood count. To be healthy, however, each corpuscle must contain a certain amount of red coloring material, or hemoglobin, which carries oxygen by combining chemically with it. Approximately a half cup of blood should supply 15 grams of hemoglobin. Anemia exists when your blood count is below 4,000,000 red corpuscles and/or 12 grams of the red hemoglobin.

Iron-deficiency anemia is common among women, children, and adolescent boys and girls but rare in men; a reason is that children grow and women menstruate. Men, however, may become anemic because of hemorrhaging, perhaps from stomach ulcers. Severe anemia often occurs in blood donors whose admirable generosity is not matched by intelligent nutrition. Anemia in general means that the body does not produce enough red corpuscles or hemoglobin. If the only deficiency is one of iron, the number of red blood cells is usually normal but the hemoglobin lacks color. The anemic person cannot be supplied with sufficient oxygen; energy production decreases, and he experiences weakness, perhaps dizziness, shortness of breath on exertion, consciousness of a pounding heartbeat, or palpitation, and fatigue which may become a continuous dead-tiredness. The fingernails are often brittle and show longitudinal ridging. Such persons are literally colorless, listlessly lacking in vitality. Since too little oxygen reaches the brain, they cannot think clearly or quickly and they forget easily. Yet when an adequate diet is adhered to and well absorbed, the amount of hemoglobin and the number of red corpuscles soon become normal.

Aside from the iron needed for hemoglobin, iron is an important part of numerous enzyme systems and of myohemoglobin, or hemoglobin of the muscles.

The greatest single cause of iron-deficiency anemia is the refining of breads, cereals, and sugar. Although much has been said about the iron in "enriched" flour, only 6 milligrams per pound is added, and relatively little flour is now "enriched"; whole-wheat flour contains approximately 18 milligrams per pound. Brewers' yeast and wheat germ are both excellent sources, supplying per ½ cup 18 and 8 milligrams, respectively. I used to recommend that iron be obtained from blackstrap molasses stirred into milk. Then I saw a child of three whose parents, superinterested in nutrition, had given him directly from the tablespoon a fourth cup of blackstrap daily. The child had never been allowed to taste candy even at Christmas, but his teeth were decayed to the gum margin. Since then

I have been afraid to recommend blackstrap. Perhaps I can no longer take the ribbing. The blackstrap gags have become shopworn. The following, written before a geologist, Dr. Natland by name, left for Arabia, is no isolated example.

> Camel's milk, boiled goat, dates and cheese,
> Poor Nat will starve if he can't eat these;
> Sun-warmed, fly-specked and sprinkled with sand,
> Sounds like a diet Adelle Davis had planned.

In a mixed diet—not mixed with sand—only about 50 per cent of the iron is absorbed even by a healthy person; the remainder is lost in the feces. In experiments in which anemia was treated with single foods, liver was found to produce the most hemoglobin, kidneys second, apricots third, and eggs fourth. Many foods which contained as much or more iron failed to be good blood builders. Part of the iron in leafy vegetables is held in insoluble compounds which cannot be absorbed. In general, the softer the texture of any food containing iron, the more complete the absorption.

When iron-containing foods are digested, the freed iron must dissolve in hydrochloric acid from the stomach before it can pass through the intestinal wall into the blood. Since approximately two-thirds of all anemic persons lack this acid, much nutritional anemia cannot be overcome unless acid is supplied along with adequate iron. Foods which contain acids, such as buttermilk, yogurt, sour fruits, and citrus juices, aid the absorption of iron. Even the drinking of sweet milk increases iron absorption because milk sugar is converted into lactic acid by intestinal bacteria. Conversely, refined carbohydrates decrease iron absorption both because they stimulate the flow of alkaline digestive juices and because they do not support the growth of valuable intestinal bacteria. Persons with stomach ulcers, anemic from loss of blood, cannot absorb iron while taking alkalinizing preparations.

Most inorganic iron is well absorbed, even iron rust. An old medical treatise entitled *Self-help for People in Remote Places* suggests for "the disease of pale ears" soaking rusty iron shavings in vinegar-water overnight and drinking the water. An ancient treatment of anemia was to stick rusty nails into a sour apple, allow it to stand overnight, remove the nails, and eat the apple.

Many iron salts and perhaps all used medically in treating anemia destroy vitamin E. If they must be taken, have the iron after one meal and the entire day's quota of vitamin E at least 8 hours later. I find liver, yeast, wheat germ, and eggs far more effective in correcting anemia, however, and that iron salts are not needed. Pork liver, incidentally, is tremendously rich in iron.

A small excess of iron can be stored in the liver, the bone marrow, and the spleen to be used at times when the diet is inadequate. The person suffering from an iron deficiency is anemic only because he lacks such a store.

Provided vitamin E is adequate (p. 150), the life span of red corpuscles is three to four months. They are then withdrawn from circulation by the spleen and liver and are broken down by enzymes. The iron is used again and again in building other corpuscles. Most authorities believe that healthy women after menopause and adult men need no dietary iron. The non-iron parts of broken-down hemoglobin are excreted in bile and are known as bile pigments. These pigments give the color to the stools and urine; during jaundice, when red blood cells may be destroyed rapidly or bile cannot reach the intestine, they color the eyes and skin.

Iron requirements are especially high during adolescence, when the blood volume increases rapidly, and during pregnancy. The needs of non-pregnant women vary with the losses during menstruation. Many women have excessive menstrual flow for years without realizing that it is excessive. Cumulative menstrual losses, pregnancies, and the long use of deficient diets cause anemia to be prevalent in women at and after the menopause. Besides causing needless fatigue, mental confusion, and depression, anemia can bring about such forgetfulness that these women often become convinced they are losing their minds.

The National Research Council recommends 15 milligrams of iron daily for adolescents and women and 10 milligrams daily for men. Any diet adequate in protein and all the B vitamins supplied by natural sources will be more than adequate in iron. If anemia does persist after a sound nutrition program supplemented with vitamin B_6 and E is adhered to, a physician should certainly be consulted.

A blood analysis tells a physican many things; it usually tells you little that you could not learn by examining yourself carefully before the mirror. If your ears and if your forehead, neck, and skin not hidden by rouge have a glow of health, you can assume that you are not anemic. You have one of the fundamental attributes of genuine beauty and probably the vivacity which helps to make up the intangible qualities known as charm and personality.

Too little iodine can be even worse than a lack of iron. When iodine is undersupplied in the mother's diet during pregnancy, the baby fails to develop normally; if the deficiency is quite severe, he may become an idiot, or cretin. When a severe lack of iodine occurs later in life, myxedema results. I have seen only one case each of these abnormalities and, please believe me, one of each is too many. The child, the first of wonderful parents, is eighteen months old, sluggish, disgustingly fat, still toothless, and covered with eczema; so many behavior problems are developing that the conscientious young mother is already nearly insane. Her physician told me, "Her troubles haven't even started yet."

I hesitate to tell of the other case, it is so unbelievable: a woman of perhaps forty-eight, unable to leave her home. I saw her on a sweltering day in August. A daughter opened the door and took me to the living room where the mother sat on a davenport, wearing a heavy winter coat, her knees covered with a blanket, a small gas heater burning at her feet, and every door and window in the room tightly closed. One could scarcely breathe in the room. The woman was stuporous, her eyes were glassy, and her movements and thinking were inconceivably sluggish. The condition had come on gradually. Her physician had given her thyroid, but she had failed to consult him again when the cumulative effect of repeated doses had made her extremely nervous and had caused frightening heart palpitations. She had stopped the thyroid weeks before. A small amount of iodine daily could have prevented both conditions and all others like them.

Iodine is needed by the thyroid glands, situated on either side of the windpipe. These glands secrete an iodine-containing hormone known as thyroxin, which can be produced in normal amounts only when adequate iodine is supplied. Thyroxin has a profound effect upon growth, mental and physical development, and the maintenance of health throughout life. Although minute amounts of iodine are found in all parts of the human body, it is concentrated in the adrenal cortex, the ovaries, and particularly the thyroid gland, which soaks it up like a sponge.

Thyroid activity is measured by analyzing the blood for protein-bound iodine. A normal basal metabolic rate, or BMR, means that energy is produced as it should be. Healthy persons with such a BMR have iodine values of

4 to 8 micrograms for each half cup (100 cc.) of blood. Individuals with less than 4 micrograms of iodine are receiving too little of this nutrient to feel energetic. It must be remembered, however, that low blood sugar or an under-supply of protein, vitamin B_1, or any one of several other nutrients decreases energy production.

A partial or severe lack of iodine causes goiter, or en-largement of the thyroid glands. The enlarged glands often use the limited iodine supply more efficiently than can normal glands; hence the amount of thyroxin produced may remain the same. Aside from a slight fullness and perhaps a mild pressure in the neck, there may be no other symptoms. The swelling in the neck may be so slight as to go unnoticed; yet every person, in my opinion, should learn to detect even a small goiter. Stand before a mirror and turn your head as far as you can from side to side; if you can scarcely see the ligaments in your neck as you turn your head, your thyroid glands are probably some-what enlarged, and your iodine intake should be increased.

Whenever iodine is undersupplied, cells in the thyroid gland break down and hemorrhage. If the deficiency con-tinues over a prolonged period, these cells are gradually replaced by large amounts of bulky scar tissue totally unable to produce the thyroid hormone. Iodine alone can-not rebuild such a gland; vitamin E must be taken daily with iodine if health is to be restored. When persons with underactive thyroid glands have been given daily both 4 milligrams of iodine and 600 units of vitamin E, the amount of iodine taken up by the gland and the quantity of thy-roid hormones in the blood have each increased almost immediately and markedly.

Because the thyroid gland controls the speed at which all body activities occur, an undersupply of thyroid hormone results in fatigue, lethargy, a feeling of coldness, loss of sex interest, slowed pulse, low blood pressure, and a ten-dency to gain weight rapidly on few calories. Even mild iodine deficiency is associated with a high incidence of thyroid cancer, high blood cholesterol, and death from heart disease. When a deficiency already exists, more iodine is needed than can be obtained from iodized salt alone. Sub-stances found in peanuts, untoasted soy flour, and vege-tables of the cabbage family can combine with iodine, pre-venting it from reaching the blood, and thus increase the iodine requirement. Four milligrams of iodine daily, the amount supplied by a teaspoon of kelp, is usually adequate to correct thyroid abnormalities.

In 1917, Drs. David Marine and O. P. Kimball gave iodine twice a year to 2,190 girls in Akron, Ohio; only five developed goiter. Among an untreated group of 2,300 girls, almost 500 relatively severe goiters developed. After this classic study iodized salt was made available; not one case of goiter should ever again have occurred. Yet recent surveys revealed that 55 per cent of the girls and 30 per cent of the boys in the Cincinnati schools had goiter; in Minnesota, 70 per cent of the girls and 40 per cent of the boys; in Portland, Oregon, 40 per cent of the girls and 22 per cent of the boys. In Cleveland, the incidence of goiter was found to be exactly the same as it was before iodized salt was put on the market. This valuable salt was not and is not being used. Figures like these are disgraceful. The ignorance and apathy which allow such abnormal conditions to be so widespread are likewise disgraceful. The amount of goiter among adults is not known, but the University of Michigan Hospital recently reported having removed more than 600 goiters during one year.

The chief source of iodine is the ocean. The only parts of our country where adequate iodine may perhaps be obtained without using iodized salt is a narrow strip along the Atlantic Seaboard, around the Gulf of Mexico, and in regions which in recent geologic ages formed the floor of the ocean, such as parts of Kansas, South Dakota, Utah, western Texas, and New Mexico. Foods grown on these soils usually contain some iodine. Other soils, although near the coast, contain little or no iodine. No food is a reliable source except ocean fish and sea foods. Even fresh-water fish in Minnesota are said to develop severe goiters. Many cities on the Pacific Coast use melted-snow water which is iodine-free; despite nearness to the ocean, iodine deficiencies are common.

Iodized salt, approved by the American Medical Association, contains the amount of iodine that occurs naturally in unrefined ocean salt. When iodized salt is used throughout life, the iodine needs are supplied. No harmful effects can result from using this salt because iodine is lost continuously in urine, perspiration, and even exhaled air. Harm caused by not using it runs into millions of dollars; yet only 15 per cent of the salt now purchased even in the goiter belts is iodized. Furthermore, we buy much food already salted, prepared by companies so uninterested in health that iodized salt is not used. Yet so great is the contribution of this nutrient to health that the compulsory iodization of all salt seems to be the only answer. Wherever this step has been taken, as in Switzerland and Austria, goiter and most thyroid problems have disappeared.

The iodine requirements are increased in early childhood, puberty, and adolescence, during pregnancy and lactation, and particularly at menopause, but little is known of the quantities desirable. It is during menopause that goiters most often grow to be huge. Additional amounts of iodine appear not to be needed at these times if iodized salt has been used continuously for years; the thyroid gland traps and stores iodine for future safety. If this valuable salt has not been used constantly, some form of iodine should be taken to meet current needs and make up the deficiency. A few drops of Lugol's solution taken daily in a little water or milk has long been given to correct goiter, but it must be obtained on prescription. Despite the ease of prevention, every year millions of people who fail to obtain a normal supply of iodine pay for their neglect through a lack of mental and physical efficiency and alertness; thousands more, through pain and misery.

Before the thyroid glands can become normal again, an adequate diet supplemented daily with both iodine and vitamin E must be maintained for many months. Even large goiters can, however, often disappear in time. Most physicians have so rarely, if ever, seen persons on such diets that they usually recommend surgery. Then lifelong thyroid medication becomes necessary, once preventable at no extra cost merely by using iodized salt.

Toxic goiter is a condition which appears to occur when the liver has been so damaged that it cannot produce enzymes necessary to inactivate any thyroid hormone not needed; hence the hormone accumulates, causing the activities of all body cells to be accelerated. The person with a toxic goiter is therefore nervous, high-strung, overactive, and usually underweight; he has a rapid pulse, may be frighteningly aware of each heartbeat, and his body requirements for all nutrients skyrocket. It has been pointed out that his symptoms are identical to those of a person severely deficient in magnesium, which he may indeed lack. If he can obtain 2 to 6 milligrams of iodine daily with a high-protein diet generously supplemented with magnesium, calcium, and all vitamins, the liver damage can be overcome and health rebuilt without surgery.

Sometimes taking 50,000 units of vitamin A after breakfast and dinner for a single month (with vitamin E to prevent its destruction) corrects toxic goiter, though this quantity of vitamin A can be toxic and must not be continued for a prolonged period. I recall a girl with toxic goiter whose hands trembled so badly that she could not write, attend school, or even feed herself. In addition to the high vitamin A and a diet adequate in all nutrients, I emphasized vitamin B_6 and magnesium because of the tremor. In less than 24 hours her tremor stopped and her pulse dropped from 150 to 75. Within a few weeks she had no sign of a thyroid problem and has had no recurrence during the intervening years.

A thyroid gland not adequately supplied with ordinary food iodine avidly absorbs the highly toxic radioactive iodine from fallout, leaving the gland particularly susceptible to cancer and precancerous nodules. Such cancers and particularly such nodules increased markedly in several Western states years after bomb testing in Nevada was discontinued. Some countries are still testing bombs, and because our earth turns, the stratosphere over those countries is over ours before a day passes. Fallout, therefore, is still a problem. If the thyroid gland can obtain adequate iodine, none of the radioactive material is absorbed and no harm is done. Harvard physicians found that Massachusetts children absorbed radioactive iodine rapidly unless given a daily supplement of 1 or 2 milligrams of iodine. Their research indicates that adults would probably need at least 3 or 4 milligrams of iodine daily. In Japan, abnormalities of the thyroid do not exist; their per-day intake from iodine-rich seaweed averages 3 milligrams. It is difficult indeed for Americans to obtain this desirable amount.

Unfortunately our Food and Drug Administration limits iodine in any daily supplement to no more than 0.15 milligrams, about a twentieth of the amount needed for protection against fallout. Physicians have often considered 300 milligrams of iodine daily a small amount, and as much as 2,400 milligrams has been given daily to children for five years without recognized toxicity. Even kelp tablets are allowed to supply only 0.15 milligrams each; hence they are valueless unless you wish to swallow 20 or more daily. A teaspoon of powdered kelp daily would meet the requirement and is not too unpalatable when added to tomato juice or buttermilk. I add it to well-seasoned salads, soups, and casserole dishes.

The person on a sodium-free diet can use neither iodized salt nor sodium-rich kelp; he cannot possibly maintain health unless he obtains a prescription for iodine. At times when I have had no prescription, I have taken a tiny bit of ordinary tincture of iodine daily, merely touching the glass rod which comes with the bottle to the surface of a little water or milk. An entire drop of such medicinal iodine is said to supply 40 milligrams. Although much iodine is lost in the urine soon after it is taken, one drop a week is probably adequate. At present, for my own needs, I take each week a 100-milligram tablet of potassium iodide obtained on a prescription written by a kindly dentist.

The edict of the Food and Drug Administration limiting iodine supplementation to 0.15 milligrams was handed down without consideration of the decreased use of iodized salt or the increased need caused by fallout. Certainly this edict is destructive to health, yet it has the power of law. Perhaps if all humanitarian readers of this book would write the Food and Drug Administration at Washington, urging that this edict be withdrawn, American health would improve. In the meantime, my advice is to use only iodized salt and, if your requirements are high, obtain additional iodine in any way you can.

CHAPTER 24

THERE MUST BE A BALANCE

THERE ARE THREE NUTRIENTS, POTASSIUM, SODIUM, AND chlorine, which we need daily in quite large amounts. They are important in keeping the body fluids near neutrality; they determine the amount of water held in the tissues; they attract nutrients from the intestines into the blood and from the blood into the cells by means of maintaining what is known as osmotic pressure; and they have many other duties. These minerals are essential parts of the glandular secretions. Potassium helps in sending messages through the nervous system. Chlorine is used in forming hydrochloric acid in the stomach. These three nutrients are excreted daily in the urine, the amount being equal to that ingested by a healthy person.

Sodium and chlorine are amply supplied by table salt, sodium chloride. Potassium is widely spread, occurring in vegetables, fruits, whole grains, nuts, and meats. It is not enough, however, for sodium, chlorine, and potassium to be adequate at all times; sodium and potassium must be in balance, each with the other. An excess of sodium, for example, causes much-needed potassium to be lost in the urine. The reverse is equally true: an excess of potassium can cause a serious loss of sodium. For example, herbivorous animals have such a high intake of potassium that they can retain little sodium; they die unless they can get salt. In early America, such animals were known to have walked hundreds of miles to salt licks, hazarding dangers of every type.

Both because most people enjoy their foods well salted and because many fewer vegetables and fruits are being eaten than formerly, the problem now is that too little potassium is obtained and too much is lost in the urine. It is by no means easy to maintain this needed balance between sodium and potassium, yet it is extremely important. Each person should know when to increase his sodium intake and when to limit it; and how and when to increase the potassium in his diet.

Under normal conditions, a healthy person runs little risk of deficiencies of sodium and chlorine. In extremely hot weather, however, so much salt can be lost through perspiration that death may result. Death from salt deficiency occurred during the first years of work on Boulder Dam and similar projects. During the blistering summer of 1933 I corresponded with an engineer who was working on Parker Dam. Each letter contained some such note as, "We had a wonderful cook but he died yesterday of heatstroke." The symptoms of sunstroke also are now recognized as caused largely by loss of salt through perspiration.

A lack of salt causes symptoms varying in severity from mild lassitude, weariness, or hot-weather fatigue, common during heat waves, to heat cramps, heat exhaustion, and heatstroke, familiar to people who work in iron foundries, furnace or boiler rooms, and industrial plants such as steel or paper mills. Even persons who play tennis or take similar exercise in hot weather may suffer from heatstroke. The symptoms of heatstroke are nausea, dizziness, exhaustion, vomiting, and cramps in the legs, back, and abdominal muscles or any muscles being used at the time. Without salt, the more water drunk, the worse the condition becomes. Persons working in extreme heat are often advised to take a salt tablet with each drink of water. During extremely hot weather, some well-salted food should be served with each meal.

There are a few other times when the sodium, or salt, intake should be kept high. The adrenals, if healthy, produce a hormone, aldosterone, which holds sodium in the body whenever it is needed. During stress, aldosterone production is accelerated and larger amounts of sodium are purposely retained, causing an increase in the blood pressure. This temporarily elevated blood pressure, in turn, helps to force nutrients into the tissues to meet the increased energy demands of stress. If the diet is so inadequate that the adrenals become exhausted, aldosterone can no longer be adequately produced, sodium is not retained, and the blood pressure cannot be increased but actually falls below normal. Nutrients can no longer be forced quickly or efficiently into the tissues. As a result, fatigue and exhaustion may be severe and constant. Such a situation occurs in Addison's disease, glaucoma, and Ménière's syndrome, where the adrenals are exhausted, and to a lesser extent in arthritis, allergies, and all illnesses helped by cortisone or ACTH, the pituitary hormone which stimulates the adrenals to produce more cortisone.

In general the blood pressure, if known, can serve as a guide to the desired salt intake. If the blood pressure is low, indicating adrenal exhaustion, well-salted foods should be eaten; at times it is even wise temporarily to take a half teaspoon or more of salt stirred into water at each meal. When the blood pressure is high, you know that salt is being retained and that additional sodium could be harmful. Early-morning fatigue usually indicates abnormally low blood pressure, in which case the antistress program (p. 224) should be followed to build up the adrenals at all possible speed. As soon as the fatigue has disappeared and the blood pressure has increased to normal, which usually takes about two weeks, salt should again be used only in moderate amounts.

Far too often, however, the sodium intake is excessive not only from table salt but also from baking soda, baking powder, drinking water, sodium nitrates used as food preservatives, and the sodium obtained from no less than 300 food additives. The kidneys, if healthy, can throw off much of this excess, but if the kidneys have been damaged or are diseased, if one is taking ACTH or cortisone, or if stress causes the production of one's own ACTH or cortisone to be far above normal, so much sodium is held in the body that a severe and dangerous potassium deficiency can occur. In such cases foods high in sodium should be avoided: catsups, cold meats, canned soups, TV dinners, salted nuts, prepared mixes containing soda, and many other foods. At the same time home-cooked dishes should be well salted with a potassium-chloride salt substitute, and perhaps three servings of cooked vegetables eaten at both lunch and dinner.

In countries using little salt, high blood pressure is virtually unknown, but in Japan, where the diet is high in dried, salted fish, the major cause of death is strokes from high blood pressure resulting from excessive sodium intake. In our country, infants receiving ½ cup of commercially canned meats and vegetables daily have been found to have the highest amount of sodium in the blood ever recorded in man (6.2 m.eq./kg.); their kidneys are too immature to excrete these excessive amounts of salt added to please the adult taste. Dr. L. K. Dahl, who has spent years studying the relationship of the sodium intake to high blood pressure, has found that, in all age groups, the greater the sodium

intake, the earlier and more numerous are deaths caused by
hypertension. By feeding baby rats canned meats and vegetables prepared for infants, Dr. Dahl has produced high
blood pressure which was fatal in four months. The earlier
these salty foods were given, the more quickly the abnormal blood pressure developed and the higher it was elevated.[1] Although this research was done several years ago,
the sodium content of canned baby foods has not been decreased, and pediatricians are still advising young mothers
to give them to their infants.

Many scientists now postulate that these salted overcooked foods being forced on infants, who should be
allowed no added salt, will cause dangerously high blood
pressure later.[2] During this past year I have planned nutrition programs for two 11-year-old girls and one 13-year-
old, each of whom has suffered severe strokes associated
with high blood pressure. At the time, my secretary clipped
a note to a diet she had just typed: "Here's a forecast of
things to come." The mother of one of these little girls
wrote me that the child had had difficulty in chewing, and
that her diet for the first three years had consisted largely
of canned baby foods. Food for an infant or small child
can be quickly prepared in a liquefier, using portions of
fresh meats and vegetables cooked for the family and
before salt is added.

Perhaps the greatest harm done by an excessive sodium
intake is that it causes such a serious loss of potassium
from the body. Potassium, by activating many enzymes, is
essential for muscle contraction. Without it, sugar (glucose)
cannot be changed into energy or into body starch (glycogen) to be stored for future energy. When sugar cannot be
utilized or glycogen held in the cells, energy production
comes to a standstill. Like a motor out of fuel, the muscles
can no longer contract, and paralysis or partial paralysis
results. Nor is that the only harm done. Under normal
conditions potassium stays largely inside the cells and is
balanced by sodium outside the cells. If potassium is deficient, however, sodium enters the cells, taking with it so
much water that many cells actually burst. The result is
water retention (edema), damage to muscles and connective tissue, and extensive scarring.

Members of certain families are known to have an un-

[1] L. K. Dahl, *Nature*, 198 (1963), 1204.
[2] J. Mayer, "Hypertension, Salt Intake, and the Infant," *Post-
graduate Medicine*, XLV (1969), 229.

usually high hereditary requirement for potassium. If this nutrient is not generously supplied them, they frequently suffer from paralysis which starts with the legs and creeps upward and lasts from a few hours to several days. Until the cause was understood, sooner or later this paralysis was usually fatal. It can be corrected immediately, however, by a potassium injection or in half an hour by potassium taken by mouth. Volunteers with this family trait have actually lived in a laboratory for months while scientists have studied them, discovering facts which apply to all of us. These investigators found that the amount of potassium in the muscle cells dropped so far below normal that paralysis from the neck down was produced in 24 hours if these persons ate candy or any refined sweets; if they were allowed salty foods such as crackers or potato chips; or if they were given cortisone, ACTH, or a diuretic, which caused large amounts of potassium to be lost in the urine. Such paralysis, however, could be completely prevented merely by restricting the sodium intake. In giving ACTH or cortisone they were simulating the conditions of stress which cause one's own pituitary and adrenal glands to produce these hormones in increased amounts.

Most people have experienced some type of partial paralysis resulting from a lack of potassium in muscle cells. For example, after the severe stress of abdominal surgery, the potassium in the muscles of the intestinal walls often becomes so low that partial paralysis may last for days. Without movement to mix food with digestive enzymes and juices and bring it into contact with the absorbing surface of the intestinal walls, foods cannot be digested and absorbed but merely ferment, supporting the growth of millions of putrefactive bacteria. So much gas is formed that gas pain can become excruciating. I am convinced that faulty diet, stress, and high sodium intake combine to cause millions of persons to suffer from gas and indigestion resulting from such partial paralysis induced by potassium deficiencies. Similarly, a study of 655 cases of infant colic showed that this abnormality occurred only when the blood potassium was unusually low; and that colic could be corrected almost immediately by potassium injections or in a few hours by potassium given by mouth. (Canned baby foods should not be given a colicky infant; their high sodium content would cause still more potassium to be lost in the urine and the colic to become worse.) Still another example resulting again from the stress of surgery is the paralysis of the muscles in the urinary bladder, making it impossible to pass urine without a catheter until potassium is given or the stress is passed.

Merely by giving a diet of refined foods supplemented with other essential nutrients, deficiencies of potassium have been produced in humans. These persons quickly developed listlessness, fatigue, gas pains, constipation, insomnia, and low blood sugar; their muscles became soft and flabby, their pulse weak, slow, and irregular. These symptoms are suffered continuously by millions of Americans. Because potassium is supplied in so many foods, it is difficult to realize that deficiencies actually exist. People are now eating relatively few fruits and vegetables, the richest sources. When vegetables are soaked and/or boiled and the water discarded, the potassium is thrown away. In addition to potassium deficiencies brought on by sloppy cooking methods and by our high consumption of refined foods, they are produced by diarrhea and vomiting as well as by stress, a high salt intake, and such medications as ACTH, cortisone, and diuretics already discussed. Taking aspirin and many other drugs or drinking excessive amounts of water or alcohol increases the urinary losses of potassium still more.

Whenever potassium in the cells is low, the blood sugar is also low. Hypoglycemia, or low blood sugar, has become a major health problem in the United States, causing fatigue, irritability, foggy thinking, and many other unpleasant symptoms. The stress of low blood sugar itself causes still more potassium to be lost in the urine. Persons suffering from hypoglycemia who were given 2 to 5 grams (2,000 to 5,000 milligrams) of potassium chloride daily have been afforded "a remarkable degree of protection"; the blood sugar quickly increased and all symptoms disappeared. Eating salty foods, however, caused both the blood potassium to decrease immediately and the blood sugar to drop, bringing with it the all-too-familiar exhaustion. Whenever the blood sugar is low, dietary emphasis must be on immediately increasing the potassium intake, restricting sodium, and rebuilding the adrenals by following an antistress program (p. 224). Unfortunately, these features are usually omitted from diets purporting to correct hypoglycemia; and though the standard recommendations of frequent high-protein meals devoid of coffee and refined carbohydrates are excellent, they do not permanently correct the abnormality.

Since a lack of potassium allows sodium and water to

pass into the cells, increasing the intake of this nutrient often corrects edema, or water retention. Weight-conscious American women, however, wishing to be quickly rid of every possible pound, beg their physicians for "water pills," which they consider to be harmless. Approximately 36 million prescriptions for such diuretics—known to induce serious potassium deficiencies—are now being written annually. Though the urine output is temporarily increased and pounds lost (a pint of water weighs a pound) the cells again retain water because of an even more severe lack of potassium. Still more diuretics are taken. The resulting potassium deficiency causes the blood sugar to drop until exhaustion becomes unbearable; dexedrine or other amphetamines are then obtained to give the desired pickup. Because amphetamines make nerves tense and sleep elusive, prescriptions are then obtained for tranquilizers and sleeping tablets. Millions of American women are caught in this vicious circle. Their adolescent sons and daughters tell the school counselors, "Pushers? What do we need with pushers? Mom's medicine chest is full of reds and whites, uppers and downers. We can get all we want." The children are blamed, not the mothers who failed to improve their diets; not the doctors who wrote prescriptions without making nutritional recommendations.

High blood pressure, though usually caused by excessive salt intake, has also been produced both in animals and in human volunteers by diets deficient in potassium; and high blood pressure has been successfully treated by giving patients large amounts of potassium chloride daily. For years physicians recommended a disgracefully inadequate diet of nothing but fruit, sugar, and unsalted white rice which reduced blood pressure because it supplied 20 times more potassium than sodium. Any varied diet of palatable unrefined foods could be equally effective because equally rich in potassium. In one study, individuals eating salt to taste excreted nine times more potassium than when they selected less salty but equally appetizing foods. Anyone with high blood pressure, therefore, should certainly limit sodium intake; all labels should be read, and foods containing preservatives avoided. It is particularly important, however, that all foods be chosen for their high potassium content.

By far the greatest harm done by a potassium deficiency is probably its effect upon the heart. It has long been known that heart attacks are often associated with a low blood potassium and a low potassium intake. Furthermore, every type of experimental animal deficient in potassium suffers extensive damage and degeneration of the heart muscles not unlike the infarcts found after human heart attacks. These muscles show masses of dead cells, numerous small hemorrhages, much inflammation, areas of scar tissue, and calcification often accompanied by kidney damage. Such degeneration of the heart muscles can be seen as early as the second week of a potassium-deficient diet. Because magnesium is necessary to keep potassium in muscle cells, similar changes occur when magnesium is deficient. Without adequate magnesium, the potassium leaves the cells, creating in them an artificial potassium deficiency. Since potassium is essential for energy to be produced, even a momentary lack of either potassium or magnesium can cause the heart to stop beating, resulting in death from a "heart attack."

It now appears quite possible that a lack of potassium in the coronary muscles may be the major cause of death from heart disease in humans. Certainly from the cradle on, the American intake of sodium is excessive, thus producing potassium deficiencies even when this nutrient may be liberally supplied in the diet. That potassium deficiencies are brought on by dietary inadequacy, excessive sugar intake, stress, and such medications as ACTH, cortisone, and diuretics has been definitely proved. The fact that a lack of potassium can cause partial or even complete paralysis in man is also well established. What happens if such paralysis occurs in a heart muscle for even a few moments? The result appears to be the same in humans as in all experimental animals: death from a heart attack.

Dr. Eörs Bajusz, a professor in the medical colleges at both the University of Montreal and the University of Vermont, has written an excellent book, *Nutritional Aspects of Cardiovascular Diseases*,[3] dealing with the relationship of potassium and magnesium deficiencies to heart attacks. In it Dr. Bajusz points out that although patients may die suddenly from what appears to be the result of a typical thrombosis (clot) or coronary occlusion (arteries plugged with cholesterol) "the most careful search" during autopsies of many persons dying of heart disease has failed to reveal either. Furthermore, autopsies have shown that persons having had no heart attacks but dying from other causes often have heavier cholesterol deposits and worse atherosclerosis than individuals whose deaths were brought on by heart failure; that circulation had not been interrupted

[3] Philadelphia: J. B. Lippincott Company, 1965.

because new blood vessels had frequently formed around arteries completely plugged with cholesterol; and that such patients often had no history of heart disease. Of 1,000 autopsies of persons who died following sudden or relatively sudden heart attacks, few clots were found, and these appeared to be the result rather than the cause of the attack. Other studies have revealed that when men under 50 years old have died of heart attacks, 63 per cent have died during the first hour of the first attack and 77 per cent have died before a physician could reach them. Research convincingly indicates that such sudden deaths, in animals and humans alike, are caused by a lack of potassium in the cells of the heart muscles. Dr. Bajusz believes that an adequate diet not only can prevent such deaths but may offset the hereditary tendency to heart disease.

Much still must be learned before the complicated causes of heart deaths are fully understood, but there can be no doubt that potassium and magnesium deficiencies play a role, perhaps the major one. What have appeared to be inconsistencies are falling into place like pieces of a jigsaw puzzle. For example, it is an established doctrine that persons with high blood cholesterol are susceptible to death from heart disease; yet animals kept on such inadequate diets that their blood vessels become plugged with cholesterol do not die suddenly of heart failure, unless deficient in magnesium. The widespread magnesium deficiencies may prove to be the common denominator: a lack of magnesium allows both the blood cholesterol to become excessive and potassium to leave the cells. Many statistics indicate that it is high sugar intake rather than too many saturated fats which predisposes persons to heart attacks; sugar decreases cell potassium. Other researchers believe that our disgraceful death rate from heart disease is caused largely by clots resulting from vitamin-E deficiencies, pointing out that such deaths were unknown prior to 1910, when vitamin E was first discarded by "improved" methods of refining grains (ref. 3, p. 151); these same methods cause tremendous losses in magnesium and potassium. My opinion is that heart disease is caused by a combination of many factors, but that a lack of potassium and magnesium in the muscle cells is probably responsible for the sudden deaths of ambitious young men under tremendous stress.

How can such deaths be prevented? If health is to be maintained, one should have at least 5,000 milligrams of potassium daily provided the salt intake is no more than one teaspoon. Americans, however, consume an average of one to 5 teaspoons of salt daily, or 4 to 20 grams; for each additional teaspoon of salt eaten, the potassium intake should be increased about 5,000 milligrams. Your daily intake of this nutrient should be computed and the best sources of potassium learned by using the tables starting on page 273.

If you find your potassium intake is too low, increase your consumption of fruits and vegetables, and try to have a cooked green leafy vegetable daily; avoid all refined foods, especially sweets; decrease your sodium intake; and try to reduce the amount of stress you are under. Make sure you get adequate magnesium daily, and increase the amount if any alcohol is drunk. Because my husband looks upon many vegetables with a jaundiced eye, I fill all of our salt shakers with a mixture of equal parts of table salt and a potassium-chloride salt substitute. If a dependable source of iodine is available, potassium chloride can be used alone instead of salt.

Enteric-coated tablets of potassium chloride, dissolving in the small intestine, have caused intestinal ulcers. For this reason, supplements containing more than 180 milligrams of potassium are sold only on prescription. Tablets furnishing 180 milligrams are available, but 28 would be needed to furnish a day's minimum potassium requirement; I swallow a small handful if my blood sugar is low or if I have foolishly eaten too many salted nuts. Many physicians, however, believe that potassium chloride should never be taken in tablet form but only dissolved in a solution. A teaspoon of potassium chloride salt supplies approximately 4,000 milligrams of potassium; though far from palatable, it can be stirred into water and taken by anyone who cannot obtain adequate amounts of this nutrient from foods. A potential heart patient would be wise to take such a supplement, especially when under stress.

In a recently published book which is used as a reference in training medical students and dietitians, I find this statement: "Potassium is especially abundant in both plant and animal tissues and does not need particular consideration" (p. 599 of ref. 1, p. 198). Such an attitude is typical of many busy physicians untrained in nutrition. We can, therefore, expect unnecessary suffering to continue and sudden deaths from heart attacks to bring more untold tragedies for many years to come.

CHAPTER 25

HOW FIRM A FOUNDATION?

ALL UNREFINED FOODS GROWN ON GOOD SOIL CONTAIN MIN-erals necessary to the normal life processes of animals and humans and to the plants themselves. Besides the minerals already discussed, there is a group spoken of as trace minerals, needed only in small amounts.

Cobalt forms part of vitamin B_{12}; as little as three micrograms of vitamin B_{12} daily can prevent pernicious anemia. This small amount could have kept thousands of people from suffering from fatigue which tortured every cell in their bodies and prevented a crippling paralysis from dooming them to a stumbling and falling existence and finally a bedridden living death during the years before Drs. George R. Minot and William P. Murphy found that raw liver could control the disease. Thousands of cattle, sheep, and other animals, grazed on land deficient in cobalt, especially in Florida and Australia, sickened and died from a crippling anemia. Deaths like these could be prevented if a few pounds of cobalt were added to each acre of land. Such anemia, however, was never confined to Florida or Australia. Studies conducted at the University of Florida Agricultural Experiment Station showed that 81 per cent of the children living in the area suffered from anemia, just as did the animals; 50 per cent showed definite anemia, whereas 31 per cent were borderline cases. When the land is deficient, the plants grown on that land are deficient; the animals which eat the plants are deficient; the people who eat the animals and the plants are deficient. It cannot be otherwise.

Another trace mineral, copper, plays a role in many enzyme systems and is essential to the production of ribonucleic acid (RNA), part of the nucleus of every cell. It aids in the development of bones, brain, nerves, and connective tissue and in the functions of the nerves and brain. A deficiency decreases the absorption of iron and shortens the life span of red blood cells, thus causing anemia. In animals, a lack results in porous bones, loss of hair, skin rash, a degeneration of the covering of the nerves (demyelination), and in heart damage and sudden death from heart failure. Copper also plays a role in pigment formation; black animals, lacking copper, become gray. Similarly, graying in humans has long been known to be associated with anemia. Copper-deficiency symptoms are also quite common in plants. "Swayback" disease occurs in lambs grazed on copper-deficient soil, and anemia in ewes; both conditions may be prevented by adding copper to the soil. A deficiency of this nutrient is rarely recognized in humans, but anemia in infants and children which was not corrected by iron has disappeared soon after copper was included in their diets.

Copper is richest in the least popular meats: liver, kidney, and brain. Smaller amounts are found in dry beans, peas, whole-grain breads and cereals, and green leafy vegetables provided they are grown on fertile soils. Like many other nutrients, copper is usually adequate if only unrefined foods are eaten.

Deficiencies of another trace mineral, zinc, are commonly recognized in crops and stock foods over most of the United States. Even when zinc is not actually lacking from the soils, deficiencies are caused by chemical fertilization saturating the soil solution to such a degree that zinc cannot dissolve in it or be absorbed by the plants. Because of this situation, zinc is customarily added to feed for stock, though it is rarely included in supplements for humans. The only reliable food source seems to be shell fish. Severe zinc deficiencies can also be produced by a diet excessively high in phosphorus. Such a diet, consumed by huge numbers of Americans, inhibits zinc absorption.[1]

A lack of zinc interferes with the formation of the nucleus, or of both RNA and DNA, of each cell in our bodies. Zinc is normally found in all human tissues, and is especially concentrated in the eyes and sperm. It is essential for the synthesis of body protein and the action of many enzymes. An undersupply in animals and humans alike causes a loss of fertility, low resistance to infections, slow healing, and a skin abnormality similar to psoriasis. The offspring of animals deficient in zinc often have thalidomide-like defects and abnormalities of the eyes, kidneys, brain, and bones.

[1] M. G. Wohl and R. S. Goodhart, *Modern Nutrition in Health and Disease*, 4th ed. (Philadelphia: Lea and Febiger, 1968), p. 390.

The dramatic results obtained when ill persons have been allowed zinc supplements would indicate that deficiencies are far more widely spread than is yet recognized. Dr. Walter J. Pories and co-workers of the School of Medicine and Dentistry at the University of Rochester, New York, found that when 200 milligrams of zinc sulfate were given three times daily to severely burned persons, to patients after surgery, and to individuals whose wounds had refused to heal, rapid healing took place. Blood cholesterols also dropped and patients with atherosclerosis improved. Even when the zinc supplement was continued for more than 3 years, no toxicity occurred. Where zinc deficiencies are severe, as in Egypt and Iran, growth and sexual development is so interfered with that the testicles and penis remain abnormally small and pubic and facial hair does not grow; yet zinc sulfate given as a daily supplement has brought development of the external genitalia and normal growth even in older boys. One young man, 20 years old, grew 5 inches in 14 months.

When foods are grown on good soils, nuts and green leafy vegetables are especially rich sources of zinc. This nutrient, however, is easily lost if cooking water is discarded. Even after being obtained, it is excreted in the urine if excess liquids or alcohol are drunk or diuretics taken.

Manganese is another nutrient needed to activate numerous enzymes in the animal body and presumably in humans as well. It aids directly in utilizing fats and is also necessary before cholin can help utilize fats. Its richest sources are wheat germ, nuts, bran, green leafy vegetables, and unrefined breads and cereals grown on healthy soils. If soils are high in iron or chemical fertilizers are used, little manganese can be absorbed into plants; hence deficiencies occur both in such plants and in the animals feeding on them. A diet high in phosphorus reduces the absorption of manganese. The daily requirement is not known.

Animals deficient in manganese show retarded growth, hyperactivity, abnormal bone structure, joint deformities, poor equilibrium, and uncoordinated movements; females become sterile and males impotent. In some animals, increasing the intake of cholin and inositol can prevent the deficiency symptoms. By increasing the manganese intake during pregnancy to above normal, certain congenital hereditary defects, which occur in animals given "adequate" manganese, can be completely prevented. The young of females slightly deficient in manganese develop abnormalities similar to the human disease myasthenia gravis; and the animal version of this illness sets in progressively earlier with each deficient generation. It has been suggested that a lack of manganese is also related to lupus erythematosus. Both lupus erythematosus and myasthenia gravis are said to be increasing rapidly.

Dr. Emanuel Josephson[2] has reported the complete recovery from myasthenia gravis by persons who had adhered for a few weeks to an adequate diet supplemented with 50 milligrams of manganese at each meal. He found manganese to be "remarkably non-toxic." I recently had lunch with Mrs. Donald Kempton of Horse Shoe, North Carolina, who has recovered after having myasthenia gravis for 27 years. Once interested in nutrition, she supplemented her diet not only with manganese but also with large amounts of cholin, inositol, vitamin E, and other nutrients. This attractive woman looked so healthy that I assumed her illness had never been serious. "How sick were you?" I asked rather lightly.

"My death certificate was made out," came the amazing answer. "Couldn't move a muscle, and the doctor was convinced I couldn't possibly live."

Some scientists say it has not been proved that humans need manganese, but Mrs. Kempton and Dr. Josephson would disagree with them.

Chromium, still another trace element, is essential before the body can utilize sugar normally. There is evidence that diabetes may be caused, in part at least, by a deficiency of this nutrient. Animals lacking chromium develop severe eye abnormalities. Some have diabetic-like symptoms with high blood sugar whereas others have extremely low blood sugar. Hypoglycemia, or low blood sugar, in humans has been promptly corrected by giving only 250 micrograms of chromium daily. Like other trace minerals, chromium is often deficient in soils and/or is not available if chemical fertilizers are used. Unless a person is fortunate enough to obtain foods grown on healthy, naturally mineralized soils, it would appear wise to supplement the daily diet with mixed minerals furnishing cobalt, copper, manganese, zinc, and perhaps chromium.

I am convinced that the trace minerals already discussed are far more important to health than most people realize, and that our diets are far more deficient in them than is generally appreciated. One reason for my belief is that in any agricultural library you can obtain books with beauti-

[2] E. Josephson, *Thymus, Manganese, and Myasthenia Gravis* (Chedney Press, 1961).

ful colored pictures of deficiency symptoms of vegetables, fruits, and other plants which we and animals use as food.[3] You can see those same deficiency symptoms in the food in every market: the split stalks of celery; the cracked cores of cabbage and cauliflower; the uneven ripening of apricots and tomatoes; yellow margins on the spinach; rusty streaks in the lettuce; those signs and dozens more. Such symptoms occur only when the plant is deficient in one mineral or another.

There are a number of trace minerals which can be either valuable or harmful to health depending on the amount obtained. In fact, all trace minerals can be toxic if taken in excess. Arsenic, well known as a drug and a poison, may be important in human nutrition. Relatively large amounts are found in the liver and blood, particularly before birth. Aluminum occurs in the human body and in the bodies of animals which have never eaten food prepared in aluminum utensils; minute amounts of it, too, may be essential. Bromine is found in human blood; in a type of insanity known as manic depressive, the amount of bromine in the blood falls to half the normal quantity and increases only upon recovery from the disease. Tin, silver, nickel, and mercury are also found in human tissues; their functions, if any, are unknown.

Though some persons claim that we need traces of fluorine, it appears not to be a dietary essential. Generations of rats remain as healthy and with as good teeth without fluorine as those given fluorine. Authorities by no means agree that fluorine benefits the teeth, and the danger of toxicity is ever-present. In 1962, our Public Health Department reported that the children in Newburgh, New York, where water was first fluoridated, had slightly more decay *after fluoridation than before*. In Baltimore, Maryland, where water has been fluoridated since 1952, rampant decay has steadily increased. In Puerto Rico not only has tooth decay increased since fluoridation of the water supply, but 64 per cent of adolescent boys have mottled, permanently stained teeth from fluoride excess, the ugly brown spots ruining every smile.

Fluorine has been shown to be harmful to many of the body's enzyme systems; and drinking fluoridated water has become a common cause of allergies. It increases the brit-

[3] *Hunger Signs in Crops, a Symposium* (Washington, D.C.: National Fertilizer Association, 1952); Frank A. Gilbert, *Mineral Nutrition of Plants and Animals* (Norman, Oklahoma: University of Oklahoma Press, 1948).

tleness of teeth and bones. There is some indication that it may damage the chromosomes. Without fluoridation, ever-increasing amounts of fluorides reach us as pollutants in air and water. In 1963 *The American Journal of Diseases of Children* emphasized editorially that fluorine was always a potential poison; that to add it to a water supply was unnecessary, unwise, wasteful, and needlessly expensive; and that it should not be given to older children or adults. Dr. Philip Chen, professor of chemistry, has pointed out that when water is fluoridated, some of the fluorine com-bines with magnesium to form magnesium fluoride, an insoluble salt which cannot be absorbed by the intestine; thus fluoridation can produce a deficiency of magnesium, a nutrient supplied all too meagerly.[4] Since potassium leaves the cells when magnesium is deficient, it would not be sur-prising to find that deaths from heart disease have increased in areas where the water is fluoridated. This fact was not once considered when fluoridation became a political issue. Certainly the choice as to whether fluorine is to be included in the diet should be left to each individual and not be imposed upon him by having the entire water supply fluori-dated at great cost to the taxpayer.

The trace minerals, like calcium and iron, cannot be absorbed until they are first dissolved in the hydrochloric acid of the stomach. As we have seen, this acid is frequently undersupplied or absent, especially when the B vitamins are inadequate. Poor absorption, therefore, can lead to deficiencies.

A friend of mine, who has made a hobby of vegetable raising, has composted his soil. In flavor and beauty his vegetables so far surpass those purchased at the market that you can scarcely recognize them as the same. His soil was analyzed at the Foundation for Agricultural Research, whose report states: "With one or two exceptions, this soil is in excellent condition. It shows evidence of repeated com-posting." My friend tells me that his soil ranked high in comparison with thousands of others analyzed by the foun-dation. This far-above-average soil, however, contained one-fourth as much phosphorus, one eighth as much sulfur, one-tenth as much copper, less than one-twentieth as much cobalt, one-fortieth as much boron, less than one-fortieth as much zinc, one-sixtieth as much iron, and one-eightieth as much manganese *as are considered to approach the ideal.*

[4] P. S. Chen, *Mineral Balance in Eating for Health* (Emmaus, Pennsylvania: Rodale Books, Inc., 1969), p. 103.

Although this soil is less than two miles from the Pacific Ocean, it contained no detectable iodine. If this is far-above-average soil, what are our market vegetables, fruits, and grains being grown on?

It is not merely the mineral content of the soil which determines the nutritive value of foods grown on that soil. Many other factors enter in. There must be minerals, of course, although plants seemingly flourish when many deficiencies exist; if minerals are not in the soil, they cannot possibly be in the plants. To build genuine health in plants, however, there must also be humus, or decaying plant material, which serves as food for bacteria, fungi, and molds. Furthermore, these minerals must first be changed to ionized form by soil bacteria and so held in the soil moisture. The soil fungi, which grow into the roots of plants, pick up the dissolved minerals and thus feed them to the plants. This co-operative situation between fungi and plant roots is known as the mycorrhiza relationship. If all minerals are generously supplied, the plants, so fed, remain healthy and resist disease. Their protein, mineral, and vitamin contents are high. They can support the health of animals and of people. Thus was all the food grown on the well-mineralized virgin soil of young America; such food helped make great men of our forefathers. The nutritive value of their food was limited only by the natural supply of minerals in the soil.

Then mass production came and with it the use of chemical fertilizers: natural rock treated with concentrated sulfuric acid, now sold as superphosphate; the pure chemicals ammonium sulfate and potassium sulfate, which is spoken of as potash. These chemicals dissolved in water as easily as sugar in a cup of coffee. They saturated the soil moisture, making it difficult or impossible for the less easily dissolved iron, copper, magnesium, zinc, and other trace minerals to stay in the soil solution. The excessive amount of sulfur, accumulating from repeated applications of chemical fertilizers, became toxic to the mineral-transferring fungi. The importance of humus was often overlooked; the already existing humus was used up, and little or none was returned to the soil. The valuable bacteria and fungi cannot grow without humus to feed them. Minerals may be in the soil, but without massive numbers of bacteria and fungi they cannot be dissolved; without life-sustaining humus, fungi no longer grow into the plant roots. The soil was gradually depleted of natural minerals which were taken into the plants, shipped to markets, passed through human bodies,

and thrown into the sea or rivers as sewage. Lands became
mineral-poor.

Still the plants grow; they look green and bulky but can
no longer support optimum health. Bugs and worms and
aphids multiply; Sir Albert Howard[5] pointed out that bugs
and worms destroyed only the unhealthy, the sooner to
return soil-rebuilding humus to the land. It now appears
that the soil molds produce aureomycin, streptomycin, penicillin, and other antibiotics, which bugs, worms, and aphids
do not enjoy; hence they will not eat healthy plants. Without sufficient humus, molds cannot grow to produce enough
antibiotics; the insects come. Their destruction is costly
to the producer. Every year more kinds and more pounds
of sprays and poisons are poured onto our foods, now
800,000,000 pounds annually of arsenic alone. Arsenic is
one of the many chemicals used to produce experimental
cancer. Bees, needed to pollinate blossoms, are destroyed
by poison sprays. Valuable bugs, needed to eat harmful
bugs, are likewise killed. The poison sprays drop to the
ground, dissolve in the soil solution, and are carried into
the very core of all our foods. The housewife tries to wash
them off, but no amount of washing can remove them
because they are *inside* each plant cell.

The protein content of our food and the food of animals
has decreased and continues to decrease still more. The
mineral content of foods is apparently only a fraction of
what it used to be or of what it could or should be. The
vitamin content varies with the health of the plant. Fresh
foods no longer have keeping qualities. Flavor is gone; there
is little joy left in eating. I talked to a Frenchman from the
provinces, an architect from a village in Mexico, an English-
man lecturing in American universities, an engineer who
had lived in the north of China. All asked the same question, "What's wrong with American food? You eat and eat,
and it doesn't fill you up. It has no flavor." These people
had been used to better foods. Our grandparents were used
to better foods. I wish everyone could be used to better
foods. As soon as the entire population of America wants
better foods, we can have them.

For four years I raised all of our own vegetables and
much of our fruits in soil composted and mineralized without chemical fertilizers. The worms in the compost piles
looked like plates of spaghetti. Bugs and aphids were no
problem; no disease which I could recognize invaded the

[5] *The Soil and Health* and *An Agricultural Testament* (Devin-Adair
Company, 1947).

garden. The flavors of these foods were superb. People say that flavor is due to freshness, but it is not freshness alone. Many times I have brought in too much and kept the excess in the refrigerator, using it later when I was busy or the garden was muddy; the marvelous flavors were retained. The quantities we ate were unbelievable; often the children had to be told to stop eating vegetables. Later I was too busy to put in a garden; I bought the best vegetables I could find and cooked them the best I could; we tasted them and threw them out. The fruits were not much better. Most of the time I can have shipped to me vegetables and fruits grown in rebuilt soils without commercial fertilizers or poison sprays. They are not fresh when they reach me, but they are still delicious.

In a city where I go to lecture live a doctor and his wife, both wonderful people; I have stayed with them so often that they used to file my bedsheets under D. Frequently when I was there, the three of us talked far into the night. The doctor's specialty is agriculture, the health-starts-in-the-soil variety. He told us:

"No virgin soil has ever been found to contain all the essential minerals in amounts now known to be somewhere near optimum in producing the health of plants, animals, or humans. Experiments are carried on in which land is rebuilt with minerals and humus; the protein content of alfalfa grown on such land has already been increased from the average of 9 per cent to 32 per cent. The protein content of other foods is increased correspondingly. No one yet knows the upper limit. The quantities of the cobalt, copper, and other trace minerals can be multiplied in our foods, yet they never reach the point of toxicity. Plants grown on such soil stay healthy, free from the dozens of diseases which have changed agricultural journals into medical magazines and treatises on poison sprays.

"There are a number of experimental farms where soils have been improved to known standards for minerals and humus for several years. Animals grazed on such land were injected with the most virulent types of bacteria; a week or two later, the blood of these animals showed not one sign that bacteria had been injected. Illness could not be produced in them, not even Bang's disease or the dreaded hoof-and-mouth disease or any of dozens of diseases which plague stockmen. The milk, meat, eggs produced by animals ranging on such soil, and the vegetables, fruits, and grains grown on such soil may produce in man a degree of health, the potential of which is not known.

"Land built up with minerals and humus can surpass any virgin soil ever found. On an acre or less, a person can raise much of the food needed by a family and have a whale of a good time doing it. The land's available. The know-how is. If that know-how were applied, the rewards for humans would be tremendous."

We talked of the great leaders who have done so much for the build-health-improve-flavor type of agriculture: Sir Albert Howard and his fascinating work in India (ref. 5, p. 204); Lady Eve Balfour, who started the successful "whole-food" movement in England; the late Louis Bromfield, whose experiences in rebuilding worn-out land are so vividly described in his books *Pleasant Valley* and *Malabar Farm*. He had bought several worn-out farms in Ohio; the wise men said the land could not pay taxes. This author had no degrees in agriculture and did not consider himself a farmer; he had lived in France and watched the peasants there, and he had ideas and was willing to study and work. He changed that eroded, worn-out land into a paradise where springs, long dried up, bubbled again, with lakes where you could swim on hot days and where delicious fish almost jumped into the breakfast frying pans. He let wild roses and berries grow along fence rows. Small animals hid there to have their babies; hunting was always good. Quail and other birds nested in the bushes, feeding their young on worms and insects which the educated wise men said must be killed with poison sprays. The paradise he created became a mecca; thousands of farmers made pilgrimages to learn wholesome farming methods which the money they had spent on taxes had not given them. This author did tremendous good for nutrition, which starts with the soil.

Then we spoke of Mr. J. I. Rodale, who also had refused to believe the wise men who said it could not be done. He had manufactured electrical equipment in New York City. Somehow he became interested in farming and moved onto worn-out land in Pennsylvania; he believed in soil bacteria, compost heaps, and lowly earthworms. When his health and the health of his family improved as his soil improved, it occurred to him that other people might want to know about his methods. This man had the courage to stick to his convictions, although the agricultural colleges said that what he said was poppycock. Several of these colleges set out to prove him wrong. Can you guess what they are finding out? That he has been right all along. Through his magazine on organic gardening and farming and books on composting and related subjects, Mr. Rodale has taught millions of Americans to be aware of wholesome food and thousands more how to raise it. Such leaders are all too few.

We talked on, seemingly of agriculture, but actually of health, the kind of health which could be built on a small amount of land by a family which loves the earth; and the degree of health which lays the foundation for character, courage, integrity, serenity, graciousness, and love in the home. Such health could be obtained by a nation educated to the need for genuinely good food.

CHAPTER 26

THE PERFECTION THAT IS YOU

LET US NOW SEE HOW ALL NUTRIENTS HELP THE BODY BY imagining that we can watch one of your cells. Let us say that you are in perfect health; therefore all the processes of this cell are perfect.

The cell is the shape of an egg. Foods can pass through its walls just as spilled juice might pass through a tablecloth. Every moment from birth until death there is poured in and sucked out a continuous surf of blood plasma, or tissue fluid. The incoming surf is pushed in by the force of the blood pressure from capillaries branching from arteries; the outgoing surf is withdrawn by the attraction of the tiny particles of a protein, albumin, in the capillaries joining the veins. The incoming wave carries fresh supplies; the outgoing wave removes wastes.

We can see through this ever-moving fluid as a diver can observe sea life about him when he walks the floor of the ocean. As we gaze into the cell itself, we see endless particles in fantastic and ceaseless motion. First we notice the business center of the cell, the nucleus. It is made of amino acids from the proteins you have eaten and of nucleic acid, obtained perhaps from yeast or liver; with the help of at least three B vitamins (biotin, pantothenic acid, and vitamin B_6) these substances are formed into what are known as nucleotides; they in turn are combined into genes and chromosomes carrying your hereditary pattern, the life program of this cell. Surrounding the nucleus are ever-changing clusters of protein particles, or molecules, formed into what are known as colloids; these protein clusters make up the tissue of the cell, the cytoplasm. The whole, or the nucleus and cytoplasm together, is called protoplasm.

There is so much to observe that we scarcely know what to look at first. Before us are molecules of fat and glucose, both combined with phosphorus; bits of the body starch, called glycogen, made up of dozens of glucose molecules; tiny globules of the fat-like materials cholesterol and lecithin. We see every known vitamin and mineral.

Our eyes fall on the worker ants in this amazing anthill, the carpenters who build, the demolition crews who tear down; these workers are the enzymes. Your genes carry the blueprint of the enzymes in your body; it is by enzymes that heredity is made possible. If you have blue eyes and brown hair, some of your enzymes are different from those of a person having hazel eyes and black hair. All enzymes are made of protein, but many also contain a vitamin and/or a mineral, such as magnesium or cobalt. They have been named according to the work they do, just as a family might originally have been named Smith because the father worked as a blacksmith.

We watch an enzyme family called phosphatase breaking phosphorus free from molecules of glucose and fat, thus beginning to change them into energy. By the help of other enzymes containing vitamin B_1 or pantothenic acid, the particles of carbon, hydrogen, and oxygen which form the sugar and fat are torn apart. Hod-carrier enzymes containing vitamin B_2 take oxygen from the blood cells and carry it to the fat or sugar. Still other enzymes, this time containing vitamin C, pick up the hydrogen freed as the food is broken into its component parts. With the help of these and other enzyme families, oxygen from the air is combined with the carbon, hydrogen, and oxygen which once formed sugar and fat and which are changed into carbon dioxide and water. By this process energy is liberated; all energy, in turn, is changed into heat.

We observe many other enzyme families; ones which tear down the genes of old cells and rebuild genes for new cells, the nucleotidases. The enzymes containing vitamin B_6 are demolishing and rebuilding bits of the protein cytoplasm. Still others containing pantothenic acid are building or demolishing the unsaturated fatty acids combined with proteins, which together form the lumber for this amazing house. Other enzymes are breaking worn-out protein into sugar, fat, and nitrogen-containing substances. There is the enzyme family of glycogenases, quickly changing glycogen into sugar to replenish that used in energy production; and there are other enzyme families, hundreds of them.

We next notice little telegraph messengers, the hormones, racing in and out of the cell. A messenger from the thyroid glands, thyroxin, helps to determine how much energy is needed and to keep the temperature at the point at which the cell can function best and the worker enzymes can be most efficient. We see another messenger from the pancreas, insulin, aiding the cell to change the sugar not needed for immediate energy into glycogen or fat. Still another messenger from the adrenal glands, cortisone, stands by to break body protein into sugar and fat if sufficient glucose is not supplied. A messenger called adrenaline (epinephrine) is here from the adrenals to speed up the change of glycogen into sugar in case large amounts are needed quickly, as during anger or fear, to produce energy required for fight or flight. Even messengers have come from the sex glands to affect the life of this cell and all cells of the body.

Our eye now catches our old friends, the minerals. Here is phosphorus, both free and combined with protein and fat as part of the cell structure. Calcium is here ready to help relax the cell when rest is required, and potassium is waiting to stimulate it into greater activity when the need arises. Here is chlorine, which originally came from table salt; like the shuttle from Times Square to Grand Central, it shifts continuously in and out of the cell, thereby aiding the body in removing carbon dioxide. Here are all the trace minerals, the catalysts, or speeder-uppers; they are the traffic cops which keep all traffic moving at a fantastic speed. Movement can take place without them, but it is slow and the traffic jams. Here is cobalt in the vitamin B_{12} portion of certain enzymes; iodine is part of thyroxin; zinc is helping the messenger insulin; here are magnesium, manganese, and all the other minerals, each helping the cell to function.

Just outside the cell wall is sodium, which may have originally come from meat or table salt. In some way not understood, sodium carries on a lifelong duel with potassium, largely inside the cell. This mysterious duel is apparently fought over the water supply. When the sodium appears to be winning, the cell contains more water, but potassium is withdrawn and excreted in the urine; when potassium wins, much sodium and water are lost. The referee for this duel appears to be a messenger from the outside of the adrenal glands, aldosterone.

Perhaps with the help of these duelists and of calcium and vitamin C, this cell has an amazing power of selectivity. If poisons, harmful chemicals, allergens, and/or bacterial toxins are carried in the tissue fluid, this healthy cell refuses to let them enter. On the other hand, if the nutrition is good, the tissue fluid carries every nutrient to this cell; the cell invites whatever nutrients it needs to enter, withdraws what it wants, and leaves the remainder to be carried on to other cells. When too little of a nutrient is supplied, the cell adjusts itself as best it can; when too much is given, the cell fights back but is sometimes defeated.

Every nutrient has its own duties; yet each works cooperatively with the others. Vitamin E helps linoleic acid, linoleic acid helps vitamin D, vitamin D helps phosphorus, phosphorus helps calcium, calcium helps vitamin C, ad infinitum. No nutrient plays a hermit role.

Many activities which take place in this cell are brought about by other substances; although neither the activities nor the substances are described here, both are known and understood by scientists. There are still, however, myriads of unknown activities and unknown substances which scientists have yet to understand.

This cell with all its processes and activities, multiplied by billions and billions, is you. The degree to which this cell can maintain its ideal structure and can carry on its normal functions is the degree of your health. A seemingly minor lack of a single nutrient or of many nutrients can damage the structure and/or interfere with its functions; a severe deficiency of one or more nutrients can bring about disaster. It is the amount of nutrients supplied to the cell itself which determines the state of your health. Malnutrition does not necessarily mean a faulty diet or even faulty absorption; it means only that less than enough of one or more nutrients reaches the cell.

The sum total of all the never-ceasing activities of all the cells is spoken of as metabolism. When these hundreds of activities, although still carried on at fantastic speed, are at their slowest, as when you lie motionless not even digesting food, the total is called basal metabolism. A lack of any nutrient or nutrients can slow down the activities of the cells; less food is needed, and unwanted weight may be gained. Only when all nutrients are generously supplied can the activities of the body be maintained at ideal speed and the metabolism remain normal.

All other parts of your body are but servants of the cell. The heart, for example, which people think of as important, only makes it possible for supplies to reach the cell and wastes to be removed. The arteries, veins, and thousands of miles of capillaries are mere pipes through which supplies and wastes are carried. The lungs are slaves which supply oxygen and throw off carbon dioxide; the kidneys are slaves which purify water and remove the wastes freed by the tearing down of worn tissue; the urinary bladder is merely a reservoir. The digestive tract is nothing more than a mechanism for changing food into the form which the cell can utilize. The bone marrow is a slave which produces blood corpuscles to carry oxygen, and the spleen is the graveyard for these corpuscles when their usefulness is spent. All of the glands are slaves which produce hormones to help regulate each cell's activity; the master gland, the pituitary, is in turn a slave which supervises the functions of the other glands and of each body cell.

The most important slave of all is undoubtedly the liver. This organ is the storage house which holds fats, sugars, and proteins coming from the digestive tract, ready to supply them to the cell the split second they are needed. It is largely in the liver that toxic substances which might damage the cell are rendered harmless; here the nitrogen-containing waste products from worn-out cell proteins are broken down; the protein albumin, needed to collect urine, is made here, and still other proteins, the antibodies, which destroy bacteria, are produced. The liver makes the fat-like substances lecithin and cholesterol; it likewise produces the bile necessary to aid the digestion of fats and the absorption of vitamins A, D, E, and K; it stores not only these vitamins but also minerals such as iron, copper, and the trace elements; it forms and stores the body starch glycogen. By the help of insulin, it largely controls the amount of sugar in the blood, withdrawing sugar when the supply is generous and changing it into body starch or fat or, when the supply runs low, changing the starch back into sugar and spilling it into the blood. When no food is eaten and all the stored glycogen is used up, cell proteins are torn down into sugar and fat; the liver again withdraws sugar from the blood and feeds it back once more as needed. This servant produces enzymes capable of inactivating the hormones which would otherwise accumulate to the extent that the cell might be injured. In spite of all these duties and many others, this master servant has only one purpose: to help maintain, regulate, and protect the life of the cell. Like the nutrients, all of these slaves co-operate with each other.

Although the structure and activity of every cell in the body are similar in that each must have oxygen and food and from each waste must be removed, the cells themselves are differentiated; their hundreds of duties vary endlessly. The cells of the muscles are the body's pulleys; their cytoplasm is so made that it can contract, and by each cell contracting in harmony, muscles are shortened and movement is made possible. The cells which make up the bones attract minerals and solidify them to give form to the body. The cells of the glands are manufacturers, turning out hormones. Thus is the function of groups of billions of cells each differentiated to make up the separate structures of the body.

Foods can be selected which will supply all the nutrients known to be needed by each cell. If these foods are grown on good soil and eaten in as nearly their natural state as possible, the nutrients still unknown can probably be furnished. Digestion and absorption, if faulty, can be improved; the destruction of nutrients in the digestive tract and the blood and losses of those nutrients from the body can be prevented. The well-nourished body can protect itself from bacterial invasion and can detoxify foreign materials which gain access to it. My belief, therefore, is that every person, if intelligent enough and financially able to obtain a completely adequate diet, can achieve perfect health provided irreparable harm has not already been done.

Dr. Szent-Györgyi, who was given the Nobel Prize for his early work on vitamin C, pointed out that when he was a medical student, everything appeared to be always wrong with the body. There were so many diseases that it seemed impossible to learn them all; he tells how he flunked examinations covering this subject. Later, when getting his doctorate in biochemistry, or the chemistry of the body, which is the study of health, he was amazed to find that this time everything was so right, so very right. Probably there never has been a person who has studied the detailed mechanisms which make up health who has not felt as did Dr. Szent-Györgyi.

In fact when one considers the healthy body as a functional structure of billions of cells having hundreds of separate purposes, yet each working co-operatively in perfect unison with absolute harmony and almost inconceivable synchronization, so far surpassing the most delicate machinery made by man, one cannot help being reminded of the philosophers who argue that there is only one perfection, and that perfection is God. Regardless of the religious skepticism of any person when he starts to study the workings of the healthy body, he usually soon agrees with the philosophers and realizes simultaneously that only disease is manmade. The God-made perfection is health, and potentially this perfection is you.

CHAPTER 27

LET'S NOT BE PART-SMART

ONE FREQUENTLY HEARS THE STATEMENT THAT ALL NU-
trients should come from good wholesome food. Of course
they should. It is extremely difficult, however, to get good
wholesome food. Certainly our overprocessed, overrefined
American diet, diluted with soft drinks, imitation juices,
candy bars, and "quick-energy" cereals, has little or no relationship to wholesomeness.

Selecting the best food available and preparing it by the
best methods known are both extremely important. Selection
and preparation determine the degree of health you enjoy.
Food supplements may help, but food itself is far more important. Let us suppose you do obtain wholesome food and
bring it into your kitchen. Losses of 60 to 100 per cent of
certain vitamins and many minerals can occur during food
preparation. One can predict with fair accuracy both the
sickness expectancy and the life expectancy of a family by
observing the wife's cooking methods.

Neither careful food selection nor preparation should be
minimized. In my opinion, however, the best of both can
still not assure health although the absence of either can
and usually does assure illness. As I see it, we are caught in
a double-squeeze play. We must have nutrients to maintain
health. Most of us, however, live sedentary lives; we can use
few calories. The desired nutrients come in packages with
undesired calories. We cannot obtain the nutrients because
we cannot use the calories; this is the first squeeze play. Because of the stresses of modern-day living, our nutritional
requirements are extremely high, perhaps higher for our entire population than ever before in history. Because our
foods are overprocessed and overrefined, our chances of
obtaining these nutrients from foods are extremely low,
lower for our entire population than ever before in history;

this is the second squeeze play. We are caught like trapped animals, and like trapped animals, we are suffering.

People are different from the experimental animals in a nutrition laboratory. Such animals are put on diets adequate in every respect except for one requirement, which may be only partially undersupplied. All other nutrients are generously supplied, their sources checked and double-checked. Even then the animals' health gradually changes to disease, and their life span is shortened. People's diets are often partly inadequate in from 20 to 40 nutrients simultaneously. A few nutrients may be severely lacking; others only slightly so. Just as the scientist produces ill health in experimental animals, so do people produce ill health in themselves. The principal difference is that, with these animals, illness is planned and expected; with people, illness is dreaded but expected.

Instead of having the clean-cut, single-deficiency symptoms discussed in the previous chapters, persons usually suffer from multiple deficiencies, with symptoms superimposed upon each other. For example, an individual uninterested in nutrition may suffer from symptoms of a severe lack of several amino acids and many B vitamins intermingled with the symptoms of milder deficiencies of vitamins C, D, and E and of calcium, iron, iodine, and the trace minerals; during certain hours of the day the symptoms of low blood sugar may become more severe than any others. Such deficiencies, however, are not too difficult to correct.

As I see it, every day you do one of two things: build health or produce disease in yourself. There is, of course, a sliding scale ranging from the most perfect health which you as an individual can attain, through all degrees of semi-health and semi-illness, to serious disease. Your choice of foods can largely determine where on this scale you will fall. Neither sickness nor health is a matter of chance.

The problem, however, is less simple than merely selecting and preparing food. The reason nutrition is not applied and may never be applied is largely psychological. We enjoy foods; our pleasures are few enough; if the only foods we feel we can enjoy are the refined and/or processed ones, we will fight to keep them, thus fighting to hold our few pleasures. We as a nation have become so malnourished that we crave sweets as an alcoholic craves drink. This craving is being bred into our children from the very day of birth when, instead of being given life-saving colostrum, the child is offered sugar water in a hospital nursery, which is soon changed to a formula often prepared from solids containing

50 per cent or more refined sugar. Later, limited budgets, radio-and-television blarings, tired mothers, kids' parties, Girl-Scout-cookie sales, and a hundred other forces combine to perpetuate this craving for sweets. People will fight to satisfy these cravings. The cravings themselves must be prevented if health is to be built.

Unpleasantness at meals often makes us dislike the food served at those times; many of these unpleasantnesses come early in life and are forgotten, but the food dislikes remain. I shudder to think of the future eating habits of a nation of individuals who, as babies, grope eagerly for warm nipples and instead have cold, hard spoons forced into their tiny mouths; of babies given formulas lacking many nutrients and stuffed with oversalted, overheated canned foods, producing ill health from the day of birth on. Later, flavors may improve, but beside the children sit giantesses, urging, scolding, prodding, nagging. The children are too young to understand that the well-meaning mothers are concerned only about their health. They become too tense to eat at meals and satisfy their hunger by eating between meals, when only junk is available, their low blood sugar urging them to eat the sweets they have already been trained to love so much. These are only a few of the psychological reasons why good nutrition may never be applied.

Let us now suppose that sound dietetics is put into practice. The best food available is obtained and prepared by the best methods known. If this food happens to be disliked, if fatigue is too great, if unpleasantness occurs during the meal, if worries are carried to the table, if the food is said to be health-building and you better eat it or else, or if fears of indigestion are harbored, the flow of digestive juices is decreased or inhibited. Few enzymes are produced. This excellent food, deliciously prepared, stays partly or wholly undigested; most of the nutrients supplied never reach the blood. For example, fecal analysis of a group of successful businessmen revealed quantities of undigested meat fibers. Such factors as worry, fatigue, and perhaps the stress of competition combined to prevent their five-dollar steaks from digesting. Relaxation and graciousness should reach their height before any meal. The mother who arranges her table as best she can, whether with pottery on clean enamel, or with lovely linen, silver, crystal, flowers, and candles, is building health as surely as the one who selects and prepares food carefully. Any person who wishes to apply nutrition must keep these many psychological and physiological factors in mind before becoming too optimistic about the results expected.

There are two major rules to follow in planning a nutrition program for any person, young or old, well or ill. First, every known requirement must be adequately supplied. Second, except for correct cooking, foods should be eaten in their natural state as nearly as possible; fresh foods should always be selected in preference to frozen or canned, unrefined foods used and refined ones avoided. Certain foods are the best sources of each body requirement. A summary of such foods, supplying nutrients in most concentrated forms, can give a basis for a day's dietary:

1. A quart of milk, which can be in the form of whole milk, preferably certified and not homogenized, buttermilk, yogurt, fortified milk, or skim milk drunk at the same meal when fat is obtained; or any combination of these milks, making a total of one quart. If health is seriously desired, eight ounces of yogurt should be eaten daily.

2. Whole-grain breads and cereals used as weight and activity permit; wheat germ used in cooking or added to cereals. Yeast and/or liver daily if requirements for the B vitamins are high. Granular lecithin as a source of cholin and inositol. The high phosphorus content of yeast and lecithin must be balanced by sifting or stirring thoroughly into each pound of both ¼ cup of calcium lactate and 1 tablespoon of magnesium carbonate or other magnesium salt; or purchase yeast to which calcium and magnesium have already been added. Both brewers' and torula yeasts are excellent.

3. Some dependable source or sources of vitamin A: green and yellow fruits and vegetables, liver, cream, butter, or margarine; capsules of vitamin A for adults when requirements are high and/or cannot be met by food; liquid fish-liver oil for children.

4. Whole citrus fruits, eaten preferably with white of the rind; or 8 ounces of fresh, unstrained orange or grapefruit juice or 12 ounces of canned or frozen juice; if frozen, select brands without added sugar.

5. A dependable source of natural vitamin D, preferably liquid cod-liver oil for children, concentrated fish-liver oil in capsule form for adults.

6. Iodized salt used to the exclusion of any other; a reliable source of iodine must be found (p. 183) if a low-sodium diet is adhered to.

7. One or two tablespoons of cold-pressed vegetable oils

used as salad dressings, in cooking, and as seasoning on cooked vegetables; preferably soy, peanut, safflower, or corn or a mixture of these oils or 2 to 4 tablespoons of unsalted nuts (50 per cent oil); keep oils refrigerated.

8. Uncooked vegetables in salads at lunch and/or dinner; 3 or more cooked vegetables, one green leafy such as chard, kale, or beet tops. Use starchy vegetables when calorie requirements are high.

9. Two or more fruits in addition to juice. Yellow fruits are preferable to colorless ones, raw to home-cooked, home-cooked to frozen, frozen to canned, and unsweetened to sweetened.

10. Two servings or more of meat, fowl, fish, eggs, cheese, or a high-protein meat substitute. Glandular meats, such as liver, sweetbreads, heart, and kidneys, served twice each week or more often. Some type of sea food several times a week. If cholesterol is high, limit beef and lamb to three servings per week; avoid pork; and increase fish and fowl each to five servings weekly if desired.

Now let us turn the tables and see that we have a dependable source of every body requirement:

1. Vitamin A: colored fruits and vegetables, cream, butter or margarine, eggs, and liver; fish-liver oil or vitamin-A capsule.

2. The B vitamins: yeast, liver and/or wheat germ; whole-grain breads and cereals; read label to make sure brown dye is not added to bread; separate B vitamins obtained from milk (B_2), green leaves (B_2 and folic acid), meats (niacin), lecithin (inositol and cholin).

3. Vitamin C: citrus fruits or juice; smaller amounts from any fresh raw fruit or vegetable; supplemented by ascorbic acid tablets if needed.

4. Vitamin D: fish-liver oil or capsule of natural vitamin D; vitamin-D milk.

5. Vitamin E: wheat germ, unrefined soy oil and other vegetable oils; natural alpha tocopherol acetate in capsule form.

6. Vitamin K: produced by intestinal bacteria; need be no concern to a healthy person if diet is adequate in milk and unsaturated fatty acids and no oral antibiotics have been taken; intestinal bacteria are increased by eating yogurt.

7. Bioflavonoids: citrus fruits, especially pulp and white of rind; helpful but not essential when massive doses of vitamin C are used.

8. Linoleic acid or essential unsaturated fatty acids: vegetable oils, such as safflower, corn, soy, peanut, and cottonseed; nuts and unhydrogenated nut butters.

9. Calcium: milk (whole or skim), buttermilk, yogurt and/or pep-up; bone powder and/or calcium tablets or tablets of calcium and magnesium combined.

10. Phosphorus: milk, eggs, cheese, meats; all unrefined and unprocessed foods.

11. Iron: liver, yeast, wheat germ, meats, egg yolks, whole-grain breads and cereals.

12. Iodine: iodized salt; powdered kelp.

13. Magnesium: fruits, grains, and vegetables, especially green leafy ones, if grown without chemical fertilizers; ¼ to ½ teaspoon powdered or 2 or 3 tablets of magnesium carbonate, magnesium chloride, dolomite, or magnesium sulfate (Epsom salts), alone or combined with calcium.

14. Potassium: fruits, vegetables, meats, fish, nuts, unrefined grains; if a reliable source of iodine is available, potassium chloride can be mixed with equal parts of table salt and kept in all salt shakers.

15. Trace minerals: sea foods; liver, green leafy vegetables, and egg yolk are usually dependable sources; unrefined foods grown under biological soil conditions; tablets of trace minerals or preparations of sea kelp.

16. Proteins: fortified milk or pep-up, yeast, fresh, canned, and powdered milks, yogurt, buttermilk, cheese, meats, game, fowl, fish, eggs, soybeans and soybean flour.

17. Bulk: fruits, vegetables, whole-grain breads and cereals.

18. Liquids: milk, fruit juices, soups, all beverages; any amount of water you may wish to drink.

Such a simplified method of checking is only superficial. Each requirement must be adjusted to the needs of the individual, the amounts of nutrients depending upon such factors as weight, activity, and degree of health.

It is not enough that all nutrients be supplied in a diet. If maximum health is to be built or maintained, these many nutrients must be furnished *at the same time*. This need can most easily be met by fortified milk, or pep-up, which may be prepared in a liquefier or with an electric or hand mixer. Combine and beat:

2 egg yolks or whole eggs (unless cooked preferred)
1 tablespoon granular lecithin
1 tablespoon vegetable oil or mixed vegetable oils

1½ teaspoons calcium lactate or 4 teaspoons calcium gluconate or 1 teaspoon of bone meal
¼ cup yogurt or 1 tablespoon acidophilus culture
2 cups of whole or skim milk
¼ to ½ cup of yeast fortified with calcium and magnesium
(p. 176)
¼ to ½ cup non-instant powdered milk or ½ to 1 cup instant
powdered milk
1 teaspoon pure vanilla or ½ teaspoon cinnamon or nutmeg
½ cup frozen, undiluted orange juice
magnesium carbonate, oxide, or other magnesium salt

Pour into a container and add the remainder of a quart of
milk; cover and keep refrigerated. Stir before using.

Other ingredients may be added: ¼ cup of soy flour
and/or wheat germ will still further increase the protein
content; 1 teaspoon of granular kelp can supply iodine;
banana, crushed pineapple, or any frozen, undiluted fruit
juice can vary flavor and furnish more calories. If milk is
not well tolerated, fruit juices or pure yogurt, predigested
during the culturing process, can be used as a base. When
the entire quantity is to be drunk immediately by a family,
¼ teaspoon of a magnesium salt should be added for each
person, but magnesium changes the flavor if the drink is
allowed to stand. Magnesium may be obtained from a tablet
or stirred into an individual serving of pep-up. If low
calories are desired, only skim fresh and powdered milk,
yeast, calcium, magnesium, and yogurt can be combined
with 1 teaspoon of oil, and the fruit or juice omitted.

Persons who have digestive disturbances or are ill should
take no more than ¼ cup of pep-up at each meal and/or
mid-meal at first; even this small amount should be sipped
through a straw to prevent air-swallowing. If the drink is
well tolerated, amounts may be gradually increased. Individuals suffering from acute infections or ulcers or under
severe stress would do well to take ⅔ cup of this fortified
milk (together with perhaps 50 milligrams of pantothenic
acid and 1,500 milligrams of vitamin C) every 2 or 3 hours
around the clock, even when they awake at night; if supplements furnish their other nutritional requirements, no foods
need be eaten temporarily. For most persons, however, a
single cup of pep-up at breakfast does much to increase
their general vitality. In other respects, their menus may
be quite conventional.

Since breakfast determines the amount of energy you have
for the day, it should be high in protein and supply some fat
and carbohydrates, although *it need not be a large meal.*

Lunches should likewise be high in protein and moderate in carbohydrate and should contain some fat. Dinners or suppers can be perhaps more graciously served but, calorically speaking, they should be no larger than breakfast or lunch. All meals should be delicious. The daily menus may be somewhat as follows:

BREAKFAST

Orange or grapefruit or fresh citrus juice or a vitamin-C tablet with other juice or fruit

¼ pound liver, chops, steak, ground lean beef, kidneys, mixed grill, fish, or other meat; or eggs with another protein as ham or sausage, or cheese omelet, or eggs scrambled with powdered skim milk and/or cheese, or an egg served with melted cheese on toast (bacon I consider an appetizer rather than food); or wheat germ and middlings or any whole-grain cereal cooked in milk and/or with powdered milk added; or waffles, hotcakes, or muffins made of high-protein ingredients

whole-grain toast or bread if desired; cheese or peanut butter used instead of butter or margarine if enjoyed

milk or milk drink, preferably pep-up

coffee if you must, preferably decaffeinized, perhaps made by adding hot milk instead of water to instant varieties

take immediately after eating, if used: capsules or tablets of vitamins A, C, D, E, and the B vitamins; calcium, magnesium, and trace minerals; enzymes and/or hydrochloric acid if digestion is below par

LUNCH

Eggs, cheese, meat, fish, fowl, or cream soup; or natural peanut butter or other protein sandwich

green salad with oil dressing or cooked vegetables seasoned with oil or mayonnaise or vegetables in soup

milk, skim or whole, yogurt, buttermilk, or fortified milk

whole-grain bread and butter or margarine, if desired

fruit, if desired

capsules or tablets if used

MIDMORNING AND/OR MIDAFTERNOON

Milk, fortified milk, yogurt, or buttermilk, or fruit or fruit juice; nuts and/or cheese if more calories are desired

DINNER OR SUPPER

Soup or fruit or fish cocktail if desired

meat, fish, fowl, or meat substitute such as eggs, cheese, or waffles with creamed ham or tuna

green vegetable salad tossed with unrefined vegetable oil

one or more cooked vegetables, including a green leafy one
whole-grain bread and butter or margarine if calorie require-
    ments are high
milk, buttermilk, yogurt, or pep-up
fruit, cheese, and nuts if desired
capsules or tablets if used

AT BEDTIME

Milk or milk drink or yogurt

Such a dietary is only a suggested outline. In order to allow considerable freedom of choice, much more food is
listed than any person would care to eat. This outline, however, can be used as a basis in planning menus for almost
any person regardless of age or degree of health. I usually
have fruit or fresh juice, eggs, pep-up, and decaffeinized coffee for breakfast. My husband's favorite breakfast is fresh
fruit or yogurt covered with frozen, undiluted orange juice,
and a whole-grain cereal cooked with wheat germ and
powdered milk. Unless I am invited out, I have only salad
and fortified milk or yogurt for lunch; if there is no time to
eat, I have nothing except a glass of yogurt or pep-up.
Afternoon snacks I particularly enjoy; I usually have fruit
or a glass of yogurt or milk. Our suppers are skimpy, perhaps only milk-soup or cottage cheese with salad, milk, and
fruit; or yogurt with fruit and homemade bread. Even when
I entertain, I serve only meat or meat substitute, a cooked
vegetable, tossed salad, whole-grain bread, milk, and fruit.
I occasionally make custard, cheesecake, or some other
dessert.

The objection is sometimes made that such a dietary is
expensive. I consider it the reverse. No money is wasted on
junk; little or none is needed for medical or dental bills.
Thousands of people who could afford adequate diets live
on markedly inadequate ones. Persons who have little
money also spend tragic amounts on "foods" which can
never produce health. At least two-thirds of the items in our
food markets are not worth carrying home, let alone paying
for.

Unfortunately there is an ever-growing list of so-called
foods marketed solely to make money, their purveyors having not the slightest concern with the resulting illnesses they
produce even in infants and children. Indeed, they loudly
deny that disease is produced, though vast masses of scientific evidence prove the contrary. If health is to be built,
foods containing no nutrients, or which have been robbed

of nutrients, must be largely avoided: all soft drinks, regardless of how sweetened; imitation fruit juices, or "fruit drinks"; powdered fruit ades; foods overloaded with refined sugar, as candies, jams, and most commercial desserts, especially those made with gelatin; white rice; most packaged, or prepared, cold cereals; foods made with refined flour, as breads, crackers, bakery products, package mixes, and noodles, macaroni, and spaghetti; bread with dye or "caramel coloring" added, made with "wheat" flour instead of unrefined 100 per cent whole-grain flour; refined oils obtained by extraction with chemicals; hydrogenated fats such as solid cooking fats, hydrogenated peanut butter (with no oil on top), and processed cheeses; foods cooked with hydrogenated fats, as potato chips, corn snacks, and most commercially fried fish and potatoes; foods containing coconut oil or other saturated vegetable fats, as imitation milks, imitation sour creams, liquid and powdered cream substitutes, and some "filled milks"; foods to which excessive amounts of preservatives have been added, as cold meats, precooked potatoes, catsup, and many precooked but unfrozen foods; overheated, oversalted, and overpriced baby foods; and the highly salted cereal tidbits designed to be served with drinks.

Many of the foregoing foods may not be particularly harmful in themselves, but all satisfy the appetite and crowd out the foods which can build health. I find that wonderful mothers who rarely bring these nutritionally robbed foods into their homes invariably have beautiful children. A father told me recently that he was explaining to his ten-year-old daughter that the peanut butter she was eating contained a large amount of sugar and hydrogenated fat and could produce heart disease whereas natural peanut butter helped to reduce blood cholesterol. The alert youngster replied, "If you loved me and believed what you are saying, you wouldn't allow me to eat this peanut butter."

There are millions of children now growing up who because of being permitted overrefined foods are robbed of beauty that they want so much and that is their birthright; and many will hate parents who cared too little to see that they ate wholesome food. Even when junk foods are avoided, it is difficult to meet all body requirements unless one can obtain produce grown organically on fertile soils. Furthermore, nutritional requirements vary widely with individuals and often with entire families; and all requirements except perhaps calories are increased for every person during times of stress. Nutritional supplements can never substitute for wholesome food, but they can furnish nutrients in quantities not readily obtainable even from carefully selected diets.

People frequently ask me what supplements I take even though my requirements may vary widely from theirs. I use fresh citrus fruits and yeast and/or liver daily as my sources of bioflavonoids, vitamin C, and the B vitamins; and eat yogurt almost daily to supply bacteria which can produce vitamin K and still more B vitamins. For years I have taken after breakfast a capsule containing 25,000 units of vitamin A and 2,500 units of vitamin D, both from fish-liver oil; 200 or 300 units of vitamin E, or d-alpha tocopherol acetate distilled from soy oil; a tablet supplying 5 milligrams of iodine taken daily or one furnishing 100 milligrams taken once a week; and 500 milligrams or more of vitamin C, the quantity varying with the amount of stress I am under. After each meal I take three tablets of calcium combined with magnesium and trace minerals, and sometimes a tablet of magnesium oxide alone to balance the calcium in milk. If I have eaten salty food, am under considerable stress, or have allowed my blood sugar to drop, I add three or more tablets of potassium chloride, 180 milligrams each. Besides yeast or liver, I take after each meal 2 B-complex tablets supplying in the course of a day 1,000 milligrams of both cholin and inositol. These two B vitamins are so important that I believe no B-complex tablet should be sold without furnishing this quantity for each 5 milligrams of B_1, B_2, and B_6 they contain.

Severe stress, such as actual sickness, causes the need for all nutrients to skyrocket, especially for pantothenic acid and vitamin C. Persons frequently take supplements regularly while well but discontinue them during illness, when they are most needed. Because little food can be eaten at such a time, enough supplements should be taken to furnish *all vitamins and minerals in larger than usual amounts* until recovery is complete. In addition to such supplements, I recommend that the ill person follow an antistress program consisting of 50 or 100 milligrams of pantothenic acid and 1,000 or 2,000 milligrams or more of vitamin C taken with ⅓ or ½ cup of fortified milk, or pep-up, every 2 or 3 hours around the clock, including when one awakes at night. The more frequent feedings and larger amounts of vitamins should be taken if the illness is acute, as for example during mononucleosis, hepatitis, a severe allergy attack, or any virulent infection. This program should be continued until definite improvement occurs. As soon as more food can be eaten, fresh liver, a cooked green leafy vegetable, and wheat germ should be obtained daily to supply the antistress vitamins.

Persons frequently ask me how long they should take supplements. I am sometimes tempted to answer, "Until you get tired of good health." As I see it, supplements should be continued as long as the nutrients they furnish are not being obtained from any other source. I expect to take supplements as long as I live, though I wish I might get all nutrients from foods.

The question of whether natural or synthetic vitamins are preferable is a controversial one. I prefer natural sources when they are practical. Vitamin A from fish-liver oils is more effective than the water-soluble variety, and natural fish-liver-oil vitamin D is less toxic in large amounts than is the artificially produced irradiated ergosterol. Many scientists have reported that natural vitamin E, or d-alpha tocopherol acetate distilled from soy oil, has consistently produced better results than synthetic vitamin E. Tablets of natural vitamin C, perhaps from rose hips, usually furnish 100 milligrams or less of bioflavonoids; 1,000 milligrams of bioflavonoids, however, can be obtained by eating the white part of an orange rind. Chemically, the synthetic vitamin C and all the B vitamins are identical to the natural ones. Furthermore, it is often impossible to obtain the quantity of a vitamin desired from a natural source, especially the huge amounts of vitamin C recommended by Dr. Klenner (p. 136). In general, it seems wise to use natural sources whenever you can, but to be willing to use synthetic ones whenever you need to.

The most frequent mistake people make when first interested in nutrition is to emphasize a single nutrient or supplement, expecting it to clear up some particular problem. This attitude comes from identifying supplements with drugs. To build health, ten amino acids from complete proteins, linoleic acid from oils, and some fifteen vitamins and fifteen minerals must be included in the diet, preferably at the same time. No one nutrient can carry the load of another, none can pinch-hit for another. Unless every one of these requirements is obtained, improvement in health should not be expected. Furthermore, regardless of how unlike individuals may be, and even illnesses or abnormalities may differ, if health is to be restored, these same forty nutrients must be amply furnished in the diet of every person.

Because many of these nutrients are difficult to obtain in adequate amounts from foods, supplements are often necessary.

Supplements should be kept, perhaps on the dining table, in a divided plastic box such as those sold for fish flies. When left in bottles, they are too easily neglected, too time-consuming to sort out, and too often identified with drugs.

Despite claims to the contrary, there is no all-in-one capsule which can meet body requirements. Supplements about which such claims are made usually contain excessive amounts of the cheaper B vitamins and little or none of the nutrients which are expensive or bulky. Their labels are purposely misleading, often listing such items as 100 milligrams of liver or lecithin, written with the knowledge that few users would realize a serving of liver would weigh approximately 112,000 milligrams, a tablespoon of lecithin about 15,000 milligrams. Unfortunately such supplements give a false sense of security, as do yeast tablets and capsules of lecithin, of unsaturated fatty acids, and of wheat-germ oil claiming to be a source of vitamin E. Ninety yeast tablets equal a heaping tablespoon of yeast; and some 18 capsules of lecithin daily would supply the amount scientists have used to reduce blood cholesterol. These foods are valuable, but the quantity obtained in a tablet or capsule is too small to be significant. Even most protein supplements, which are usually mixtures of yeast, powdered milk, and soy flour, are rarely worth the expense; the ingredients are cheaper purchased separately.

To determine what supplements you need, write down everything you eat for a day, or better still, for several days, then use the tables of food composition (pp. 276-303) to analyze your dietary intake and compare it to the recommended daily allowances (pp. 274-275). These allowances are quite low and were designed only for well persons whose diets have presumably been adequate. Anyone who has been ill or whose previous diet has been inadequate needs much larger quantities of all nutrients except calories. If you find you are getting too little of any nutrient which could be obtained from ordinary foods, adjust your intake accordingly. Supplements are needed only when your requirements cannot be met by food. Unfortunately, figures are not available for many nutrients, and others vary so widely with soil conditions that they have little meaning.

Before buying any supplement, read labels and compare potencies and prices of various brands. Products shipped across a state line are inspected by the Food and Drug

Administration. No company wishes its reputation marred by government citations; therefore the potencies stated on the labels of products marketed for some time are usually reliable. The prices vary widely, however, even for products prepared by the same manufacturers. The cheaper product is often excellent.

There is little value in improving your nutrition if your digestive system is so below par that the food is not efficiently digested or absorbed. If your tongue shows the symptoms discussed on page 66 or if you get gas from taking yeast, milk, or other nutritious food, you can be sure, unless you are eating too fast and swallowing air (p. 163), that your digestion is not functioning normally. Sipping all cold liquids through a straw often reduces gas tremendously. Hydrochloric acid tablets, usually labeled as "glutamic acid hydrochloride," if taken with each meal temporarily, may make you more comfortable; and magnesium carbonate or dolomite should be used as a supplement rather than magnesium oxide (p. 176). Tablets of digestive enzymes with bile are also often advisable. One physician I know tells his patients to take five of each kind of these tablets after each meal; if no gas occurs, to decrease to four, three, two, and finally one of each, increasing the amounts again if gas recurs. Such a procedure is excellent, but I usually advise only one tablet of each after each meal, to be increased later if trouble with gas persists. Both the acid and enzymes should be stopped as soon as digestion appears normal, or in about a month after a good nutrition program is initiated.

The overweight person obviously has no trouble in digesting and absorbing food; hence he needs neither hydrochloric acid nor enzymes. If he gets gas, it is because he is eating too rapidly or too much; usually he is doing both.

There are two approaches to improving the diet when nutrition has been neglected. The cautious approach is to increase the amounts of supplements and such foods as yeast, yogurt, or fortified milk gradually; thereby you can prevent digestive upsets and give yourself a chance to cultivate a taste for these foods. Improvement may be slow, but this method is safest for persons without supervision. The other approach, which can end in disaster or spectacular improvement, is to take enough supplements to saturate the tissues and large amounts of foods supplying proteins, B vitamins, and other nutrients for a few days, then decrease the amount drastically when body needs have been met. I use the latter method but have sometimes regretted it. Persons who consume more nutrients than their bodies need lose much through their excreta.

I take vitamin pills and recommend them, but I still disapprove of them. If wholesome foods were available, supplements would rarely be needed except for vitamin D. Few people can obtain wholesome food. By wholesomeness, I mean the kind of food our grandparents and all our ancestors before them ate at every meal. Just plain food. Fruits, vegetables, and grains grown on naturally mineralized, naturally composted soil untouched by smog, chemical fertilizers, and poison sprays. Milk from healthy animals grazed on green pastures (most such milk need not be pasteurized, and its hormones, enzymes, and steroids are not destroyed; if "pasteurization" is necessary, it can be done by the natural methods of souring or changing into yogurt). Eggs laid by hens allowed to run on the ground, gathering worms and scratching in manure piles rich in bacteria-produced vitamin B_{12}, vitamin K, and many other nutrients. Fertile eggs produced by hens kept with roosters (such eggs are rich in hormones which commercial eggs lack). Meats from animals which have not been castrated. Foods which have not been refined or processed.

Although such foods have been eaten by billions of people who have lived and died, this degree of wholesomeness is no longer practical. As I see it, thousands of adults and millions of children in our country have never once had one mouthful of genuinely wholesome food; not one sip of delicious medically certified raw milk or one bite of delightful freshly stone-ground, 100-per-cent-whole-grain bread or cereal or of unbelievably good organically grown fruits and vegetables. My critics once selected the foregoing sentence for ridicule, claiming it to be false, yet I am still convinced that it is completely true.

Everything we eat is tinkered with in one way or another. With every tinkering come losses, some small and unavoidable, some large and avoidable; the cumulative amount of these losses is staggering and crippling. It is we who are staggering, we who are being crippled. We must do the best we can, but our best can be none too good. Supplements, therefore, appear to be necessary.

One should constantly be aware that a certain balance seems to exist between the various nutrients in the body, as in the case of the B vitamins. Furthermore, the absorption, utilization, and/or retention of one nutrient often depend upon the presence of another. For example, it is silly to take calcium if you fail to obtain enough fat and/or vitamin D to absorb and use that calcium; and it must be balanced with half as much magnesium. It is useless to spend money on vitamin A unless vitamin E is available to prevent its destruction. These problems are largely taken care of automatically when natural foods are eaten. The overall picture, however, should be kept constantly in mind.

It seems to me that the situation is much like boxes inside of boxes. Each box should be seen as a whole and in relation to each other. The smallest box, let us say, represents the whole of nutrition from the proper preparation of the soil, through the harvesting, handling, processing, and marketing of food; the careful selection which makes it possible for each of the 40 body requirements to be met; the scientific preparation and gracious serving of that food; the pleasantness and relaxation necessary to assure digestion and absorption; and the factors which must be controlled to prevent destruction of nutrients in the body and losses through the excreta.

The next larger box might symbolize the body as a whole, all its parts and organs functioning co-operatively. Health is not of a part of the body but of all the cells together. Whether recognized or not, disease is not of a part but also of every body cell. The third box could be symbolic of the body needs as a whole, such as love, worthiness, peace of mind, psychological adjustment, relaxation, and personal recognition as well as the needs for exercise, sleep, fresh air, sunshine, and warmth. The next larger box might represent the individual in relation to his environment, family, friends, work, hobbies, and recreation. The largest box could symbolize this individual's personal philosophy, religion, convictions, ethics, prejudices, and morals, which in turn determine the part he plays in the world about him. Nutrition, seen in such light, becomes a small part; yet it remains a vital part.

A doctor friend of mine calls persons only part-smart who fail to see nutrition as a whole and its relation to the world about us. When an individual takes vitamin B_1 or a physician gives injections of vitamin B_{12}, either is granting that nutrition has a little value; since some 40 nutrients are considered essential, he is approximately one-fortieth part-smart. Wonderful physicians have made such outstanding contributions by their clinical research with vitamins B_1, B_2, and niacin that they have become famous; yet these brilliant men are still, nutritionwise, only part-smart. The person who fails to see the value of soil bacteria, the losses caused by refining, the psychological factors involved in food choice and/or absorption or any other fragment of the picture is, in his opinion, only part-smart. The individual who perhaps harms nutrition most is one who exaggerates its importance; he is often neurotically part-smart. The man who has not yet realized that nutrition plays a role in his ability to be a good husband and father, to make a good income, or to enjoy recreation, or that it can influence his thinking and feeling is, nutritionwise, not even part-smart.

Personally applied nutrition is a means to an end, a means which need be remembered only a few minutes daily during the remainder of your life. The end goal is health in all its aspects, a type of physical health which can help to form a basis for mental, emotional, moral, and spiritual health. Such a goal is valueless unless you do something worthwhile with the health you attain. If a high degree of health, however, increases your mental alertness and emotional stability and can thus give you the moral courage to live up to your spiritual convictions, then you will find your work fulfilling, your fun rewarding, your goals tantalizing, and the world about you both a good place to live and a better place because of your presence. Then only will nutrition have reached its personal goal.

Dr. Rountree has pointed out that the goal of nutrition is growth of body, mind, and conscience. She states that the possibilities of improvement of family, community, and world conditions through better food and the use of nutritional knowledge for man's welfare make up a vision all must catch; that nutritional knowledge alone is of little value but that what you do with this knowledge is all-important. She reminds us that undernourished bodies are tied up with self-centered, pessimistic minds and that malnourished people are not interested in abstract ideas like democracy. She writes: "Nutritional knowledge can give us a sense of mastery over life, help balance the budget, reduce medical costs, maintain the right architectural propositions for social success and long life, improve the sense of humor, promote efficiency in home, school and business and make us better able to take it. Nutrition well taught will make people glory in the American way of life."[1]

It seems to me that the person who can be ever mindful of such a concept of health is, nutritionwise, no longer only part-smart.

[1] Jennie I. Rountree, "Nutrition in Health Education," *Modern Nutrition*, V (1952), 7.

CHAPTER 28

PERSONAL REWARDS OF GOOD NUTRITION

WHEN A GOOD NUTRITION PROGRAM IS CONSCIENTIOUSLY followed, other problems often disappear. They are rather like happiness, which comes as a by-product of unselfishness but is elusive if sought directly. No one can say what nutrients or combinations of nutrients have brought about the change. Probably the improved psychological outlook which comes with feeling better helps as much as anything.

It has been known for years, for example, that persons who drink excessively suffer from multiple nutritional deficiencies. Dr. Roger J. Williams, professor at the University of Texas, and other scientists have shown that the desire to drink, in itself, can be caused by nutritional deficiencies; and that adequate niacin amide appears to be particularly important in overcoming the desire to drink.

Many experiments have been conducted, the general gist of which is as follows: Large numbers of rats are given the choice of four beverages: water; 3 per cent alcohol, representing beer; 10 per cent alcohol, comparable to light wines; and 50 per cent alcohol, suggestive of hard liquors. Each rat is kept in a separate cage, its liquid consumption measured daily. All the animals are given the same "normal" diet. Under such treatment, some rats become teetotalers; others land on skid road. Then the abstainers are put on an inadequate diet, perhaps partially lacking one or more B vitamins. The excessive drinkers are given a superior diet containing far-above-normal amounts of certain nutrients, especially the B vitamins. Before long, the teetotaler rats start drinking, and many land on skid road. All the skid-road rats drink less, and many become teetotalers. When offspring of the teetotaler rats and the skid-road rats are offered their choice of drinks as were their parents, like father like son, they become abstainers or drunkards.

A number of conclusions have been drawn from such experiments. First, there is no such thing as a "normal" diet. What is normal for one person may not be normal at all for another. Second, the need for greater than so-called "normal" amounts of certain nutrients is a hereditary need. When these excessively high nutritional requirements are not met, the person with such needs becomes susceptible to certain abnormalities to which Dr. Williams has given the name "genetotrophic diseases," of which alcoholism is one.[1] If the nutrition is adequate for each individual, however, such diseases need not appear in any generation. Another conclusion is that alcoholism might be partly prevented if our national diet were improved. The third conclusion to be drawn from the experiments is that if persons who have the compulsive urge to drink excessively are given far-above-average amounts of B vitamins, especially niacin amide, and are treated with understanding, their desire for liquor may decrease.

Although an undersupply of B vitamins appears to be a major cause of alcoholism, the blood-sugar level is also of extreme importance (ref. 3, p. 24) in preventing the craving for alcohol. Although Alcoholics Anonymous deserves no word of criticism, its members suffer unnecessarily by being unaware of the value of good nutrition. They wash B vitamins from their bodies by drinking tremendous quantities of coffee. They lower their blood-sugar levels by over-stimulating their insulin flow with quantities of sweets. They merely change crutches from alcohol to tremendous quantities of coffee, sugar, and tobacco, causing their already exhausted adrenals to become even more exhausted. Since they ignore the simple rudiments of good nutrition, without either dietary or psychological help, it is surprising indeed that as many give up alcohol as do. Certainly nutrition is only one part of this problem. But it is indeed an important part.

Dr. Williams in his book *Alcoholism: The Nutritional Approach*[2] tells of the dozens of persons who have written him of their success in giving up alcohol after improving their nutrition. Frequently persons have sent me similar reports, most of them stating that as long as they took large amounts of all the B vitamins, and especially yeast and liver daily, they had no desire to drink. Some

[1] R. J. Williams, *Nutrition Reviews,* VIII (1950), 257.
[2] Austin, Texas: University of Texas Press, 1959.

years ago a brilliant young man, whose life was being ruined by excessive drinking, wanted me to plan a diet for him because of a skin rash, though he emphatically declared he had no intention of giving up alcohol. The adequate diet I recommended was heavily supplemented with B vitamins, magnesium, and calcium. Even before the rash disappeared, he had given up drinking and he has not touched liquor since.

Many psychological factors such as self-hatred, self-destructiveness, and emotional immaturity resulting from early deprivations make it difficult for an alcoholic to adhere to a good nutrition program. If he can follow a health-building diet, the chances are that his alcoholic intake will decrease. One friend who works with Alcoholics Anonymous tells me that she carries with her tablets supplying 500 milligrams each of niacin amide, others of calcium and magnesium, and still others furnishing all the B vitamins; she gives two tablets of each of these every three hours to persons trying to remain sober. She tells me that these individuals notice great improvement in a remarkably short time.

A physician once asked me to plan menus and supplements for a "home" where men stayed who were trying to give up liquor. To maintain normal blood sugar and to repair liver damage, I suggested six small, high-protein meals daily free of all refined carbohydrate. At each meal and mid-meal pep-up was served or eggnog fortified liberally with yeast, lecithin, calcium, and magnesium. Dishes of assorted tablets were placed on each table: magnesium with calcium; B complex high in inositol and cholin; vitamin C with pantothenic acid; and capsules of vitamins A, D, and E. The men were told that this program was designed to help them feel better during the sobering-up process but that they could participate or ignore it as they wished. We were met with grateful co-operation. The doctor reported that within three days he could notice a marked change, especially in the men's dispositions. The fights which usually occurred had stopped. The men found they had no problem in staying sober as long as they did not eat elsewhere.

When the main problem has been alcoholic depression, 1,000 milligrams of niacin amide taken with each meal and before bed and/or between meals has been used with great success. Large quantities of niacin amide have been continued for years with no recognizable toxic effects, but I believe such huge quantities are rarely needed if the entire diet is adequate. It has been reported that unpleasant LSD trips can be stopped by giving 1,000 milligrams or more of niacin amide. The severe psychosis of delirium tremens, however, is said to be caused by a magnesium deficiency; and the hallucinations, convulsions, tremors, clouded thinking, mental confusion, and muscle weakness have disappeared within hours after magnesium has been given.

Weakness, trembling, and mental depression are also symptoms of drug withdrawal. The addict, knowing little of nutrition, usually develops multiple severe deficiencies; the resulting discomfort causes him to continue drugs and is largely covered up by them. Drugs destroy huge amounts of vitamin C, already undersupplied; hence it is not unusual now to find teen-age youngsters who have lost teeth from scurvy.

Only last week I was asked to suggest supplements for a man who had repeatedly tried to give up drugs—amphetamines, tranquilizers, sleeping tablets—which for eleven years he had taken at the rate of 300 to 500 doses per month. Each time the intense suffering of withdrawal had defeated him. Six hours after his last dose, he was already depressed and experiencing intense weakness; his entire body trembled as if it would shake to pieces. The next day the weakness and trembling were both worse and the depression "simply terrible." He could not walk or even dress himself without help. Supplements were then started and taken faithfully at each "mealtime" (he was unable to eat) and before bed: 1,000 milligrams of niacin amide, suggested because of the depression; 25 milligrams of vitamin B_6, 500 milligrams of magnesium carbonate (2 tablets), and 1,000 milligrams of calcium (2 tablets of bone meal) were all given to alleviate the shaking; 2,000 milligrams of vitamin C to help detoxify the drugs; and 2 B-complex tablets and an antistress tablet supplying 100 milligrams of pantothenic acid. Because it is largely predigested, yogurt was to be eaten at each meal as soon as he could tolerate food. For two days there was no noticeable improvement except that he slept well for the first time since stopping drugs. The next two days, however, brought a marked change. By the fifth day all depression was gone, he looked like a new person, and he walked vigorously for three miles without tiring.

The wonderful work of rehabilitation centers for alcoholics and drug addicts could be far more successful, prevent untold suffering, and decrease the return to alcoholism and addiction if they both applied and taught sound nutrition.

Because most foods which are especially nutritious—fruits, vegetables, sea foods, lean meats, cheese, eggs, and milk—are not high in calories, the person who seriously applies sound nutrition is rarely overweight. Through the years a number of obese persons who wanted to reduce when they came to me have been too ill to be put on reducing diets.

"Let's forget about reducing for at least three months and concentrate on building health," I would tell them. "You'll feel like working and exercising by that time, and reducing will be easier."

Many of these persons were so malnourished that I recommended 150 grams of protein daily for them temporarily: large servings of fish, fowl, or meat, with liver daily if they enjoyed it; a quart of fortified milk, yogurt, cottage cheese, and an egg daily; and a green salad at each lunch and dinner tossed with a teaspoon of cold-pressed oil. Usually they took two or three tablets each of mixed minerals and B-complex vitamins and 500 milligrams or more of vitamin C after each meal; and vitamins A, D, and E in capsules daily after breakfast. I asked them to forego starchy vegetables, cereals, concentrated sweets, and rich desserts; certainly refined foods had no place in their health-building regimes. Their menu plans followed those on pages 221-222. They used decaffeinized coffee unless too exhausted to live without a stimulus.

Some of these people gained weight for a week or two; then they complained they could not eat so much. Their blood sugar was high; they had no craving for sweets. When the diet is adequate, fewer calories are desired. By the end of three months they had lost weight; some phoned or came in to ask, "How can I stop losing?" One was a seventy-six-year-old woman who had been in a wheelchair for years with arthritis; she had weighed 186 pounds; now she is 40 pounds lighter and walks well with a cane. Another was a man with heart disease, his legs swollen to twice their normal size; now his weight is exactly as he wants it, and all heart symptoms are gone. I shall never forget a middle-aged woman, whose brilliant mind worked sluggishly, and who had huge varicose veins covered with elastic stockings; she had a history of repeated attacks of gout. Three months later I did not recognize this woman: she had been transformed into an alert, slender person with a new vivacious personality and without a visible varicose vein or a tinge of gout. There are many others.

Finally it dawned on me that this method was the way every person should reduce. My advice now is: Throw away your bathroom scales and calorie charts; forget about reducing, but never forget about building health. When health comes, you cannot keep yourself from exercising; you will work twice as hard without fatigue; you will find yourself wanting to go skiing or dancing or walking or swimming, your own vitality urging you into activity. Weight loss will come slowly perhaps, but if you adhere to the program, it will come. And it will be a permanent loss.

There are many people who want to reduce, but their principal hunger is subconscious. Eating is a substitute for love. The child first experiences love as his mother feeds him, at the same time cooing, singing, and caressing him. The happy old-fashioned mother loved and nursed her baby perhaps 1,500 times. Under these circumstances any child soon associates love with food; later, if love is withdrawn, overeating becomes a compensation. People who suffer in this way can usually be helped only by a competent psychiatrist.

To say that obesity is caused merely by consuming too many calories is like saying that the only cause of the American Revolution was the Boston Tea Party. There are many causes. One, I suspect, is that our foods are so depleted of the nutrients which starved bodies crave that overeating is due to a physiological compulsion to obtain them; even that usually fails to supply the nutrients longed for by the tissues. Another cause is that people often eat too little rather than too much; the basal metabolism drops far below normal; there is no energy for work or play, none to be turned into heat. When few calories are used, few are needed. Such people sit, sluggish as lizards sunning themselves, gaining weight on tiny meals and becoming more miserable with each added pound.

If you have repeatedly tried to reduce and failed, I would recommend that you join the Weight Watchers, who have had phenomenal success with such persons. The diet recommended by this organization was planned by the head of the New York Public Health Department, the late Dr. Norman Jolliffe, who designed it to reduce high blood cholesterol and prevent heart attacks. It is adequate except for linoleic acid, easily supplied by 1 or 2 teaspoons of vegetable oil daily, which Dr. Jolliffe himself would have added had he lived until later research was done. Canned tuna, however, supplies some oil. To maintain high blood sugar during the day, part of the large amount of protein allowed at dinner should be eaten instead at breakfast. Because persons who have long tried to reduce have multiple deficiencies, I am convinced that supplements should be taken at least until ideal weight is achieved. Aside from these points, any nutritionist would give the Weight Watchers a wholehearted blessing.

Another reward of nutrition is gaining weight, if that is desired. Once I planned a diet for a man who weighed 121 pounds and who wanted so much to gain; later he asked for a reducing diet. Not long afterward, an extremely tall, ill man came to see me; he then weighed 155 pounds and he, too, wished to gain. A year or so later he weighed 210 pounds and wanted to reduce. I still know both of these men. Although gaining was no problem and a reducing diet was planned for each of them, neither has reduced.

For years I have refused to make out a gaining diet for anyone. When faulty digestion and absorption are corrected, when nerves and muscles are relaxed to the extent that energy is no longer needlessly wasted and sound sleep is induced, the underweight person gains easily without increasing his calorie intake. A gaining diet usually causes him to put on too much weight.

There is another problem which almost invariably disappears if nutrition is taken seriously over a considerable length of time. For me, the most striking example of this problem is a woman I saw first when she was twenty-nine. She was underweight, pale, and listless; her hair was stringy; tension lines cut her forehead; and fatigue was stamped on her face. Her blood count and blood pressure were both low. She had trouble with constipation and hemorrhoids and was "miserable from gas." The radio and youngsters made her "fly off the handle." She had severe headaches about twice a week. My notes say, "Can't sleep; stays up all night at least once each week to be sure she can sleep the next night." She told of several miscarriages. Because of tumors her uterus had been removed shortly before I saw her.

Three years later, when this same woman came to a series of lectures I was giving, she had become my idea of genuine beauty. She reminded me of a racehorse being held back at the starting line. Her eyes were bright and flashing, her skin had both color and glow, her figure was the kind any woman might envy. Her hair was resilient and amazingly alive. Her face was animated; it glowed with health even in repose. After these lectures, a group of us often went to her home for "coffee," meaning a near-smörgasbord of cold meats, cheeses, and dark breads. I usually sat watching her, fascinated. Every time I saw her, I asked myself how any person could have met her and not been immediately struck by her beauty. I knew the answer perfectly well. Before this woman applied sound nutrition, she was *not* beautiful.

Too much "beauty" is only cosmetic-deep, though that is better than no beauty at all. The person who is satisfied with cosmetic-deep beauty has, in my opinion, low standards. Beauty should be at least vivacity-deep. It is better still if it can be both vivacity-deep and character-deep. Before I die, I hope mine can be soul-deep. Sound nutrition is absolutely essential for vivacity-deep beauty, a form of beauty which, I believe, any semi-healthy individual at any age can have provided it is wanted badly enough. When persons are seriously malnourished, as far too many of them are, those who could have character-deep beauty are often so ill and mentally confused and self-centered because of their illnesses that they fail to achieve this higher form of beauty. When malnutrition is severe, it prevents the serenity and calmness which in my opinion are essential ingredients of that rare and intangible quality I think of as soul beauty.

Another problem which often disappears after dietary improvement has to do with sexuality. Let us grant that perhaps 95 per cent of such problems are psychological, and consider only those which may be nutritional. Probably every nutrient plays some role in stimulating normal hormone production or in maintaining the health of the prostate, the uterus, and the penial and vaginal passages, all essential before mate relationships can be fulfilling.

Many people have told me that after dietary improvement their sexual difficulties have disappeared; a few say a contemplated divorce was forestalled. These reports have covered many varieties of sexual problems. Several were cases of impotence; others, of restoration of libido, or sexual desire. A young husband complained one month that his wife had no sex interest and the next that she had too much. A sixty-year-old widower told me that he felt much better when eating an adequate diet but that he could no longer do so; he would gladly follow the diet again as soon as he remarried. Many reports had to do with prostate infections which had interfered with sexual expression; others concerned eczemas on the genitalia or Manila albicans infections in the vagina or penis resulting from the use of aureomycin, streptomycin, or other antibiotics. Whatever the improvement was, it came as a by-product of dietary help sought for other reasons.

Worry over possible inability to express sexual love seems to be a masculine trait. These fears might disappear if men understood more fully the relation of nutrition to sexual function. For example, the pituitary gland, situated at the base of the brain, produces gonadotrophic hormones which in turn stimulate the gonads—testicles or ovaries—to produce other hormones necessary for normal sexual activity. The gonadotrophic hormones are made of protein; the sex hormones, of protein and fat-like substances known as steroids. If the diet is seriously inadequate in protein, fat, the B vitamins, or almost any nutrient, the pituitary and/or the gonads are unable to produce these hormones in adequate quantities. For example, I was amused to find that scientists had studied the vitamin-C content of the pituitary gland before and after male rabbits were bred. When the diet lacks vitamin C, the animals do not care to breed. If the diet is adequate, the pituitary is saturated with vitamin C before breeding but depleted of the vitamin afterward. Anyone who has bred a rabbit will admit that this is rapid utilization of a nutrient.

Studies of men in prison camps, of the conscientious objectors in the starvation experiments at the University of Minnesota, and of numerous clinical investigations show that libido decreases or disappears when the nutrition is inadequate. On the other hand, as long as even an average degree of health is maintained, glands rarely become abnormal. I know of no man who worries about the function of his thyroid, pancreas, or adrenal glands; if they become abnormal, he knows he can obtain thyroxin, insulin, or cortisone from his physician. Testosterone is also available, but it is probably never needed when the nutrition is adequate.

If neither psychological nor nutritional problems exist, sexual function is probably maintained as long as is health itself. A doctor told me of his Danish grandparents. At the age of eighty-seven, his grandfather, after working in the garden all morning and eating a hearty lunch, had quietly passed away while sitting in his chair. Grandmother, considerably younger, outlived him many years. Once when the women of the family were gathered with their sewing, someone asked the grandmother at what age, in her opinion, men became functionally unable to express love through sexual union. Grandmother answered softly in Danish, *"Aldrig"*— which means never. This same doctor, speaking of the importance of maintaining adequate nutrition in order that the sexual relationships may be fulfilling, then remarked, "It's putting money in the bank which will be a pleasure to spend."

Now I come to the you-won't-believe-it problem which sometimes disappears, the problem of growing older. Actually I am convinced it need not be a problem at all. There are people—not many, but a few—who seem to grow younger instead of older.

One day on a television program I may show you some of these people. For all of you doubting Thomases I could supply names and addresses, except in one case. This is a woman of eighty-two who enjoys tremendously the fact that most people think she is sixty; she works half-time as a secretary, flitting about like a hummingbird. There is Mr. G., now eighty-six, who talks about having fun on borrowed time; he loves to garden, and once when I was entertaining, he turned our house into a florist shop and in addition brought a camellia corsage for each guest. Mrs. S. must be nearly eighty by now. It is unbelievable that one person can do as much good as she does; I know how much she helps people because she sends many to me for nutritional advice. She was ill and old when I first saw her 15 years ago; now she is active and young and vibrantly alive.

Mrs. L. is one of the most amazing of this group. I would bet that in 12 years she has swallowed no morsel of food which does not build health. Her figure is that of a thirty-year-old. I tell her I should pay her to visit me instead of vice versa. She is particularly amazing because she is a crack skier and is on the ski patrol, skiing down the slopes with stretchers, helping to carry youngsters who have broken bones. She does not worry about breaking bones, nor does she need to.

One of my favorites is Mrs. H. She came to me because of pernicious anemia, exhausted, depressed, her mouth and tongue so sore she could hardly eat. Her life had been hard, money always scarce. Before child-labor laws were passed, she was taken out of school and forced to work in the New England woolen mills, leaving home when it was still dark in the morning and returning after dark at night. There was little love and few bright spots in her life until she was sixty-eight; then a childhood sweetheart found her, a wonderful physician whose record is in *Who's Who*. A friend and I poured coffee at their wedding, a big occasion with the brightest bunch of oldsters I have ever seen assembled; we laughingly said we were the only persons present who could hold a coffee cup without shaking out its contents. This woman sent me a report of her physical examination from Johns Hopkins Hospital: "Although this patient claims to be seventy-four years old, she has the body of a fifty-year-old woman." She and Dr. H. are now spending happily-ever-after summers in Vermont and winters in Florida. Dr. H. asked me to visit them in Vermont. I said I could not decide when to come; I wanted to be there for maple-syrup making but also for autumn colors. His answer was graciousness at its height: "If you can come only once, come in the spring and stay till the fall."

I wish you could all meet Mr. and Mrs. R., people whom it seems God must have made especially for each other. He is seventy-six; she, seventy-two. She had been crippled with arthritis for years, and he had the usual old-age symptoms: a tremor, fatigue, some shortness of breath, trouble with his eyes, years of hay fever and sinus infection, both still troublesome. The arthritis scarcely bothers her any more; his symptoms, too, have gradually cleared. Both are now amazingly active. She is busy with a grandchild who lives with them, with Spanish classes and social gatherings. Mr. R. holds down what could be considered three full-time jobs. He is president of a building and loan association, which takes a great deal of his time; he operates three oil wells which require as much attention as spoiled children; and he has gardened their acre of land since their Mexican gardener, an old man of forty, became ill. Besides these activities he plays 18 holes of golf twice each week. I remarked that he probably played with men 20 years his junior, and he said they were sometimes 30 years younger than he. If you want to taste really good homemade bread, you should drop in to see them, as I frequently do.

And lastly, there is Dr. P., who earned his Ph.D. at Columbia half a century ago. He and his family lived in Shanghai for years, then in Manila, where he was caught at the outbreak of World War II. He spent the war years in the terrible Santo Tomas Prison. His health was broken then, and recovery was never complete; heart attacks followed and then polyneuritis, the American term for beriberi. His pain was too excruciating to be deadened by opiates. Although he was given B vitamins by many physicians, he became worse and was not expected to live. As a last resort, his wife and daughter came to see me. Fortified milk, liver, wheat germ, all three in small amounts at first, large quantities of pantothenic acid, which had not been given before, calcium tablets to help deaden pain, vitamin pills of every letter, tablets of enzymes and hydrochloric acid to digest the food combined to turn the tables; his recovery was spectacular. Since childhood, Dr. P. has had a wonderful voice, and singing had been his joy. He sang solos at churches, clubs, and weddings. His voice failed with his illness, but now he believes it is stronger than ever; again he is singing for churches and clubs and weddings. Just before he left for Manila to be an executive of an insurance company, he sang to me a song he said he had especially selected. It was "I'll Be Loving You Always." And if I could have held back the tears, I would have sung the same song to him.

These are young people, every one of them. The good health they enjoy, however, is no mere happenstance. Every person in this group takes his nutrition seriously, not just occasionally but at every meal of every day and year after year. The rewards are pretty wonderful. With these people there is no gap between the generations. Each one of them is an inspiration, almost a vision of what could be for possibly every human being. They remind you again that aging may not be a "natural" process but the result of years and years of cumulative nutritional deficiencies. I tell them that they make me look forward to my nineties.

Are you looking forward to yours?

CHAPTER 29

HOW GOOD IS OUR NATIONAL HEALTH?

THOUSANDS UPON THOUSANDS OF PERSONS HAVE STUDIED disease. Almost no one has studied health.

Years ago Dr. Weston A. Price traveled the world over, examining people untouched by so-called civilization. He investigated groups in a then-isolated part of the Swiss Alps, in northern Italy, on the Isle of Man, in the New Hebrides, Australia, New Zealand, central Africa, the South American jungles, the north of Canada and Alaska and on various islands in the South Pacific. The foods of many of these peoples were limited indeed. In some cases their diets were largely meat or fish without vegetables or grains; in others, vegetables and grains without meat or fish; they appeared to have nothing in common. These peoples, however, had two things in common: their diets met every body requirement; and the know-how for refining foods was lacking. The latter allowed the former to be so.

Dr. Price told of his findings in a book, *Nutrition and Physical Degeneration.*[1] He tells of people with erect posture, unbelievable endurance, and cheerful, even dispositions. These people had excellent bone structure; their faces and jaws were so wide and well developed that their teeth were not crowded together and stayed free from decay just as their bodies stayed free from disease. The statistics concerning the incidence of cancer, ulcers, high blood pressure, tuberculosis, heart and kidney diseases, muscular dystrophy, multiple sclerosis, and cerebral palsy were zero, zero, zero in every case. Names for these diseases were unknown and unneeded. Dr. Price found no physicians, surgeons, psychia-

[1] The Price-Pottenger Foundation, Inc., 137 N. Canyon Blvd., Monrovia, California 91016, 1969.

trists, no crime, no prisons; no mental illness and no institutions for the insane, feebleminded, alcoholics, or drug addicts; no child delinquency, no homosexuality. Every mother nursed her babies; a non-functional breast was unheard of. Mental, moral, and emotional health accompanied physical health.

Sir Robert McCarrison, an English physician, investigated the health of the Hunzas, living high in the Himalayas. Their foods were limited, but their lands were composted and watered by glacial streams rich in minerals from rocks grinding on rocks. Dr. McCarrison's statistics were the same as those gathered by Dr. Price: all zeros. He could find no ulcers, cancers, heart or kidney diseases, or other illnesses; no insanity, no crime, no drug addicts, no alcoholics; no prisons, mental institutions, child-delinquency problems. Other Hunza visitors have written of the cheerfulness and endurance of these people; a runner carried a message to a nearby village only 35 miles away and returned the same day with no sign of fatigue. As mountain guides, the Hunzas scrambled surefooted over precipitous cliffs, carrying tremendous loads, laughing and singing the while.

Years ago a group of medical missionaries, Mormons by faith, collectively examined more than a million natives in central Africa; they found no disease, no cancer, no crime, no insanity, no alcoholics, no drug addicts. A similar group found none among primitive peoples in South America.

The late Dr. Michael Walsh studied Indians in an isolated district in Mexico, people without even a water supply. Their only beverage was fermented cactus juice, so rich in vitamin C that the amount allotted per person per day was equivalent to a dozen glasses of fresh orange juice. These people had never taken a bath; yet they were as free from body odor as they were from cancer, high blood pressure, heart disease, crime, and insanity.

These same investigators also studied diseases in villages only a few miles away, where white men had brought white sugar, white flour, and so-called "civilization." In such villages, Dr. Price found faulty bone structure, crowded, crooked teeth, rampant tooth decay, diseases of all kinds, crime, prisons, perversions, insanity, and sexual immorality. Dr. McCarrison found ulcers, heart and kidney diseases, cancer, high blood pressure, colitis, and tuberculosis. In Africa and South America the medical missionaries found cancer rampant among members of the very tribes who, on their native diets, had stayed cancer-free. Now these African natives are dying from a form of malnutrition called kwashiorkor; 60 per cent coming to the autopsy tables have died of cancer. In populated areas in Mexico, Dr. Walsh found every disease he had the heart to look for.

I hunted for statistics of health in America to compare with the zeros found by Drs. Price and McCarrison. All I found were records showing people suffering from diseases in huge, heartbreaking numbers. The statistics of the numbers and causes of army rejections during the Korean War and Vietnam War compared with those of World War II threw me into a depression which lasted days; the time interval is so short, the increases in abnormalities so appalling. These are not sickness figures, merely statistics of our finest young men at the height of their physical development.

Statistics can tell so little. The number of new cancer cases discovered each year tells nothing of the fear and dread in the hearts of millions of Americans who already know that someday they themselves may suffer from the horrible disease. Statistics about the "chronics" in every county and state home, people whose illnesses go on year after year, do not mention the tired underpaid nurses ready to drop in their tracks, the stinking bedpans, the raw, running bedsores, or the looks of despair on the faces from which hope was lost so long ago. Statistics of the number of elderly people sitting or lying out monotonous and/or agonizing days in the thousands of rest homes in our country do not mention the bitterness, the fear, the hopelessness in the hearts of these still fine old people; if you see enough of these homes, you wonder whether our increased life span is always to be viewed with unmitigated pride.

It is easy to find statistics on the billions of man-hours lost from work per year when 12,000,000 people per day are sufficiently sick to require medical care. These statistics tell nothing of those who suffered from minor but painful ailments, or of the millions whose illnesses were severe but who called no physician because they feared the expense or because none could come during the night when the pain was most excruciating.

There are no statistics available for dozens of things which really matter or really hurt; of exhausted mothers who, missing nights of sleep because of a sick child, must still go to an office the next day or drag themselves through mountains of housework, simultaneously caring for other children. No statistics tell of the billions of father- and mother-hours of worry or anguish endured per year; of the billions of spankings given annually to good children whose parents were irritable or frustrated; of the billions of meals ruined per year by nagging and scolding; of the billions of student-hours wasted because so many in school attendance receive too few nutrients to keep their minds alert; of the number of parents paying dentists with savings they had hoped to spend on college educations.

I could find no health statistics. What is health? It seems to be something we talk glibly about. We speak of health insurance, meaning sickness insurance; of health benefits, meaning sickness benefits; health plans and surveys, meaning sickness plans and surveys. People talk about health education, health courses, health books; I have taken the courses, read the books; you learn about vaccinations, contagion, and diseases. What health actually is, apparently no one knows; certainly it is more than freedom from disease or ability to go to work. The best definition appears to be one which a small boy used to define money: "It's something we ain't got much of."

In contrast to the primitive peoples investigated by Drs. Price and McCarrison, our country now leads the world in the number of deaths from heart disease and cancer. Strokes, high blood pressure, emphysema, diabetes, and degenerative diseases are increasing rapidly. Abnormalities once rare, such as myasthenia gravis, muscular dystrophy, scleroderma, and multiple sclerosis, have become commonplace. New diseases appear annually, mostly iatrogenic, or physician-caused, illnesses, largely brought on by the excessive use of drugs; and inborn errors of metabolism, apparently resulting from inadequate prenatal diets. Few of our people now have good bone structure; 98 per cent of the children have rampant tooth decay. Crime, alcoholism, drug addiction, and divorces are at an all-time high. More mentally defective children are born each year. In short, our sickness record is a national disgrace. It is difficult to find a single person who is radiantly healthy.

The less health we have, the less money we will have. Before Medicare, 60 per cent of the savings of people sixty years old was said to have been spent on a search for health; but 60 per cent of the people sixty years old have no savings. Their sickness bills are paid by you and me. Our taxes pay for the county and state hospitals and homes for the chronically ill, as well as for institutions for the insane and feebleminded. It is your tax money and mine which pays for schools, whether the children attend or not, are mentally alert or not, or whether the teachers are healthy or not.

In addition to the taxes, there are the fund-raising campaigns: the heart fund, the hypoglycemia fund, the cerebral palsy fund, the cancer fund, and numerous others. Money-raising has become big business, for which experts are trained. To my knowledge, no money has yet been raised for the purpose of what I call prevention. The native races studied by Drs. Price and McCarrison did not "prevent" tuberculosis by early X-rays, or cancer by free clinics where frightened people could be examined; they merely ate wholesome food.

Unless something is done and done quickly toward real prevention, we can expect still more irritability, fatigue, mental sluggishness, psychological maladjustment, faulty posture and bone structure, crooked and decayed teeth. We can expect more surgery: more tumors, cancers, gall bladders and prostates removed, more sinuses scraped, more hysterectomies performed. We can be sure of an increase in the incidence of cancer, ulcers, high blood pressure, heart and kidney diseases, diabetes, muscular dystrophy, multiple sclerosis, cerebral palsy, and many other diseases, some still unknown and unnamed. How sincerely I hope I am wrong!

Can you hear the arguments being raised? Diagnostic methods are better. People are living longer, we are told, into the heart-disease-, diabetes-, cancer-susceptible age. Granted that these arguments contain some truth, but not all the truth. Before Iron Curtain days, it was known that the Bulgarians lived to be older than other peoples in the world without these diseases. When grains were unrefined in Denmark from 1914 to 1920, people lived longer, into the "disease-susceptible age," and had fewer of these diseases. Diagnostic methods are better, yes; they are now so good that a tremendous increase in cancer among babies and small children is being diagnosed. I shall not forget a young woman sitting beside my desk, sobbing, sobbing, sobbing. Her three-year-old child, a little girl whose picture she showed me, had just died of cancer; another child of less than two and still another of scarcely five were then dying. She herself wanted to die; she said so repeatedly. Yet she came asking for help for her two dying children. I wish I could have helped her six years earlier.

Our national health began to decline at the onset of the Industrial Revolution, as families moved from self-sustaining farms into crowded cities. It declined still further with the invention of machinery for milling grains, and with each new method of refining and processing foods, each new trick for forcing hybrid crops to yield higher tonnage per acre on worn-out soil. New problems arising every year make sound nutrition more difficult to apply or prevent its application. The fact still remains, however, that unrefined foods can be selected if one wishes to eat them; that in every case the world over, when foods have been unrefined, diets have been adequate, health has been built, and no supplements have been needed; and that physical, mental, and social degeneration has occurred in proportion to the amount of refined foods eaten.

We must someday face the fact that disease is produced in humans in exactly the same way as it is produced in laboratory animals: by inadequate diets. We must also realize that social problems are caused in part by inadequate diets. Science has shown that alcoholism can be produced by a lack of B vitamins; half of all traffic accidents, half of all arrests by the FBI are associated with the excessive use of alcohol. Dr. Hoffer and persons using his methods (ref. 1, p. 87) have helped to bring thousands of hopelessly insane schizophrenics back to health through improved nutrition. Though most schizophrenics harm no one, our most atrocious crimes are committed by schizophrenics. The rate of suicides among schizophrenics is extremely high, yet suicides have not occurred after their nutrition has been improved. Poor nutrition can bring on such bickering, irritability, and self-centeredness that marriages fail; and impotency has now become common among forty- and even thirty-year-olds. If one watches what schoolchildren are eating—or not eating—one can easily understand why so many are using drugs.

Alcoholism, crime, insanity, suicides, divorces, and drug addiction cannot be separated from the nutrition of a people. Furthermore, we can expect all of these social problems to continue to increase, involving ever larger per cents of our population, unless our nutrition is markedly improved. I am not saying for a minute that faulty nutrition is the *only* cause of these social ills. Many psychological and sociological problems are involved, but inadequate nutrition is still a vital factor which has received, as Dr. Margaret Mead puts it, "nearly total inattention."

How good—or how bad—is our nutrition? First one must have a standard by which to judge. The Food and Nutrition Board of the National Research Council–National Academy of Sciences, a private organization supported by industry, suggests that, to maintain health, persons should have certain quantities of several nutrients, spoken of as the Recommended Daily Allowances, or RDA (pp. 274-275). It is doubtful whether these allowances are actually sufficient to maintain health; certainly they are inadequate for any person whose health is below par. For example, the RDA of vitamin C is 30 to 80 milligrams, small indeed compared to the amount Dr. Klenner has found necessary to get arthritics out of their wheel chairs. The RDA of 9 to 20 milligrams of niacin certainly did not help Dr. Hoffer to send schizophrenics from mental hospitals back to college. The recommended amounts of most other nutrients are all equally low. Yet studies of the nutrition of thousands of Americans show that their diets do not begin to meet even these low standards.

Dozens of national nutritional surveys, recently reviewed,[2] considered the adequacy of 7 of the 40 essential nutrients: calcium, iron, and vitamins A, B_1, B_2, C, and niacin. Analysis of the food intake revealed that thousands of people, huge per cents of those studied, obtain far less than the pitifully low Recommended Daily Allowances. The diets of thousands more supplied less than half the nutrients suggested by these allowances, and of still other thousands, even less than a fourth of the RDA. Whenever the protein intake was determined, it was usually found to be low. Whether we wish to face it or not, persons obtaining such diets are rapidly producing disease in themselves, and indeed are already suffering from many abnormalities.

None of these surveys, however, were of poor families; they were of people living in small urban communities and surrounding rural areas near universities where the studies were made. No survey revealed the horrors of diets eaten in city ghettos or rural poverty areas. None considered the intake of magnesium, potassium, vitamin E, cholin, and many other nutrients equally essential but more often deficient than the ones studied. No survey included pregnant women, ill persons, hospital patients, or alcoholics, whose diets are all known to be remarkably inadequate.

To report such studies is to become bogged down in statistics. In general, women and especially teen-age girls had poorer diets than men and boys; their intake of calcium, iron, and vitamins A and B_2 was appallingly deficient. Blood analysis showed a heartbreaking amount of anemia and deficiencies of vitamins A, B_1, B_2, and C and carotene. Farm families, few of whom bothered to raise their own food, were usually fed no better than city dwellers. Persons having a high income were better fed than those with little money, yet a large per cent of them still had poor diets.

2 T. R. A. Davis et al., "Review of Studies of Vitamin and Mineral Nutrition in the United States (1950-1968)," *Journal of Nutrition Education*, I (1969), 41.

Particularly tragic and certainly the most inexcusable is that infants under a year of age are being given appallingly deficient diets. Their intake of nutrients was often found to be less than half or even a fourth of the Recommended Daily Allowances required to maintain any degree of health.[8] The younger the infants, the more deficient were their diets. Infants from poor families, whose mothers had not graduated from high school, received more calcium and vitamins B_1, B_2, C, and D than ones whose mothers held college degrees and whose fathers were on university staffs;[4] the poorer mothers could not afford pediatricians who, untrained in nutrition, keep infants on inadequate commercial formulas and so much canned baby food that milk is crowded out. Such inadequate diets have produced the allergies, infections, skin rashes, convulsions, and dozens of other abnormalities so common among American infants. In North Africa, in the Orient, and in every country of Europe, I have been charmed by the beautiful, beautiful healthy babies, yet I rarely find one in a hundred in America. It is now known that if the diet is inadequate during the first few months, especially in protein, magnesium, or vitamin B_6 or E, the brain cannot develop normally. In our city, the IQ of schoolchildren is said to have decreased 9 points in the last twenty years; I suspect the decline during the next twenty years will be much greater.

The combined studies on our national dietary adequacy (ref. 2, p. 249) conclude: "Nutritional problems in the United States affect virtually all age groups and segments of the population." By blood analyses, these combined surveys indicate that 48 million Americans suffer severe nutritional deficiencies; and that the diets of 24 million do not even supply *half the amounts of nutrients* deemed to be essential to health. Thus literally millions of Americans are producing diseases in themselves.

In January, 1969, Dr. Arnold Schaefer gave to the Select Committee on Nutrition and Human Needs of the United

[8] V. A. Beal, "Nutritional Intake of Children: Calcium, Phosphorus, and Iron," *Journal of Nutrition*, LIII (1954), 499; ". . . Thiamin, Riboflavin, and Niacin," *ibid.*, LVII (1955), 183; ". . . Vitamins A and D and Ascorbic Acid," *ibid.*, LX (1956), 335; R. Rueda-Williamson et al., "Growth and Nutrition of Infants," *Pediatrics*, XXX (1962), 639; H. A. Guthrie, "Effect of Early Feeding of Solid Foods on Nutritive Intake of Infants," *ibid.*, XXXVIII (1966), 879.

[4] Beal, Guthrie (see note 3); L. J. Filer, Jr., et al., "Intake of Selected Nutrients of Infants in the United States: An Evaluation of 4,000 Representative Six-Month-Olds," *Clinical Pediatrics*, II (1963), 470; III (1964), 633.

States Senate the first report of a national nutritional survey undertaken by the Department of Health, Education, and Welfare.[5] During examinations of 12,000 persons, the committee had discovered "an alarming prevalence" of malnutrition. A third of the children under six and vast numbers of adults were found to be anemic. Another third of the youngsters showed vitamin-A deficiencies. Iodine deficiencies were prevalent and a huge increase in goiter was noted; surgery for goiter removal was increasing rapidly. X-ray examinations showed much retarded bone development. The amounts of vitamins C and D in the blood of children were found to be far "less than acceptable levels." Not infrequently teen-agers, their teeth decayed to the gum line, were unable to chew. Even several cases of the disease resulting from extreme protein starvation, kwashiorkor, were found. The data "yielded definite signs of malnutrition in an unexpectedly large number of persons"; and the situation was described as a "terrible crisis." The point was stressed that malnourished children cannot learn and malnourished adults cannot work.

A large per cent of the families investigated by Dr. Schaefer's committee were poor by our standards. Compared to the healthy persons investigated by Drs. Price, McCarrison, and others, they would be considered wealthy. The very fact that these people are alive shows that they have obtained food. Why should any country allow its food to be so refined that it can produce disease? Dr. Schaefer is quoted as saying that these people need food, not supplements. He had apparently overlooked the fact that they have become extremely malnourished not by eating supplements but by eating what Americans call food.

The Department of Agriculture made national nutritional surveys in both 1955 and 1965.[6] Only half of our people had appallingly inadequate diets in 1955. Ten years later nearly two-thirds were deficient in protein, calcium, vitamins A and C, and all other nutrients considered except iron. During a mere ten years the consumption of such junk foods as soft drinks, sweet bakery products, and packaged cereals had increased tremendously. The intake of whole milk, cheese, and fresh fruits and vegetables had markedly decreased. There was also a decrease in the use of whole-

[5] *The Food Gap: Poverty and Malnutrition in the United States* (Washington, D.C.: Government Printing Office, 1969).
[6] *Dietary Levels of Households in the United States, Spring 1965,* Agricultural Research Series (Washington, D.C.: U. S. Department of Agriculture).

some starchy foods such as dry beans, legumes, potatoes, and whole grains which for generations had kept persons relatively healthy even with little money to spend for food. Still other studies have shown that American diets became much worse between 1960 and 1968.

Regardless of which survey is quoted, and there are a surprising number of them, Americans are not healthy; and they are obviously becoming less healthy each year. The question is: What, if anything, are we going to do about it?

CHAPTER 30

IT IS EASY TO BELIEVE

WHO HAS NOT HEARD THAT AMERICA IS THE BEST-FED NATION in the world? This statement has been made so many thousands of times that large segments of our population undoubtedly believe it. When anything is represented time and again as a fact, one unthinkingly accepts it as truth. Being abundantly fed with refined foods, however, does not make a nation best-fed.

For decades, dozens of such misleading statements have been endlessly repeated as part of the propaganda of the 100-billion-dollar-a-year food industry. The smallest comment concerning the value of nutrition is a criticism, direct or implied, of this industry which allows nutrients to be lost during food processing in order to increase profits. Awareness of nutrition decreases sales, hence is not to be tolerated. The propaganda, therefore, must convince the public that our nutrition is adequate; that nutrients discarded in food processing are only minor losses; and that devitalized foods—the big profit-makers—actually build health. If we are now to survive, however, we must distinguish truth from falsehood.

The enormous power of the food processors is almost beyond comprehension. Millions upon millions of dollars spent for lobbyists sway state and federal lawmakers to the food refiners' advantage. These powerful industrialists control the food advertising of every radio and TV outlet, every newspaper and magazine. They pay for hundreds of "feature articles" which seemingly give innocent and factual information, though designed to increase sales and to keep under cover facts detrimental to them. The food processors are aided by the powerful drug interests, which have immense influence on physicians through advertising in medical journals; a nation of healthy individuals uses few drugs.

If people can be convinced that America is indeed the best-fed nation, however, and that refined foods really "build champions," sales will not decrease. Tremendous wealth can still be made annually at the expense of our health and the health of our children.

Dr. Arnold Schaefer (ref. 5, p. 251) has said with masterful understatement that the food industry is contributing to the malnutrition in the United States. The food industry has caused and is causing our national malnutrition. Fewer devitalized foods would be purchased, of course, if everyone appreciated the value of nutrition; no one is forced to buy them. It should be remembered, however, that the healthy primitive races investigated by Drs. Price and McCarrison (pp. 243-244) did not select adequate diets because they were educated in nutrition; no food available to them had been raped.

Nor can one argue that the industrialists are innocent of the harm they have caused. A large soft-drink company, which has done incalculable damage to the health of Americans, ironically produces a highly nutritious protein-rich supplement which we taxpayers buy for export to "underprivileged" countries. Similarly, many companies, afraid that increased nutritional awareness will decrease their sales, are now adding microscopic amounts of vitamin B_6 and pantothenic acid to such foods as packaged cereals, again misleading the public into thinking that these additions make up for the dozens of nutrients discarded.

Let us consider the actual losses when bread is made from refined flour. The type of bread a nation uses is of extreme importance to health. It makes up a large per cent of the diet, especially of growing children and persons with low incomes. After grains are crushed into flour or cereal, however, the oil of the germ quickly becomes rancid, spoiling flavor and keeping-qualities. To grind grains daily and/or to refrigerate them decreases profits. The goal is always to make millions, not to produce health.

Americans have been told so many times that "enriched bread" is as valuable nutritionally as whole wheat that even persons of education and authority, such as physicians, dietitians, and professors of nutrition, apparently believe it. Our Department of Agriculture[1] gives figures which show that white bread, compared to whole wheat, has lost the following per cents of nutrients: calcium, 60; potassium, 74; iron, 76; magnesium, 78; linoleic acid, 50; vitamin B_1, 90;

[1] B. K. Watt et al., *Composition of Foods*, U. S. Department of Agriculture Handbook No. 8 (1963).

vitamin B_2, 61; and niacin, 80. Though only the protein of the germ, or 22 per cent, is discarded, it is rich in essential amino acids, whereas the remaining protein cannot support growth. The loss of folic acid in per cent is 79;[2] of vitamin B_6, 60;[3] zinc, 50;[4] pantothenic acid, 69; vitamin E, 100; manganese, 84; and copper, 74. I am unable to find the losses of cholin, inositol, PABA, biotin, cobalt, and other trace minerals, but one can be sure they are significant.

The statement that "enriching" white bread with vitamin B_1, niacin, and iron makes it as valuable nutritionally as the entire grain is obviously untrue. Yet the same health-giving nutrients lost from bread are also discarded during the production of packaged cereals, macaroni, spaghetti, noodles, crackers, cookies, pastries, cakes and cake mixes, stuffings, and dozens of other foods. It is not enough that wheat costing 3 cents a pound can be sold for a dollar after being robbed of its nutrients and puffed, crinkled, or popped into a cereal; the public must also be convinced that this cereal fosters athletic prowess, a non-fact directed at our malnourished adolescents and believed by all too many of them.

The nutrients lost during the past 50 years by refining wheat have been astronomical. Our local department of agriculture tells me that the production of wheat during the past ten years for human use only has averaged 30,700 million pounds, or 511.7 million bushels. If we assume that 10 per cent of the grain is used unrefined—a generous estimate—the loss of potassium in a single year would be 34,454,610,000 grams. Losses of other nutrients are comparable. These losses alone, especially of vitamin E, magnesium, and potassium, may be largely responsible for our deaths from heart disease; certainly they can determine the difference between health and disease. No nation with a sickness record as disgraceful as ours can afford such extravagance.

Another misleading practice is to add brown dye, semantically referred to as "caramel coloring," to white bread; thus it appears to be made of whole grain. It is then labeled "wheat" bread to imply that it is made of 100 per cent whole wheat. Thousands of women serve such bread, convinced they are giving their families a superior product. I have yet to see a loaf of dark bread in Minnesota, for

[2] E. W. Toepfer et al., *Folic Acid Content of Foods*, U. S. Department of Agriculture Handbook No. 29 (1951).

[3] W. H. Sebrell et al., *The Vitamins*, Vol. II (Academic Press, 1954).

[4] H. C. Sherman, *Chemistry of Food and Nutrition*, 8th ed. (The Macmillan Company, 1952).

example, the very heart of the bread basket, which was not made with dye and white flour. Equally tragic are the many communities in our southern states where no unrefined breads whatsoever are available. Preservatives are also often added to perishable flour, though excellent unrefined breads containing none are sold at health food stores and many markets. Some thirty chemicals are said to be added to white flour, but since it cannot support life of bacteria or bugs, no preservatives are needed.

The refining and/or processing of almost every food causes the loss of much or all of its nutritive value. White sugar, for example, retains not one milligram of vitamins or minerals. Furthermore, American markets are now flooded with synthetic or nearly synthetic "foods" which contain little or no nutrients. All soft drinks, imitation "fruit" ades, imitation "fruit" juices, gelatin desserts, and many other "foods" are little more than sweetened chemicals. Besides harmful preservatives (p. 270), a large per cent of foods contains so many additives—thousands are now used—that a correct label would look like the inventory of a chemistry supply room. Such additives may be harmless individually but combinations of them, which no one has investigated, could be highly toxic or even cancer-producing.

Much of the propaganda of the food processors is released through newspaper columns written by physicians and/or college professors. These readily believed voices of respect and authority have been cleverly wooed by vast sums given to numerous universities for nutritional research. Such a procedure has paid rich dividends. There are, of course, tax benefits. The "image" of the refined-food industry becomes one of public-spirited generosity. Though the research itself is excellent, the industrialists dictate the choice of research projects, set policies, help evaluate the findings, and make sure that no problem is investigated or finding published which could possibly decrease sales or detract from the propaganda that refined foods are capable of building health.

One might well ask why wonderful people in the universities are accepting money from companies whose influence on American health is so detrimental. Unfortunately, university instructors and professors become known, attain status, receive promotions, and are given salaries in proportion to the number of research papers they publish. Research is expensive. Before it can be done, money must be obtained. Often no money is forthcoming except from the refined-food industry. By giving millions to the nutrition, dietetics, and home economics departments, the refined-food and drug interests have gained tremendous control over the universities. Thus persons with education, training, and integrity become their spokesmen. If a recipient of a research fund fails to co-operate, his grant is not renewed.

The amount of money given as university research grants was recently brought into the open at the food supplement hearings conducted by the Food and Drug Administration (FDA). The popularity of food supplements showed that people were realizing their diets were not adequate, a situation which threatened refined-food sales. In 1966, the FDA proposed rulings forbidding vitamins and minerals, except for tiny amounts, to be sold without prescriptions.[5] These rules stated that no firm could represent, suggest, or even imply on a label or in advertising that a nutrient might help to prevent illnesses or to speed recovery. Neither could a firm insinuate that ordinary foods do not supply adequate amounts of all vitamins and minerals. Despite the many surveys to the contrary, no company was to be allowed to report in its advertising that a significant segment of our population suffers or is in danger of suffering from any dietary deficiency. Not one word could be mentioned that there is any loss of nutritive value because of cooking, processing, transportation, storage, or poor soil. A violation of these rulings would be a criminal offense, or felony, subject to heavy fines.

Millions of dollars of taxpayers' money have now been spent on hearings in which college professors, many also physicians, have testified that misleading and untrue statements are indeed factual. Almost without exception, the persons testifying in favor of these rulings were receiving research grants from the refined-foods and drug industries.[6] The transcript of these hearings may be read by anyone who cares to look them up.

Recently Dr. Miles Robinson, who has represented the National Health Federation at the FDA vitamin hearings, said to me, "I used to feel critical of my fellow physicians because they underestimated nutrition so much. Now I'm convinced they've been so brainwashed by propaganda that they can't help believing our foods really do supply the nutrients we need." University professors and millions of other Americans have been equally brainwashed, or con-

[5] *Federal Register,* Vol. XXXI, No. 241, Dec. 14, 1966.
[6] M. H. Robinson, *Big Brother and His Science: A Report on the FDA* (10121 Chapel Road, Potomac, Maryland 20854, 1969).

vinced by clever propaganda, that our nutrition is adequate.

One condition which makes this situation possible is that research scientists pursue knowledge for its own sake. They are not only uninterested in practical application but usually hold it in contempt as being unscientific. This typical attitude is expressed in a letter I received only yesterday from a woman who had just discovered practical nutrition. She writes, "The appalling thing is that I have spent 15 years doing research in biochemistry, carefully providing nutrients for animals, yet it never once occurred to me to apply the same principles to my own family."

The extent of the food processors' influence on university dietetics departments is shown by the foods served in hospitals throughout the country. Such food, notoriously poor, should be both delicious and nutritious. Last year a physician, head of a hospital, asked me to help his dietitian plan more nutritious meals. This young woman held a degree from one of our great universities; her technical training was excellent. Yet the first things I saw on entering the kitchen were great stacks of thawing French-fried potatoes and French-fried shrimps, already fried once in cholesterol-raising hydrogenated fat, and then to be reheated in the same variety of fat. Ample fresh foods were on the market and the kitchen was well staffed with idle women; yet most of the vegetables and fruits served were canned or frozen. Meats were overcooked at high temperatures. Greasy hot breads and pies of the chiffon variety were served at each lunch and dinner. Not a teaspoon of unrefined flour or wheat germ was in the kitchen; this dietitian was convinced that white flour is just as nourishing as the whole-grain. Refined foods were recommended throughout her manual of the American Dietetics Association, which listed not a single health-building diet, though persons coming to any hospital, already ill, need the most nutritious food possible to aid recovery. Hundreds of similarly inadequate diets planned by dietitians are sent me. These girls literally do not believe in nutrition; the propaganda that all essential nutrients can be obtained from our overrefined foods has been successful.

The control and brainwashing of university foods departments have tragic and far-reaching influence through the home economics teachers they train. During the past semester at our local high school, the children in the foods classes were taught to make pie dough, cake, cookies, biscuits, rolls, and muffins, all with white flour and hydrogenated fats. One lesson was on white-bread sandwiches of processed cheese, hydrogenated peanut butter, or cold meats having 50 per cent saturated fat. While making gelatin salads and desserts the students were told that gelatin supplied protein, but not that it lacked five essential amino acids and supplied such an excess of glycine that it could be toxic. Far from being taught nutrition, these girls, so soon to be wives and mothers, were actually taught how to produce disease in themselves and their future husbands and children. In thousands of similar foods classes across the United States, girls are being taught by attitude, implication, and actual food preparation that nutrition does not really matter. Their teachers, like so many dietitians, had been taught not to believe in nutrition.

Because millions must be made and propaganda controlled, no sphere of influence appears to have been overlooked. The mammoth food interests have now made available in many large cities a telephone service known as Dial-A-Dietitian, ostensibly run by the American Dietetics Association. It was brought out at the FDA vitamin hearings that this phone service was generously supported by the refined-food industry, which obtained much free publicity from the newspapers and magazines in which it advertises.[7] Phone them and you can be sure of having foods recommended which will make money for their processors. They can also tell you which books on nutrition you should read and which you should avoid.

It came out in the FDA hearings[8] that the food processors had arranged for the blacklisting of books which might in any way harm their colossal sales. This list of not-recommended books supplied the Dial-A-Dietitian service was compiled by a professor of nutrition at a small eastern college. It includes authors quite as well trained in nutrition as herself, such as Dr. Roger J. Williams, professor at the University of Texas, who first isolated pantothenic acid and who has helped thousands of alcoholics to give up drinking; and Dr. Carlton Fredericks, who has contributed magnificently to popular education in nutrition and whose work with cerebral palsy children is particularly exciting. Almost every writer has been blacklisted who is sufficiently humane to have tried to decrease the appalling suffering being produced by processed foods. Even half a dozen cookbooks recommending unrefined ingredients are listed as "dangerous." Certain universities, which Dr. Robinson speaks of as

[7] M. H. Robinson, *The Concerted Blacklisting of Books on Nutrition*, National Health Federation Bulletin No. 15 (1969), p. 9.
[8] See note 7 above.

"hotbeds of antinutrition," have circulated this list or similar lists of not-recommended books, and have especially urged that they be removed from the shelves of public libraries. The procedure is quite reminiscent of the book burnings under Hitler. Yet it is difficult not to believe persons of authority, integrity, and education whom one naturally respects, especially when we are told that they merely wish to protect an unsuspecting public from faddism and quackery.

Name-calling, derogatory articles, and adverse propaganda are other methods used to belittle persons refusing to recommend refined foods. We have long been called crackpots and faddists regardless of training or of accuracy in reporting research. The words "quacks" and "quackery" are now such current favorites that you can be fairly sure that anyone using them is receiving benefits from the food processors.

Only recently has it been realized that millions of malnourished Americans have little money to spend on food. Our Senate has been told that the only solution to this problem is to appropriate billions of dollars, thus giving each family enough tax dollars to buy whatever food it wishes. The food processors and persons under their influence enthusiastically endorsed such a solution, knowing full well that a large share of these tax dollars will be spent on refined foods and skyrocket profits. Since their advertising supports most of our news media, they are quickly convincing most unthinking Americans that such a solution is humanitarian.

Welfare handouts have never produced health. In a study of the nutritional status of New York schoolchildren, 73.2 per cent of the diets were judged inadequate and only 6.6 per cent excellent (ref. 5, p. 251). The report of this study states: "Those on welfare had a higher incidence of poor diets and a decidedly lower incidence of excellent diets." Furthermore, their nutrition was not improved by free school lunches.

I have before me a newspaper clipping of a New England community which set out to provide "adequate nutrition through school lunch programs for needy children." It states that, though the program was costing the community huge sums, it was met with "numerous examples of excessive negativism." The children had complained about the "dry old bologna sandwiches"; they said the soft drinks should have been chilled; and that the lunches of cheese (processed?) on stale bread (white?), a sour pickle, and a soggy brown apple were too unpalatable to eat. Milk is not mentioned. When one multiplies this example by hundreds of thousands of communities throughout America, it becomes obvious why giving money to persons unaware of nutrition will increase profits but not build health.

If the "solution" to the malnutrition among low-income families takes the form of welfare handouts, the American taxpayer can expect to pay doubly: first for the processed, health-destroying foods; second, for the medical care necessitated by the resulting ill health. Our national doctor bill has already reached $10 billion annually; the drug bill is $6 billion (ref. 6, p. 257). We can be sure both will increase.

It seems to me it is time to face the fact that producing disease in human beings is the cruelest of all possible cruelties. The amount of suffering in our nation now is astronomical. Hospitals, mental institutions, jails, drug addiction centers, all are overflowing; more are needed and still more will be needed. Each person occupying a bed in any of these institutions is suffering and has suffered, no one knows how much. Their families are suffering and have suffered, no one can imagine how much. If you hear enough people sobbing or screaming with pain, if you watch them gasping for air through seemingly endless nights, you can realize that disease-production is a cruel thing. You see cruelty in billboards tempting persons to use more soft drinks; in misleading ads on TV and radio, in newspapers and women's magazines; in inadequate formulas recommended by pediatricians; in the meals of processed foods served by tired mothers. You understand, forgive, perhaps excuse, but the fact remains that persons are being made to suffer, and to induce suffering is a cruel thing.

Where will so much suffering lead us? The power and might of a country can fall with amazing speed. Half of the people living today vividly remember the British Empire; that empire no longer exists. Hundreds of civilizations have fallen, many because of the food supply. How long can overprocessed foods maintain the United States as a world power?

When a country can be convinced that it is "the best-fed nation in the world" while millions of its people are dying and its death rate from heart disease alone drops from 11th to 37th place in a few short years, it is time to realize that we have been as completely brainwashed as if we were living behind the Iron Curtain. If this country is to survive, the best-fed-nation myth had better be recognized for what it is: propaganda designed to produce wealth but not health.

CHAPTER 31

WHEN ABILITY BECOMES
RESPONSIBILITY

MANY PEOPLE AGREE THAT SOMETHING SHOULD BE DONE about our national malnutrition. Who should do it? Some say the universities or the Department of Agriculture or of Health, Education, and Welfare. So far these organizations have done little to solve the problem.

My father used to say, "When you want something done, do it yourself." If enough persons with a do-it-yourself attitude would get interested in nutrition, amazing changes could be made. There are now, for example, several hundred groups of do-it-yourself young people who are "returning to the soil" all over America. They are growing their own foods without chemical fertilizers or poison sprays, and canning supplies for winter; some are setting out orchards. They make their own breads and cereals from stone-ground whole grains. Many raise goats for delicious raw milk and chickens to supply fertile eggs and fresh poultry. Usually their only sweets are honey, maple syrup, and unrefined molasses. One such group recently invited me to a delightful wedding where the cake was made of whole-wheat flour, nuts, grated carrots, and honey; instead of champagne and mints, carrots and apple juice and unsalted nuts were served. These young men and women are refreshingly unimpressed by the propaganda of the food industrialists.

Last year while lecturing on a number of college campuses, I found hundreds of young people sufficiently interested in nutrition to do something about it. At the University of California at Santa Cruz a large number had refused to eat the junk foods served at the college cafeteria. Instead, they were cooking in their rooms. Because of the danger of fire, school authorities had asked the cafeteria management to prepare whatever foods they wanted. When I visited them, the students interested in their health were being served a fondue of eggs, milk, and natural cheese; soy beans deliciously seasoned with celery, bell peppers, and green onions; brown rice; applesauce; and cottage cheese. An organic garden on the campus, tended with volunteer student labor, supplied radishes, carrots (cut into sticks), lettuce for tossed salad, and chard, which was deliciously steamed. Bread of soy flour and stone-ground whole wheat was served hot from the oven. Dessert was fresh oranges, apples, and bananas cut up with nuts, sunflower seeds, and wheat germ. The only sweet was a large bowl of honey. Huge quantities of yogurt and milk were being consumed.

In contrast, the menu for the other students included meat balls with white rice and chicken (fried in hydrogenated fat) with mashed potatoes; white bread, hot white rolls, and sweet white-flour muffins; two desserts of sweetened gelatin, a cornstarch pudding, and four different kinds of chiffon-type pies; and huge quantities of coffee and especially of soft drinks were being consumed. Ill health was all too obviously being produced. Unfortunately, on these same campuses I found young girls probably ruining their chances of having healthy children by fasting, following inadequate vegetarian regimes, or avoiding milk because they erroneously believed it to be mucus-forming. The fact remains, however, that never before has there been such a large group of fine young people not only interested in nutrition but with the courage to apply it, which is where everyone starts.

If you are a housewife, you begin merely by improving your own nutrition; not your husband's or children's quite yet, but just your own. Gradually, in order not to antagonize anyone, you make changes such as buying better food each time you go to market and eliminating the trash foods. You bring home fruits and nuts for the children instead of candy; you avoid the lollipops of dye, synthetic flavoring, and sugar and make delicious ones of pure juices or of yogurt, vanilla, and undiluted, frozen orange juice. You study every label and avoid chemical additives and preservatives. If fertile eggs and medically certified raw milk are not available, you find such eggs and a source of milk safe to use unpasteurized. You locate such supplies as really fresh stone-ground flour and—perhaps with your baker's help—non-instant powdered milk. You may start making homemade bread; everyone enjoys it so much that one of your daughters or even a son or your husband may make it when you are busy.

After you apply personal nutrition for a while, you find that you have twice the energy you formerly had. Energies demand to be used. I recently heard a physician say that his practice was made up largely of women, every one of whom complained of fatigue; and that their fatigue was caused by boredom. To my way of thinking, fatigue prevents people from doing interesting things and is a major cause of boredom. Energies catapult you into rewarding activities; thus life becomes more fascinating for a healthy person than a half-alive one. Radiantly healthy individuals usually become involved in many hobbies such as gardening, tennis, golf, a hiking club, dancing, or yoga exercises; painting, sculpturing, music, Great Books groups, or Little Theater; and in some type of worthwhile community work or church work. These activities come only gradually for the person whose energy level has been low.

Since you now realize that health comes from the kitchen, your first hobby is to discover the fun of cooking. You begin by learning the principles so that you can consistently cook meat which is never tough and fish which is never dry. Soon you can make unbelievably delicious salads; can prepare vegetables people really enjoy; and put genuinely health-building ingredients into desserts. You save money by making your own yogurt. Perhaps you make what the sheepherders call "pocket soup," so stiffly jellied with good meat broth and vegetables that it could be cut into squares and carried in one's pocket. Certainly you get acquainted with herbs and enjoy using them. Since you want to show off your new talents, you invite more friends to dinner.

Soon your acquaintances exclaim, "You look wonderful! What have you been doing?" They want what you now have, the sparkle, the pep, the glow a healthy person radiates. They become interested in nutrition, and before long they report that their fatigue has also given place to energy. Perhaps their leg cramps or headaches have disappeared, their constipation has been corrected, their complexion improved. They ask you to talk to other persons who have problems. Your own children bring in friends who have pimples or menstrual cramps. You have a warm glow inside, knowing that you are helping people. It makes you want to do more.

Perhaps you organize a nutrition study group which meets once a week. For a year you discuss general nutrition, have reports of current books and magazines, and invite in speakers. Later you study nutrition for infants and children, and find it rewarding to share your problems and knowledge with others. Many such groups exist in the United States.

Because you realize no housewife can expect to have a healthy family until she learns to cook delicious meals, you may offer to show friends how to make breads; you enjoy the contact and soon find that you have a nutrition cooking class in your home. Several persons I know have done that, some charging a fee. Lessons may include the 24-hour roasting of inexpensive meats, enhancing the flavor of vegetables, the use of spices and herbs, and making yogurt, fortified meat loaf, high-protein custards and cereals, cookies prepared with oil, and butterscotch brownies made entirely with wheat germ. Discussions of nutrition take place at each lesson.

The more deeply you become involved, the more you may wish to do. Perhaps you volunteer for the refreshment committee and serve really good cookies at the PTA and Women's Club teas; you improve the food at scout meetings and birthday parties; and you put some neighborly love into the church suppers. You get the soft drinks out of the Little League snack shacks, no longer willing to sacrifice children's health to make so little money. If you live in a rural district, you become interested in 4-H Clubs, an organization thousands strong to whom nutrition could be easily and wonderfully taught. If you are a man, you improve the menus at the Breakfast Club and the Rotary and Kiwanis luncheons. In case you are an executive, you realize the stupidity of paying for inefficiency produced by mid-meals of coffee, soft drinks, and doughnuts; you see that nuts, cheeses, milk and milk drinks, and fresh fruits are made available.

If you happen to love children, you show it by getting the soft-drink and candy-bar machines out of the school corridors. You eat at the school cafeteria, observe the mountains of white bread, the sweet gelatin desserts, the soaked, overcooked vegetables, and the utter lack of flavor necessary to give joy to eating. Perhaps you talk to the principal, go before the PTA and/or the school board, or merely volunteer to help.

A friend of mine, aware of sound nutrition, planned menus and frequently supervised lunch preparations in an elementary school cafeteria for the five years her children ate there. She obtained fresh vegetables, often organically grown, and saw that they were quickly steamed or baked,

never allowing their flavor to be robbed by soaking or boiling. Finger salads were served daily. Meat loaves, soups,
and casserole dishes were fortified with powdered milk,
wheat germ, rice polish, and yeast. Fish, for example, was
brushed with mayonnaise, rolled in wheat germ, and baked.
All bread was made daily of stone-ground whole-wheat
flour; it was so delicious that parents soon reported their
children refused the white styrofoam variety long served
at home. Often parents came to school to buy bread for
home use. Because much pasteurized milk was wasted, my
friend changed to medically certified raw milk; the children
enjoyed it so much that the milk consumption quickly
doubled and then tripled. Honey was used instead of sugar.
Usually dessert was fresh fruit, cheese, and dates. Occasionally spice cake, homemade cookies, or sweet muffins were
made with whole-wheat and soy flour, rice polish, wheat
germ, and powdered milk. Any child coming to school
without breakfast was allowed homemade bread, butter,
and milk at the cafeteria.

Not a penny went for trash foods or soft drinks; hence
the cost of running the cafeteria decreased. The employees
found new joy in their work; they were pleased by the
hearty appetites and the compliments which took the place
of complaints. Every teacher in the school and almost every
parent eventually gave the same spontaneous report: the
children were much easier to manage; they were more alert
and learned more quickly; grades improved; the youngsters
were happier, cried less, and fought less; the ones who had
been problem youngsters ceased being problems. Teachers
and children alike were less often ill and missed fewer days
of school. Though rare indeed, this same type of cooking
could easily be done in every school cafeteria in the United
States.

You realize that nutrition should be taught in every class-
room, from kindergarten throughout high school and even
college. You lend your books, magazines, and any material
on nutrition you have to teachers, knowing that, once interested, they will apply it, experience greater health, and soon
be helping students to feel better. In a few communities,
courses in nutrition have been started in several elementary
schools by individuals working through such an organization as the National Health Federation. You realize, too,
that every evening school should have an adult education
class in nutrition; if you cannot find a nurse or practical
dietitian to teach it, offer to teach it yourself. Perhaps you

go back to college for a few courses in foods and chemistry.

If you can get home economics teachers interested in nutrition, you may be sure they will no longer tolerate the disease-producing ingredients they so often use now. I know of one foods teacher who for years made every class a lesson in applied nutrition. She actually taught her students, so soon to be wives, how to become healthy mothers of beautiful children, who will be tomorrow's leaders, thinkers, and doers. She tells me that scarcely a day passes now that a young mother does not stop to show her an outstanding child.

Since athletic coaches are already interested in health, you help to increase their knowledge of nutrition by loaning them whatever books and magazines you have available. They get enthusiastic approval because everyone wants his team to win. An acquaintance who worked in a high school cafeteria and was interested in nutrition used the football team as an entering wedge to improve the food of all the students. She served the athletes much the same type of nutritious food already described (pp. 217-218). For a while their cafeteria had two lines, one serving foods for athletes, the other offering the devitalized foods assumed to be the children's preference. The students, however, soon discovered that the nutritious foods were far more delicious, and the second line was discontinued.

The coach was especially pleased because the football players had developed much greater endurance, were less short-winded and less fatigued. They suffered fewer injuries, and those which did occur healed faster. There was a marked decrease in illnesses, hence fewer practices missed and less school absence. The basketball team won a championship on good nutrition that year. The school physician reported that he could scarcely believe the improvement in physical stamina he found. As in the elementary school, the teachers discovered that the children learned more rapidly and were more co-operative and more cheerful; hence their work was easier. This entire procedure could also be duplicated in every high school cafeteria in our country.

In case you are a science teacher or a mother of children fond of white mice or rats, you might conduct a nutritional experiment. Put each animal or group of animals into a separate cage and give both whole-wheat bread and water; to one give milk, to another a soft drink. The cages must be set on wire, usually above a shallow pan, to prevent the

animals from reaching their feces, rich in B vitamins synthesized by intestinal bacteria. If after a few weeks the
animal or animals given the soft drink look as if they might
die, the diets can be reversed. Such a procedure shows that
the better diet cannot make up for the faulty diet obtained
earlier; and that a poor diet given later during development
is less damaging than one early in life. Instead of contrasting
milk and a soft drink, you might wish to compare stone-
ground whole-wheat bread with so-called "enriched" white
bread; a sweet gelatin dessert with custard or other milk
pudding; or a packaged cold cereal with wheat germ. The
animals must, of course, always have water. If such an
experiment is carried out at home, it could be shared at
school; or if at school, shared with other classrooms. Even
though simple, such experiments make lasting impressions
on children.

If you have ever considered opening a private school, you
should know of one in upper New York State where nutrition is successfully applied. All the vegetables used and
many of the fruits are organically grown on the school
grounds. The children help with the garden, do the milking,
grind wheat and other grains with stone burrs, and make
their own bread. They gather apples from abandoned orchards which have not been coated with poison sprays and
make applesauce and applebutter. Their only sweets are
honey and maple syrup. The mental and physical health of
these youngsters is almost unbelievable. In their studies,
they far excel students of comparable ages in the public
schools; and children in other private schools are no match
for them in athletics. I saw movies of these youngsters
showing them enjoying all sorts of activities including skiing,
mountain climbing, playing football in the pouring rain,
and going on overnight hikes where they lived off the land.
When the school first opened, it was considered essential
to have a physician and a nurse on the staff. Because no
child was ill, the physician was dropped after the first year
and the nurse after the second.

When you realize that a family that can raise some or
much of its food is far healthier than those that must
depend on city markets, you become increasingly interested
in gardening. If space is limited, you may put out chard,
a few tomato plants, and zucchini among the flowers. Most
people outside the large urban centers can plant a few fruit
trees without damage to the landscaping; I have eight such
trees in our small yard. Often an empty lot is available for
gardening where a surplus of vegetables can be raised for

freezing and canning. Many young couples, realizing that because our soils are depleted, our food animals and plants are sick, move to the suburbs especially to have a garden, a small orchard, perhaps a goat or a cow, and a few chickens. Yet one can drive hundreds of miles through the Midwest and see scarcely a garden, though ample land is available, whereas every farm family once raised most of its own food. There is, however, a wonderful organization known as the Natural Food Associates, which believes in building up the soil with natural minerals, compost, and mulches; the food thus grown is vastly more delicious than the freshest produce forced with commercial fertilizers. While there are some farms in our country producing foods by organic methods, they are all too few, especially when one realizes that almost every inch of land in America now needs rebuilding to be made truly fertile. In contrast, last year, when my husband and I drove three thousand miles through rural France, we found every home with a garden, every garden and farm with compost heaps. The flavor and beauty of their produce testifies to the fertility of their loved soil, which they have not allowed to be ravished as we have.

The more interested you become in nutrition, the more you want to help improve our national health. You can help to get new edicts or laws made or unwise old ones retracted by writing to your state and federal senators and representatives, to the Food and Drug Administration at Washington, and even to the President. I am convinced that if the tremendous number of thyroid cancers is to be decreased, laws must be passed requiring that all salt be iodized as it is in Switzerland, and that iodine supplements of 5 milligrams daily should be allowed. One should be permitted to buy PABA and folic acid (with vitamin B_{12}) without a prescription. I believe that laws should be passed forbidding bakers to add dye to bread; and insisting on truth in advertising, imposing heavy fines for half-truths and misleading statements. Antipollution laws should require that every city reclaim its sewage and treat it in order that humus may be returned to the land. Because of the large amounts of toxic fluorides in air pollutants, the fluoridation of water supplies should be discontinued, especially until its effect on heart disease has been studied (p. 202).

Certainly all labeling laws should be improved: food composition should be stated and all additives listed. You have the right to know if an ingredient given merely as "vegetable fat" is unrefined oil or saturated coconut butter; if a cold or canned meat is 50 per cent saturated fat rather than the protein you thought you were buying; and whether any protein food can support growth or has little value. Every soft drink should be required to list all its ingredients, including caffeine, on the label, whether it crosses a state line or not.

All preservatives should be clearly stated with their full chemical names rather than innocent-sounding abbreviations, such as BHA and BHT. Laws should require that no combinations of additives be allowed until tested on animals. Americans now consume an estimated three pounds of synthetic chemicals per year, the combinations of which have by no means been tested. Many food additives have been used for years before they were discovered to be cancer-producing.

If malnutrition is to be stamped out, I feel strongly that laws must be passed now forbidding the marketing of more new "foods" which contain no natural nutrients, thus discouraging the introduction of still other such foodless "foods" as soft drinks, imitation "fruit" juices, and synthetic "fruit" ades. Furthermore, it seems to me that foodless "foods" already on the market should be taxed. Why should alcoholic beverages, which are rarely given to children, be so heavily taxed while soft drinks, which have done incalculable harm to youngsters, be sold tax-free? I wish every reader would join me in demanding of his legislators that a penny tax be levied on every bottle of soft drink, every pound of white flour and refined sugar, and every package of food from which all nutrients have been removed.

You may believe that laws should be passed preventing the food processors from discarding the valuable nutrients from our breadstuffs. A friend who has been living in Iran tells me that the Shah has forbidden white flour to be used in his country. "Their bread is so delicious that every time you go to a bakery, you buy twice as much as you had planned to," she remarked. "Half you eat on the way home, the other half you save for a meal. The only place in the entire country where you can buy white flour is at the United States Embassy commissary." She told me she had never seen an Iranian with crooked teeth; and that heart disease is practically unknown. Similarly in Denmark during World War I and in England during World War II, when wheat germ was allowed to remain in all breadstuffs, such illnesses as high blood pressure and diabetes decreased, and deaths from heart disease dropped markedly despite unbelievable stress. Surely the United States can do what Denmark and England did successfully, even though the Shah's method seems un-American to us. Since our national malnutrition is becoming progressively worse, some such laws will eventually have to be passed, requiring either that wheat germ be left in the flour or that no nutrients be discarded.

You may well ask, "What laws are necessary to prevent wasting billions of tax dollars without eradicating the hunger and malnutrition of low-income citizens?" I would not pretend to have the answer to this vastly complicated problem.[1] Inexpensive solutions, however, have been found for other countries. In Haiti, for example, malnutrition was a major cause of death; severe protein deficiencies were particularly common, though fruits and vegetables were available from home gardens. "Mothercraft centers" were established to teach illiterate women how to prepare a cereal of two parts of corn mashed with one part of beans, a combination previously tested by a group of scientists in the United States.[2] The amino acids lacking in corn were supplied by those in the beans; the combination was almost as high in quality as is milk protein. This corn-and-bean-meal mush was found to be palatable and was well tolerated even by six-months-old babies. For a mere 9 cents per day, a family's calorie intake was increased by 30 per cent and iron and B vitamins by 50 per cent. Within two years, malnutrition had totally disappeared from the areas using the corn-and-bean meal. No billions had been spent, and the educational program was modest indeed. The most important factor, however, was that no trash foods were available. Another group of scientists from the United States has been equally successful in stamping out malnutrition in areas of Central America, again by the use of an inexpensive cereal mixture and the total absence of foods which have been robbed of nutrients. If we in the United States are to eradicate both hunger and malnutrition, somewhat the same steps must be taken here: some basic, inexpensive food or foods high in nutrients must be made available; persons must be taught how to use such food; and trash foods supplying no nutrients must be eliminated.

Lastly, as you have learned more about adequate nutrition, you perhaps feel it will correct certain personal problems, and wish to find a physician knowledgeable in or at least tolerant of nutrition. Thousands of persons write me

[1] N. Kotz, *Let Them Eat Promises: The Politics of Hunger in America* (Englewood Cliffs, New Jersey: Prentice-Hall, Inc., 1969).
[2] *U.S. News & World Report*, Feb. 3, 1969.

each year asking for the names of doctors specializing in nutrition. How can such physicians exist when no medical school teaches the subject? Through no fault of their own, doctors have been made to feel that nutrition is unimportant. If enough people ask such questions as "Where will the baby get linoleic acid if I give him only skim milk?" "Why aren't you allowing him any vitamin E?" "How many milligrams of pantothenic acid should I take daily until I get over my allergies?" or "Why do you recommend an antibiotic instead of vitamin C, which is never toxic?" and physicians hear enough questions which they cannot answer concerning nutrition, perhaps the subject will be taught in medical schools; thousands of practicing physicians are on the staffs of such schools.

If our nation is to survive as a world leader, there is a big job which must be done by big people, the big people sometimes mistakenly called the little people, by uncommon men so wrongly called the common man. I know of many such big people, several of whom have changed the lives of almost everyone in their communities. Without any special training, any organization, any particular leadership, and with very little money, this problem of America's malnutrition could be solved if enough people wanted to solve it. There is work for everyone; every talent is sought. Equally important are the discipline of the scientist, the humanitarianism of the clinician, and the enthusiasm of the amateur.

Nutrition is bigger than a mere study of how to produce health. It has to do with how abundantly life is lived. Francis Bacon once wrote, "A healthy body is a bounteous host to the soul, a sick body, its prison." By our actions, we can help people to be bounteous hosts or condemn them to prisons.

Every person who has the ability to see our country's need can help to fill that need. It is part of my creed—of my religion, if you like—that when you have the ability to help your fellow-man, that ability ceases to be merely an ability and becomes a responsibility. It is this responsibility which must be shouldered by the big people of America.

TABLES OF
FOOD COMPOSITION

FOODS VARY SOMEWHAT IN COMPOSITION; AND THE NUTRIENTS listed in the following tables are not more important than magnesium, cholin, pantothenic acid, and the many other items not listed. A comparison of nutrients obtained in one day with the Recommended Daily Dietary Allowances, however, often reveals many flaws in a diet. Since these allowances are designed for healthy individuals, ill ones should receive two or three times the amounts of all nutrients except sodium and possibly calories. Unfortunately, no data are available for the highly nutritious foods that can be prepared at home.

Because of people who must stay on low-sodium diets, foods are listed unsalted except when salt has been added during preparation, as in packaged cereals and canned soups. People who salt foods lightly should add 3,000 milligrams of sodium to a day's dietary, and those who enjoy well-salted foods, 7,000 milligrams. Normally the intake of potassium should be approximately the same as that of sodium; and the calcium intake should be two-thirds or more of that of phosphorus.

Both animal and vegetable fats contain large amounts of partially unsaturated oleic acid, a non-essential fatty acid that appears to be laid down in the walls of the blood vessels in atherosclerosis; therefore I have combined oleic acid with the saturated fatty acids in the following tables. When the total fat is greater than the sum of oleic acid, the saturated fatty acids, and linoleic acid, the difference represents the amount of linolenic and arachidonic acids present. The ideal amount of linolenic acid needed daily is not known, but it appears to be approximately 15 grams. To support the growth of valuable intestinal bacteria, the diet should also contain 15 grams or more of fiber.

RECOMMENDED DAILY

	Age Years from	to	Wgt. pounds	Hgt. inches	Calories	Protein gm.
MEN	18	35	154	69	2,900	70
	35	55	154	69	2,600	70
	55	75	154	69	2,200	70
WOMEN	18	35	128	64	2,100	58
	35	55	128	64	1,900	58
	55	75	128	64	1,600	58
	During last 6 months of pregnancy				+200	+20
	While nursing infant				+1,000	+40
CHILDREN	1	3	29	34	1,300	32
	3	6	40	42	1,600	40
	6	9	53	49	2,100	52
BOYS	9	12	72	55	2,400	60
	12	15	98	61	3,000	75
	15	18	134	68	3,400	85
GIRLS	9	12	72	55	2,200	55
	12	15	103	62	2,500	62
	15	18	117	64	2,300	58

Equivalents used in the following tables

1 quart	= 4 cups
1 cup	= 8 fluid ounces
	= ½ pint
	= 16 tablespoons
2 tablespoons	= 1 fluid ounce
1 tablespoon (T.)	= 3 teaspoons (t.)
1 stick butter or margarine	= ½ cup
	= 16 pats or squares

DIETARY ALLOWANCES[1]*

Calcium mg.	Iron mg.	VITAMINS					
		A units	B₁ mg.	B₂ mg.	Niacin mg.	C mg.	D units
800	10	5,000	1.2	1.7	19	70	
800	10	5,000	1	1.6	17	70	
800	10	5,000	.9	1.3	15	70	
800	15	5,000	.8	1.3	14	70	
800	15	5,000	.8	1.2	13	70	
800	10	5,000	.8	1.2	13	70	
+500	+5	+1,000	+.2	+.3	+3	+30	400
+500	+5	+3,000	+.4	+.6	+7	+30	400
800	8	2,000	.5	.8	9	40	400
800	10	2,500	.6	1	11	50	400
800	12	3,500	.8	1.3	14	60	400
1,100	15	4,500	1	1.4	16	70	400
1,400	15	5,000	1.2	1.8	20	80	400
1,400	15	5,000	1.4	2	22	80	400
1,100	15	4,500	.9	1.3	15	80	400
1,300	15	5,000	1	1.5	17	80	400
1,300	15	5,000	.9	1.3	15	70	400

[1] Report of Food and Nutrition Board, National Academy of Sciences, National Research Council, Public. 1146 (rev. ed., Washington, D.C., 1964).
* Intended to meet the needs of healthy individuals living in the United States.

TABLES OF FOOD COMPOSITION,

FOOD	Approximate measure	Wgt. in grams	Calories	Protein grams	Carbohydrate grams	Fiber grams	Fat grams	Saturated fatty acid° grams
DAIRY PRODUCTS								
Cows' milk, whole	1 qt.	976	660	32	48	0	40	36
skim	1 qt.	984	360	36	52	0	t	t
Buttermilk, cultured	1 cup	246	127	9	13	0	5	4
Evaporated, undiluted	1 cup	252	345	16	24	0	20	18
Fortified milk, or pep-up†	6 cups	1,419	1,373	89	119	1.4	42	23
High-calorie pep-up†	⅔ cup	160	155	10	13	.2	5	2
Low-calorie pep-up‡	4½ cups	1,053	738	56	62	.2	28	12
Low-calorie pep-up‡	⅞ cup	200	148	11	12	t	5	2
Powdered milk, whole	1 cup	103	515	27	39	0	28	24
skim, instant	1⅓ cups	85	290	30	42	0	t	t
skim, non-instant	⅔ cup	85	290	30	42	0	t	t
Goats' milk, fresh	1 cup	244	165	8	11	0	10	8
Malted milk								
(½ cup ice cream)	2 cups	540	690	24	70	0	24	22
Cocoa	1 cup	252	235	8	26	0	11	10
Yogurt, of partially								
skim milk	1 cup	250	120	8	13	0	4	3
Milk pudding								
(cornstarch)	1 cup	248	275	9	40	0	10	9
Custard, baked	1 cup	248	285	13	28	0	14	11
Ice cream, commercial	1 cup	188	300	6	29	0	18	16
Ice milk, commercial	1 cup	190	275	9	32	0	10	9
Cream, light, or half-and-half	½ cup	120	170	4	5	0	15	13
Cream, heavy, or whipping	½ cup	119	430	2	3	0	47	42

SOURCES: U.S. Department of Agriculture, Agriculture Handbook No. 8 and Home and Garden Bulletin No. 72. Nutritional Data: H. J. Heinz Company, Pittsburgh, Pa., 1963.

EDIBLE PORTIONS

Lino-leic acid grams	MINERALS					VITAMINS				
	Iron	Cal-cium	Phos-phorus	Potas-sium	Sodium	A	B₁	B₂	Niacin	C
grams	mg.	mg.	mg.	mg.	mg.	units	mg.	mg.	mg.	mg.
t	.4	1,140	930	210	75	1,560	.32	1.7	.8	6
0	.4	1,192	940	215	78	0	.4	1.7	.8	6
t	.1	298	270	52	19	180	.1	.4	.2	2
t	.2	570	465	102	38	780	.1	.8	.5	t
14.2	12.1	2,949	3,116	2,704	248	2,670	11.5	10.9	103.5	330
1.7	1.4	333	351	300	27	295	1.3	1.2	9.5	37
12.2	7.4	1,792	2,040	1,015	84	0	10.4	11.4	100.8	6
2.5	1.5	358	408	203	17	0	2.1	2.3	20.1	1
t	.4	968	1,160	200	72	1,160	.3	1.5	.7	t
0	.4	1,040	940	210	75	t	.2	1.4	.7	t
0	.4	1,040	940	210	75	t	.2	1.4	.7	t
t	.2	315	212	66	8	390	.1	.3	.7	2
t	.8	270	615	60	19	670	.3	1.1	.2	2
t	.9	280	212	50	19	390	.1	.5	.3	t
t	.1	295	270	50	19	170	.1	.4	.2	t
t	.1	290	260	48	21	360	.1	.4	.1	t
1	1	278	370	100	60	870	.1	.5	.2	t
1	.1	175	150	170	140	740	t§	.3	.1	t
t	.1	290	250	54	58	390	.1	.4	.2	t
t	t	130	90	95	55	550	t	.2	t§	t
1	0	82	70	65	50	1,900	t	.1	t	t

* Includes oleic acid.   t Indicates trace only.

† Made by recipe on pp. 219-220 with 2 eggs, torula yeast fortified with calcium, and a 6-ounce can of frozen undiluted orange juice.

‡ Made with torula yeast fortified with calcium. Since lecithin and milk sugar are apparently not used for calories, the total calorie content of 4½ cups is probably 425.

§ Contains less than .1 milligram.

FOOD	Approximate measure	Wgt. in grams	Calories	Protein grams	Carbohydrate grams	Fiber grams	Fat grams	Saturated fatty acid° grams
DAIRY PRODUCTS (Continued)								
Cheese, cottage,								
creamed	1 cup	225	240	30	6	0	11	10
uncreamed	1 cup	225	195	38	6	0	t	t
Cheddar, or American	1-in. cube	17	70	4	t	0	6	5
Cheddar, grated	½ cup	56	226	14	1	0	19	17
Cream cheese	1 oz.	28	105	2	1	0	11	10
Processed cheese	1 oz.	28	105	7	t	0	9	8
Roquefort type	1 oz.	28	105	6	t	0	9	8
Swiss	1 oz.	28	105	7	t	0	8	7
Eggs, boiled, poached,								
or raw	2	100	150	12	t	0	12	10
Scrambled, omelet,								
or fried	2	128	220	13	1	0	16	14
Yolks only	2	34	120	6	t	0	10	8
OILS, FATS, AND SHORTENINGS								
Butter	1 T.	14	100	t	t	0	11	10
Butter	½ cup or ¼ lb.	112	800	t	1	0	90	80
Hydrogenated cooking								
fat	½ cup	100	665	0	0	0	100	88
Lard	½ cup	110	992	0	0	0	110	92
Margarine, ¼ pound or	½ cup	112	806	t	t	0	91	76
Margarine, 2 pats or	1 T.	14	100	t	t	0	11	9
Mayonnaise	1 T.	15	110	t	t	0	12	5
Oils								
Corn, soy, peanut‡								
cottonseed	1 T.	14	125	0	0	0	14	5
Olive	1 T.	14	125	0	0	0	14	13
Safflower, sunflower								
seed, walnut	1 T.	14	125	0	0	0	14	3
Salad dressing								
French	1 T.	15	60	t	2	0	6	2
Thousand Island	1 T.	15	75	t	1	0	8	3
Salt pork	2 oz.	60	470	3	0	0	55	—

Lino- leic acid grams	MINERALS					VITAMINS				
	Iron mg.	Cal- cium mg.	Phos- phorus mg.	Potas- sium mg.	Sodium mg.	A units	B₁ mg.	B₂ mg.	Niacin mg.	C mg.
t	.9	207	360	170	625	430	.1	.6	.2	0
t	.9	202	380	180	620	20	.1	.6	.1	0
t	.1	133	128	30	180	230	t	.1	t	0
t	.6	435	390	90	540	700	t	.2	t	0
t	.1	18	170	25	180	440	t	.1	t	0
t	.1	210	190	22	370	350	t	.1	t	0
t	.2	122	100	22	284	350	t	.2	.1	0
t	.2	270	140	25	225	320	t	.1	t	0
1	2.3	54	205	129	122	1,180	t	.3	t	0
1	2.2	60	222	140	338	1,200	t	.4	t	0
1	1.8	48	175	33	9	1,180	t	.1	t	0
t	t	3	0	4	120	460	0	t†	0	0
2	t	22	0	28	990	3,700	0	t	0	0
7	0	0	0	0	4	0	0	0	0	0
11	0	0	0	t	t	0	0	0	0	0
8	0	22	16	58	1,150	3,700	0	t	0	0
1	0	3	2	9	144	460	0	0	0	0
6	.1	2	8	3	85	40	t	t	t	0
7	0	0	0	0	0	0	0	0	0	0
1	0	0	0	0	0	0	0	0	0	0
9	0	0	0	0	0	0	0	0	0	0
3	.1	3	0	0	—	0	0	0	0	0
4	.1	2	t	—	—	60	t	t	t	0
—	.4	t	t	19	1,350	0	t	t	t	0

* Includes oleic acid.
t Indicates trace only.
† Contains less than .1 milligram.

‡ Richest source of arachidonic acid.
— No data available.

FOOD	Approximate measure	Wgt. in grams	Calories	Protein grams	Carbohydrate grams	Fiber grams	Fat grams	Saturated fatty acid* grams
MEAT AND POULTRY, COOKED								
Bacon, crisp, drained	2 slices	16	95	4	1	0	8	7
Beef, chuck, pot-roasted	3 oz.	85	245	23	0	0	16	15
Hamburger, commercial	3 oz.	85	245	21	0	0	17	15
Ground lean	3 oz.	85	185	24	0	0	10	9
Roast beef, oven-cooked	3 oz.	85	390	16	0	0	36	35
Steak, as sirloin	3 oz.	85	330	20	0	0	27	25
Steak, lean, as round	3 oz.	85	220	24	0	0	12	11
Corned beef	3 oz.	85	185	22	0	0	10	9
Corned beef hash, canned	3 oz.	85	120	12	6	t	8	7
Dried or chipped	2 oz.	56	115	19	0	0	4	4
Pot-pie, 4½" diameter	1 pie	227	460	18	32	t	28	25
Stew, with vegetables	1 cup	235	185	15	15	t	10	9
Chicken, broiled	3 oz.	85	185	23	0	0	9	7
Fried, breast or leg and thigh	3 oz.	85	245	25	0	0	15	11
Roasted	3½ oz.	100	290	25	0	0	20	16
Chicken livers, fried	3 med.	100	140	22	2.3	0	14	12
Duck, domestic	3½ oz.	100	370	16	0	0	28	—
Lamb, chop, broiled	4 oz.	115	480	24	0	0	35	33
Leg, roasted	3 oz.	86	314	20	0	0	14	14
Shoulder, braised	3 oz.	85	285	18	0	0	23	21
Pork, chop, 1 thick	3½ oz.	100	260	16	0	0	21	18
Ham, cured, pan-broiled	3 oz.	85	290	16	0	0	22	19
Ham, as luncheon meat	2 oz.	57	170	13	0	0	13	11
Ham, canned, spiced	2 oz.	57	165	8	1	0	14	12
Pork roast	3 oz.	85	310	21	0	0	24	21
Pork sausage, bulk	3½ oz.	100	475	18	0	0	44	40
Turkey, roasted	3½ oz.	100	265	27	0	0	15	—
Veal, cutlet, broiled	3 oz.	85	185	23	0	0	9	8
Roast	3 oz.	85	335	23	0	0	14	13

Lino-leic acid grams	MINERALS					VITAMINS				
	Iron mg.	Calcium mg.	Phosphorus mg.	Potassium mg.	Sodium mg.	A units	B_1 mg.	B_2 mg.	Niacin mg.	C mg.
1	.5	2	42	65	600	0	t	t	.8	0
t	2.9	10	110	340	50	30	t	.18	3.5	0
t	2.7	9	145	320	100	30	t	t	5.1	0
t	3	10	158	340	110	20	t	t	5.3	0
t	2.1	7	105	350	60	60	t	t	3	0
1	2.5	8	150	320	60	50	t	t	4	0
t	3	11	180	300	62	20	t	t	4.8	0
t	3.7	17	100	60	1,200	20	t	.2	2.9	0
t	1.1	20	125	180	540	10	t	.1	2.4	0
0	2.9	10	60	190	30	t	t	.2	2.2	0
1	2.5	20	150	318	620	2,800	t	.1	3	t
t	2.8	30	150	500	75	2,500	.1	.2	4.4	14
2	1.4	10	250	350	50	260	t	.1	7	0
2	1.8	13	218	320	50	200	t	.1	5	0
4	1.9	10	220	280	58	960	t	.2	7.4	0
2	7.4	16	240	160	51	32,200	.2	2.4	11.8	20
—	2.4	9	170	285	74	—	t	.4	7.9	0
1	3.1	10	140	275	75	0	.1	.2	4.5	0
0	2.8	9	190	270	70	0	.1	.2	5	0
1	2.4	8	170	260	60	0	.1	.2	4	0
2	2.2	8	250	390	30	0	.6	.2	3.8	0
2	2.2	8	240	370	1,000	0	.4	.1	3	0
1	1.5	5	170	290	700	0	.2	.1	1.6	0
1	1.2	5	170	280	800	0	.2	.1	1.8	0
2	2.7	9	240	360	40	0	.8	.2	4.4	0
3	2.4	7	165	270	958	0	.8	.3	3.7	0
—	3.8	23	320	320	60	0	t	.1	8	0
t	2.7	9	230	400	70	0	t	.2	6	0
t	2.9	10	200	390	70	0	.1	.3	6.6	0

* Includes oleic acid.
t Indicates trace only.
— No data available.

FOOD	Approximate measure	Wgt. in grams	Calories	Protein grams	Carbohydrate grams	Fiber grams	Fat grams	Saturated fatty acid* grams
VARIETY MEATS								
Brains, beef, calf, pork, sheep	3½ oz.	100	125	10	0	0	8	—
Chili con carne with beans	1 cup	250	325	19	30	1.2	15	14
Without beans	1 cup	255	510	26	15	t	38	36
Heart, braised	3 oz.	85	160	26	1	0	5	4
Kidney, braised	3½ oz.	100	230	33	1	0	7	—
Liver, beef, sautéed with oil	3½ oz.	100	230	26	5	0	10	7
Calf, 1 large slice	3½ oz.	100	261	29	4	0	13	—
Lamb, 2 slices	3½ oz.	100	260	32	3	0	12	—
Pork, 2 slices	3½ oz.	100	241	29	3	0	11	—
Liver, desiccated see Supplementary foods								
Sausage, bologna	2 slices, ⅛ × 4"	50	124	7	2	t	10	9
Frankfurter	2, ¾ × 7"	102	246	14	2	t	20	18
Liverwurst	2 oz.	56	132	8	1	0	11	—
Sweetbreads, calf, braised	3½ oz.	100	170	32	0	0	3	—
Tongue, beef	3 oz.	85	205	18	t	0	14	13
FISH AND SEA FOODS								
Clams, steamed or canned	3 oz.	85	87	12	2	0	1	—
Cod, broiled	3½ oz.	100	170	28	0	0	5	0
Codfish cakes, fried	2 small	100	175	15	9	—	8	—
Crab meat, cooked	3 oz.	85	90	14	1	0	2	0
Fish sticks, breaded, fried	5	112	200	19	8	0	10	5
Flounder, baked	3½ oz.	100	200	30	0	0	8	0
Haddock, fried	3 oz.	85	135	16	6	0	5	4
Halibut, broiled	3½ oz.	100	182	26	0	0	8	0
Herring, kippered	1 small	100	211	22	0	0	13	0
Lobster, steamed	½ aver.	100	92	18	t	0	1	0
Mackerel, canned	3 oz.	85	155	18	0	0	9	0
Oysters, raw	6-8 med. or ½ cup	120	85	8	3	0	2	0

Lino-leic acid grams	MINERALS					VITAMINS				
	Iron mg.	Cal-cium mg.	Phos-phorus mg.	Potas-sium mg.	Sodium mg.	A units	B_1 mg.	B_2 mg.	Niacin mg.	C mg.
—	2.4	10	312	219	125	0	.2	.2	4.4	0
t	4.2	98	360	500	1,060	100	t	.2	3.5	0
1	5.9	14	365	520	1,000	130	t	.3	5.6	0
t	6	14	203	190	90	30	.2	1	6.8	—
—	13.1	18	220	320	250	1,150	.5	4.8	10.7	0
2	9	8	476	380	184	53,400	.3	4.1	16.5	27
—	14.2	13	537	453	118	32,000	.2	4.2	16.5	37
—	17.9	16	572	330	85	74,000	.5	5.1	24.9	36
—	29	15	539	390	111	14,000	.3	4.4	22.3	22
t	1.2	4	54	110	550	0	t	t	1.3	0
1	1.2	6	50	215	1,100	0	.1	.2	2.5	0
—	2.8	4	120	75	450	2,860	.2	.6	2.3	0
—	.8	7	360	244	116	0	.1	.3	5	0
t	2.5	7	180	240	90	0	t	.3	3	0
—	5.4	74	110	230	170	100	t	t	.9	0
—	1	30	270	400	110	180	t	.1	3	0
—	—	—	—	—	—	—	—	—	—	0
0	.8	38	170	100	900	—	t	t	2.1	0
5	.4	12	180	140	—	t	0	t	1.6	0
—	1.4	22	344	585	235	0	t	t	2.5	0
t	.7	11	200	510	56	0	t	t	2.6	0
0	.8	14	267	540	56	440	t	t	9.2	0
0	1.4	66	254	—	—	110	t	.1	3.4	0
0	.6	65	192	180	210	0	.1	t	1.9	0
0	1.9	221	260	—	—	20	t	.3	7.4	0
0	6.6	113	150	120	80	320	.2	.2	3.3	0

* Includes oleic acid.
t Indicates trace only.
— No data available.

FOOD	Approxi-mate measure	Wgt. in grams	Calo-ries	Pro-tein grams	Carbo-hydrate grams	Fiber grams	Fat grams	Satu-rated fatty acid* grams
FISH AND SEA FOODS (Continued)								
Oyster stew, made with milk	1 cup	230	200	11	11	0	12	—
Salmon, canned	3 oz.	85	120	17	0	0	5	1
Sardines, canned	3 oz.	85	180	22	0	0	9	4
Scallops, breaded, fried	3½ oz.	100	194	18	10	0	8	—
Shad, baked	3 oz.	85	170	20	0	0	10	0
Shrimp, steamed	3 oz.	85	110	23	0	0	1	0
Swordfish, broiled	1 steak	100	180	27	0	0	6	0
Tuna, canned, drained	3 oz.	85	170	25	0	0	7	3
VEGETABLES								
Artichoke, globe	1 large	100	8-44	2	10†	2	t	t
Asparagus, green	6 spears	96	18	1	3	.5	t	t
Beans, green snap	1 cup	125	25	1	6	.6	t	t
Lima, green	1 cup	160	140	8	24	3	t	t
Lima, dry, cooked	1 cup	192	260	16	48	2	t	t
Navy, baked with pork	¾ cup	200	250	11	37	2	6	6
Red kidney, canned	1 cup	260	230	15	42	2.5	1	0
Bean sprouts, uncooked	1 cup	50	17	1	3	.3	t	0
Beet greens, steamed	1 cup	100	27	2	6	1.4	t	0
Beetroots, boiled	1 cup	165	68	1	12	.8	t	0
Broccoli, steamed	1 cup	150	45	5	8	1.9	t	0
Brussels sprouts, steamed	1 cup	130	60	6	12	1.7	t	0
Cabbage, as coleslaw‡	1 cup	120	140	1	9	1	14	4
Sauerkraut, canned	1 cup	150	32	1	7	1.5	t	0
Steamed cabbage	1 cup	170	40	2	9	1.3	t	0
Carrots, cooked, diced	1 cup	150	45	1	10	.9	t	0
Raw, grated	1 cup	110	45	1	10	1.2	t	0
Strips, from raw	1 med.	50	20	t	5	.5	t	0
Cauliflower, steamed	1 cup	120	30	3	6	1	t	0
Celery, cooked, diced	1 cup	100	20	1	4	1	t	0
Stalk, raw	1 large	40	5	1	1	.3	t	0
Chard, steamed, leaves and stalks	1 cup	150	30	2	7	1.4	t	0
Collards, steamed leaves	1 cup	150	51	5	8	2	t	0
Corn, steamed	1 ear	100	92	3	21	.8	1	t
Cooked or canned	1 cup	200	170	5	41	1.6	t	0

Lino-leic acid grams	MINERALS					VITAMINS				
	Iron	Cal-cium	Phos-phorus	Potas-sium	Sodium	A	B_1	B_2	Niacin	C
grams	mg.	mg.	mg.	mg.	mg.	units	mg.	mg.	mg.	mg.
—	3.3	269	230	310	940	640	.1	.4	1.7	0
0	.7	160	280	340	45	60	t	.2	6.8	0
4	2.5	367	490	540	480	190	t	.2	4.6	0
—	1.4	110	338	470	265	0	t	.1	1.4	0
0	.5	20	300	350	75	20	.1	.2	7.3	0
0	2.6	98	250	205	130	50	t	t	1.9	0
0	1.1	20	250	780	51	2,000	t	t	10.3	0
4	1.2	7	300	240	700	70	t	.1	10.9	0
0	1.3	50	69	300	30	150	t	t	.7	8
0	1.7	18	43	130	3	700	t	t	.9	18
0	.9	45	20	204	2	830	t	.1	.6	16
0	2.5	44	105	320	2	290	.2	.1	1.9	15
0	1.5	15	75	306	1	t	.3	.1	1.3	0
0	4.2	112	226	420	960	t	.1	.1	1.3	t
t	4.6	74	350	750	6	0	.1	.1	1.5	0
t	3.8	19	170	514	3	40	.2	.1	1.3	t
t	3.2	118	45	332	76	5,100	t	.1	.3	30
t	1	24	44	324	64	30	t	t	.5	10
t	2.1	190	100	405	15	5,100	t	.2	1.2	105
t	1.7	44	95	400	14	520	t	.1	.6	60
9	.5	47	30	240	150	80	t	t	.3	50
t	.8	54	45	210	915	0	t	.1	.2	24
t	.8	78	50	240	23	150	t	t	.3	53
t	.9	38	55	600	75	18,130	t	t	.7	6
t	.9	43	29	410	51	13,000	t	t	.7	7
t	.4	20	19	205	25	5,000	t	t	.3	3
t	1.2	26	84	220	11	100	t	.1	.6	34
t	.5	54	40	300	80	0	t	t	.4	7
t	.2	20	18	130	30	0	t	t	.2	3
t	3.6	155	54	475	120	8,100	t	.1	.1	17
t	1.2	282	75	393	40	11,700	t	.2	1.6	75
t	.5	4	120	300	t	300	t	t	1.1	12
t	1.3	10	102	400	472§	520	t	.1	2.4	14

* Includes oleic acid.   † Largely inulin, which is not utilized in the body.
t Indicates trace only.   ‡ With mayonnaise.
— No data available.   § Salted.

FOOD	Approximate measure	Wgt. in grams	Calories	Protein grams	Carbohydrate grams	Fiber grams	Fat grams	Saturated fatty acid* grams
VEGETABLES (Continued)								
Cucumbers, ⅛" slices	6	50	6	t	1	.2	0	0
Dandelion greens, steamed	1 cup	180	80	5	16	3.2	1	0
Eggplant, steamed	1 cup	180	30	2	9	1.2	t	0
Endive (escarole)	2 oz.	57	10	1	2	.6	t	—
Kale, steamed	1 cup	110	45	4	8	.9	1	—
Kohlrabi, raw, sliced	1 cup	140	40	2	9	1.5	t	—
Lambs'-quarters, steamed	1 cup	150	48	5	7	3.2	t	—
Lentils	1 cup	200	212	15	38	2.4	t	—
Lettuce, loose leaf, green	¼ head	100	14	1	2	.5	t	—
Iceberg	¼ head	100	13	t	3	.5	t	—
Mushrooms, cooked or canned	½ cup	120	12	2	4	t	t	—
Mustard greens, steamed	1 cup	140	30	3	6	1.2	t	—
Okra, diced, steamed	1⅓ cups	100	32	1	7	1	t	—
Onions, mature, cooked	1 cup	210	80	2	18	1.6	t	—
Raw, green	6 small	50	22	t	5	1	t	—
Parsley, chopped, raw	2 T.	7	2	t	t	t	t	—
Parsnips, steamed	1 cup	155	95	2	22	3	1	—
Peas, green, canned	1 cup	100	68	3	13	1.4	t	—
Fresh, steamed	1 cup	100	70	5	12	2.2	t	—
Frozen, heated	1 cup	100	68	5	12	1.8	t	—
Split, cooked	½ cup	100	115	8	21	.4	t	—
With carrots, frozen, heated	1 cup	100	53	3	10	1	t	—
Peppers, pimientos, canned	1 pod	38	10	t	2	t	t	—
Raw, green, sweet	1 large	100	25	1	6	1.4	t	—
Stuffed with beef and crumbs	1 med.	150	255	19	24	.1	9	8
Potatoes, baked	1 med.	100	100	2	22	.5	t	—
French-fried	10 pieces	60	155	1	20	.4	7	3
Mashed with milk and butter	1 cup	200	230	4	28	.7	12	11

Lino- leic acid grams	MINERALS					VITAMINS				
	Iron mg.	Cal- cium mg.	Phos- phorus mg.	Potas- sium mg.	Sodium mg.	A units	B₁ mg.	B₂ mg.	Niacin mg.	C mg.
0	.1	5	9	80	3	0	t	t	.1	4
t	5.6	337	126	760	130	27,300	.3	.2	1.3	29
t	.9	17	60	390	2	10	t	t	.9	8
—	1	45	28	215	9	1,700	t	t	.1	6
—	1.3	130	57	260	29	8,000	t	.2	.8	60
—	.8	66	70	520	10	t	t	t	.3	85
—	1	460	100	—	—	14,650	.1	.4	1.4	120
—	4.1	50	238	505	15	40	t	t	1.2	0
—	2	35	26	260	9	1,900	t	t	.3	18
—	.5	20	22	175	9	300	t	t	.3	6
—	.9	8	105	180	400†	0	t	.3	3	3
—	4.1	308	60	510	68	10,050	.1	.2	1	60
—	.7	82	62	370	1	740	t	t	.8	20
—	1	67	88	315	14	0	t	t	.4	10
—	.4	65	12	115	2	500	t	t	.2	16
—	.4	14	7	80	1	580	t	t	.2	14
—	1.1	88	120	570	11	0	t	.2	.3	19
—	1.8	25	67	96	270	500	.1	t.	1	8
—	1.9	22	122	200	1	960	.3	.1	2.3	24
—	1.8	19	86	135	115	600	.2	t	1.7	13
—	1.7	11	89	296	13	40	.2	t	.9	0
—	1.1	25	57	160	84	9,000	.2	t	1.3	10
—	.7	9	10	50	t	800	.1	t	1.7	20
—	.4	11	25	170	t	370	t	t	.4	120
t	3	60	180	387	420	420	.1	.2	3.5	60
—	.7	13	66	500	4	10	.1	t	1.2	15
4‡	.7	9	6	510	6	0	t	t	1.8	8
t	1	45	150	654	660	470	.2	.1	1.6	16

* Includes oleic acid.
t Indicates trace only.
— No data available.

† Salted.
‡ If fried in oil.

FOOD	Approximate measure	Wgt. in grams	Calories	Protein grams	Carbohydrate grams	Fiber grams	Fat grams	Saturated fatty acid° grams
VEGETABLES (Continued)								
Potatoes, pan-fried	¾ cup	100	268	4	33	.4	14	6
Scalloped with cheese	¾ cup	100	145	6	14	.4	8	7
Steamed before peeling	1 med.	100	80	2	19	.4	t	—
Potato chips	10	20	110	1	10	t	7	4
Radishes, raw	5 small	50	10	t	2	.3	0	—
Rutabagas, diced	⅔ cup	100	32	t	8	1.4	0	0
Soybeans, unseasoned	1 cup	200	260	22	20	3.2	11	0
Spinach, steamed	1 cup	100	26	3	3	1	t	—
Squash, summer	1 cup	210	35	1	8	.6	t	—
Winter, mashed	1 cup	200	95	4	23	2.6	t	—
Sweet potatoes, baked	1 med.	110	155	2	36	1	1	—
Candied	1 med.	175	235	2	CO	1.5	6	5
Tomatoes, canned whole	1 cup	240	50	2	9	1	t	—
Raw, 2 by 2½"	1 med.	150	30	1	6	.6	t	—
Tomato juice, canned	1 cup	240	50	2	10	.6	t	—
Tomato catsup	1 T.	17	15	t	4	t	t	—
Turnip greens, steamed	1 cup	145	45	4	8	1.8	1	—
Turnips, steamed, sliced	1 cup	155	40	1	9	1.8	t	—
Watercress, leaves and stems, raw	1 cup	50	9	1	1	.3	t	—
FRUITS								
Apple juice, fresh or canned	1 cup	250	125	t	34	—	0	0
Apple vinegar	⅓ cup	100	14	t	3	0	0	0
Apples, raw	1 med.	130	70	t	18	1	t	—
Stewed or canned	1 cup	240	100‡	t	26	2	t	—
Apricots, canned in syrup	1 cup	250	220	2	57	1	t	—
Dried, uncooked	½ cup	75	220	4	50	1	t	—
Fresh	3 med.	114	55	1	14	.7	t	—
Nectar, or juice	1 cup	250	140	1	36	2	t	—
Avocado	½ large	108	185	2	6	1.8	18	12
Banana	1 med.	150	85	1	23	.9	t	—
Blackberries, fresh	1 cup	144	85	2	19	6.6	1	—
Blueberries, canned	1 cup	250	245	1	65	2	t	—
Cantaloupe	½ med.	380	40	1	9	2.2	t	—

Lino-leic acid grams	MINERALS					VITAMINS				
	Iron	Cal-cium	Phos-phorus	Potas-sium	Sodium	A	B$_1$	B$_2$	Niacin	C
grams	mg.	mg.	mg.	mg.	mg.	units	mg.	mg.	mg.	mg.
8†	1.1	15	100	775	225	0	.1	t	2.8	20
t	.5	127	122	310	450	320	t	.1	.9	10
—	.8	11	56	407	3	10	.1	t	1.2	15
3†	.4	6	38	210	200	t	t	t	.6	0
—	.5	5	53	130	4	15	t	t	.1	12
0	.4	40	35	170	4	350	t	t	.7	21
7	5.4	150	360	1,080	4	60	.4	.1	1.2	0
—	.2	124	33	470	74	11,800	.1	.2	.6	30
—	.8	8	32	480	8	700	t	.1	1.3	24
—	1.6	23	49	510	2	6,100	t	.1	.6	7
—	1	36	58	300	12	8,900	.1	t	.7	24
1	1.6	50	70	360	18	11,600	.1	.1	1.1	30
—	1.5	27	44	552	18	2,500	.1	t	1.7	40
—	.9	16	40	360	5	2,600	t	t	.8	35
—	1	17	80	540	36	2,500	.1	t	1.8	38
—	.1	2	3	160	260	300	t	t	.4	2
—	3.5	375	75	—	—	15,300	.1	.6	1	90
—	.8	62	51	345	87	t	t	t	.6	28
—	.8	75	27	140	25	2,500	t	1	.4	80
0	1.2	15	12	200	5	90	t	t	t	t
0	.6	6	9	100	1	0	0	0	0	0
—	.4	8	13	130	1	50	t	t	t	3
—	1	10	12	210	4	80	t	t	.1	3
—	8	28	37	600	2	4,500	t	t	.9	10
—	4.1	50	75	780	19	8,000	t	.1	3	9
—	.5	18	30	280	1	2,900	t	t	.7	10
—	.5	22	30	440	t	2,300	t	t	.5	7
2	.6	11	42	600	4	310	.1	.2	1.7	15
—	.7	8	44	390	1	190	t	t	.7	10
—	1.3	46	46	220	t	290	t	t	.5	30
—	.5	100	15	200	2	100	t	t	.2	30
—	.8	33	64	910	40	6,000	t	t	1	65

* Includes oleic acid.   † If fried in oil.
t Indicates trace only.   ‡ Unsweetened.
— No data available.

FOOD	Approximate measure	Wgt. in grams	Calories	Protein grams	Carbohydrate grams	Fiber grams	Fat grams	Saturated fatty acid° grams
FRUITS (Continued)								
Cherries, canned, pitted†	1 cup	257	100	2	26	2	1	—
Fresh, raw	1 cup	114	65	1	15	.3	t	—
Cranberry sauce, sweetened	1 cup	277	530	t	142	1.2	t	—
Dates, dried	1 cup	178	505	4	134	3.6	t	—
Figs, dried, large, 2 by 1"	2	42	120	2	30	1.9	t	—
Fresh, raw	3 med.	114	90	2	22	1	t	—
Stewed or canned, with syrup	3	115	130	1	32	1	t	—
Fruit cocktail, canned	1 cup	256	195	1	50	.5	t	—
Grapefruit, canned sections	1 cup	250	170	1	44	.5	t	—
Grapefruit, fresh, 5" diameter	½	285	50	1	14	1	t	t
Grapefruit juice†	1 cup	250	100	1	24	1	t	—
Grapes, American, as Concord	1 cup	153	70	1	16	.8	t	—
European, as Muscat, Tokay	1 cup	160	100	1	26	.7	t	—
Grape juice, bottled	1 cup	250	160	1	42	t	t	—
Lemon juice, fresh	½ cup	125	30	t	10	t	t	—
Lemonade concentrate, frozen	6-oz. can	220	430	t	112	t	t	—
Limeade concentrate, frozen	6-oz. can	218	405	t	108	t	t	—
Olives, green, canned, large	10	65	72	1	3	.8	10	9
Ripe, canned, large	10	65	105	1	1	1	13	12
Oranges, fresh, 3" diameter	1 med.	180	60	2	16	1	t	t
Orange juice, fresh	8 oz. or 1 glass	250	112	2	25	.2	t	—
Frozen concentrate	6-oz. can	210	330	2	78	.4	t	t

Lino-leic acid grams	MINERALS					VITAMINS				
	Iron mg.	Cal-cium mg.	Phos-phorus mg.	Potas-sium mg.	Sodium mg.	A units	B₁ mg.	B₂ mg.	Niacin mg.	C mg.
—	.7	37	30	135	8	1,680	t	t	.4	13
—	.4	18	20	270	1	620	t	t	.4	10
—	.8	34	27	150	3	80	t	t	.3	5
—	5.7	105	110	1,300	1	100	.1	.2	3.9	0
—	1.7	80	55	390	15	40	.1	t	.8	0
—	.4	35	20	110	1	90	t	t	.6	2
—	.4	36	21	105	1	50	t	t	.4	0
—	1	23	30	350	12	360	t	t	1	5
—	.7	32	35	237	2	20	t	t	.5	75
0	.5	21	54	290	4	10	t	t	.3	72
—	1	20	40	280	2	20	t	t	.4	84
—	.4	13	30	120	5	100	t	t	.3	4
—	.6	18	30	240	6	120	t	t	.4	7
—	.8	28	33	450	1	t	.1	t	.6	t
—	.2	8	13	80	4	20	t	t	.1	50
—	.4	9	15	170	5	40	t	t	.7	66
—	.7	11	12	118	t	t	t	t	.2	260
t	1.2	65	13	45	1,400	200	t	0	0	0
t	1.1	56	11	23	650	60	t	t	0	0
—	.5	50	40	300	t	240	1	t	.3	75
—	.5	27	42	500	2	500	.2	t	1	129
—	.8	69	115	1,315	4	1,490	.6	.1	2.4	330

* Includes oleic acid.   — No data available.
t Indicates trace only.   † Unsweetened.

FOOD	Approximate measure	Wgt. in grams	Calories	Protein grams	Carbohydrate grams	Fiber grams	Fat grams	Saturated fatty acid* grams
FRUITS (Continued)								
Papaya, fresh	½ med.	200	75	1	18	1.8	t	—
Peaches, canned, sliced	1 cup	257	200	1	52	1	t	—
Fresh, raw	1 med.	114	35	1	10	.6	t	—
Pears, canned, sweetened	1 cup	255	195	1	50	2	t	—
Raw, 3 by 2½"	1 med.	182	100	1	25	2	1	—
Persimmons, Japanese	1 med.	125	75	1	20	2	t	—
Pineapple, canned, sliced	1 large slice	122	95	t	26	.4	t	—
Crushed	1 cup	260	205	1	55	.7	t	—
Raw, diced	1 cup	140	75	1	19	.6	t	—
Pineapple juice, canned‡	1 cup	250	120	1	32	.2	t	—
Plums, canned in syrup	1 cup	256	185	1	50	.7	t	—
Raw, 2" diameter	1	60	30	t	7	.2	t	—
Prunes, cooked‡	1 cup	270	300	3	81	.8	1	—
Prune juice, canned‡	1 cup	240	170	1	45	.7	t	—
Raisins, dried	½ cup	80	230	2	62	.7	t	—
Raspberries, frozen	½ cup	100	100	t	25	2	t	—
Raw,‡ red	¾ cup	100	57	t	14	5	t	—
Rhubarb, cooked, sweetened	1 cup	270	385	1	98	1.9	t	—
Strawberries, frozen	1 cup	227	242	1	60	1.3	t	—
Raw‡	1 cup	149	54	t	12	1.9	t	—
Tangerines, fresh	1 med.	114	40	1	10	1	t	—
Watermelon, 4 by 8"	1 wedge	925	120	2	29	3.6	1	—
BREADS, CEREALS, GRAINS, AND GRAIN PRODUCTS								
Biscuits, 2½" diameter§	1	38	130	3	18	t	4	3
Bran flakes	1 cup	25	117	3	32	1.3	t	—
Bread, cracked wheat	1 slice	23	60	2	12	.1	1	1
Rye	1 slice	23	55	2	12	.1	t	t
White,‖ 20 slices, or a	1-lb. loaf¶	454	1,225	39	229	9	15	12
Whole-wheat	1-lb. loaf	454	1,100	48	216	67.5	14	10
Whole-wheat	1 slice	23	55	2	11	.3	1	—
Corn bread of whole-ground meal	1 serving	50	100	3	15	.3	4	2

Lino-leic acid grams	MINERALS					VITAMINS				
	Iron mg.	Cal-cium mg.	Phos-phorus mg.	Potas-sium mg.	Sodium mg.	A units	B₁ mg.	B₂ mg.	Niacin mg.	C mg.
—	.5	40	32	470	6	3,500	t	t	.6	112
—	.8	11	35	310	6	1,100	t	t	1.4	7
—	.5	9	22	31	5	1,320†	t	t	1	7
—	.5	13	30	75	12	t	t	t	.3	4
—	.5	13	29	182	3	30	t	t	.2	7
—	.4	7	28	310	1	2,710	t	t	.1	11
—	.7	26	9	150	1	100	.1	t	.2	11
—	1.6	75	15	140	2	210	.2	t	.4	23
—	.4	22	12	210	1	180	.1	t	.3	33
—	1.2	37	22	370	2	200	.1	t	.4	22
—	2.7	20	25	213	2	260	t	t	.9	3
—	.3	10	10	100	t	200	t	t	.3	3
—	4.5	60	100	810	10	1,800	t	.2	1.8	3
—	9.8	34	100	625	5	—	t	t	1.1	4
—	2.8	50	112	575	19	15	.1	t	.4	0
—	.6	12	17	95	t	80	t	t	.6	20
—	.9	40	37	190	t	130	t	t	.3	24
—	1.1	112	39	510	15	70	t	0	.2	17
—	1.3	50	34	220	3	80	t	.1	.4	93
—	1.2	20	24	157	2	50	t	t	.5	60
—	.4	33	23	110	2	420	t	t	.2	30
—	1.2	63	96	600	2	520	t	t	.2	6
t	.7	61	58	40	208	0	t	t	.7	0
—	2	25	248	480	960	0	.1	.1	3.4	0
0	.4	16	25	50	125	0	t	t	.3	0
0	.4	17	29	52	120	0	t	t	.3	0
2	10.9	318	662	720	2,655	0	1.1	.7	10.4	0
4	10.4	449	1,083	810	2,880	0	1.2	1	12.9	0
—	.5	23	54	40	144	0	t	t	.7	0
2	1.1	60	205	75	314	100	t	t	.3	0

* Includes oleic acid.
t Indicates trace only.
— No data available.
† If yellow only.

‡ Unsweetened.
§ Made with refined flour.
|| "Enriched" with vitamins B₁, B₂, niacin, and iron.
¶ Contains 4% milk solids.

FOOD	Approximate measure	Wgt. in grams	Calories	Protein grams	Carbohydrate grams	Fiber grams	Fat grams	Saturated fatty acid* grams
BREADS, CEREALS, GRAINS, AND GRAIN PRODUCTS (Continued)								
Cornflakes†	1 cup	25	110	2	25	.1	t	—
Corn grits, refined, cooked	1 cup	242	120	3	27	.2	t	—
Corn meal, yellow	1 cup	118	360	9	74	1.6	4	2
Crackers, graham	2 med.	14	55	1	10	t	1	—
Soda, 2½" square	2	11	45	1	8	t	1	—
Farina†	1 cup	238	105	3	22	0	t	—
Flour, soy, full fat	1 cup	110	460	39	33	2.9	22	0
Wheat, all purpose†	1 cup	110	400	12	84	.3	1	—
Wheat, whole	1 cup	120	390	13	79	2.8	2	—
Macaroni, cooked	1 cup	140	155	5	32	.1	1	—
Baked with cheese	1 cup	220	475	18	44	t	25	24
Muffins of refined flour†	1	48	135	4	19	t	5	4
Noodles	1 cup	160	200	7	37	.1	2	2
Oatmeal, or rolled oats	1 cup	236	150	5	26	4.6	3	2
Pancakes, buckwheat, 4" diam.	4	108	250	7	28	.1	9	—
Wheat, refined flour,† 4" diam.	4	108	250	7	28	.1	9	—
Pizza, cheese, ⅛ of 14" diam.	1 section	75	180	8	23	t	6	5
Popcorn, with oil and salt	2 cups	28	152	3	20	.6	7	2
Puffed rice†	1 cup	14	55	t	12	t	t	—
Puffed wheat,† presweetened	1 cup	28	105	1	26	.6	t	—
Rice, brown	1 cup‡	208	748	15	154	1.2	3	—
Converted	1 cup‡	187	677	14	142	.4	t	—
White†	1 cup‡	191	692	14	150	.3	t	—
Rice flakes†	1 cup	30	115	2	26	.1	t	—
Rice polish	½ cup	50	132	6	28	1.2	6	—
Rolls, breakfast, sweet	1 large	50	411	3	23	.1	12	11
Of refined flour†	1	38	115	3	20	t	2	2
Whole-wheat	1	40	102	4	20	.1	1	—

Lino- leic acid grams	MINERALS					VITAMINS				
	Iron mg.	Cal- cium mg.	Phos- phorus mg.	Potas- sium mg.	Sodium mg.	A units	B$_1$ mg.	B$_2$ mg.	Niacin mg.	C mg.
—	1.2	6	15	40	165	0	.1	t	.6	0
—	.7	2	24	200	2	t	t	t	.4	0
2	1.8	6	178	284	1	500	.4	.1	2	0
—	.3	3	56	45	90	0	t	t	.2	0
—	.1	2	19	12	110	0	t	t	.1	0
—	.8	31	29	20	33	0	.1	t	1	0
11	8.8	218	613	1,826	1	121	.9	.3	2.3	0
—	3.2	18	87	86	1	0	.4	.2	3.2	0
—	3.9	49	464	445	3	0	.6	.2	5.1	0
—	.6	11	82	276	1	0	t	t	.4	0
1	2	394	363	132	1,192	970	.2	.5	1.9	0
t	.7	74	80	62	221	60	t	.1	.7	0
t	1	16	52	—	—	60	t	t	.7	0
1	1.7	21	140	142	508	0	.2	t	.4	0
—	1.2	249	360	245	464	230	.1	.2	.7	0
—	1.3	158	159	135	470	110	.1	.1	.9	0
t	.7	157	147	96	525	570	t	.1	.8	8
4	.8	4	90	—	646	0	t	t	.7	0
—	.3	2	82	57	t	0	t	t	.6	0
—	.5	4	38	110	180	0	.1	t	1.4	0
—	4	78	608	310	18	0	.6	.1	9.2	0
—	1.6	53	244	300	6	0	.3	t	7.6	0
—	1.6	46	258	247	4	0	t	t	1.6	0
—	.5	9	44	60	329	0	.1	t	1.7	0
—	8	35	553	357	t	0	.9	.2	14	0
t	.4	42	54	56	185	70	t	t	.8	0
0	.7	28	39	34	202	t	.1	t	.8	0
—	1	46	112	100	225	0	.1	.1	1.5	0

* Includes oleic acid.
† "Enriched" with vitamins B$_1$, B$_2$, niacin, and iron.
t Indicates trace only.
— No data available.
‡ Measured before cooking.

FOOD	Approximate measure	Wgt. in grams	Calories	Protein grams	Carbohydrate grams	Fiber grams	Fat grams	Saturated fatty acid* grams
BREADS, CEREALS, GRAINS, AND GRAIN PRODUCTS (Continued)								
Spaghetti with meat sauce†	1 cup	250	285	13	35	.5	10	6
With tomatoes and cheese	1 cup	250	210	6	36	.5	5	3
Spanish rice with meat†	1 cup	250	217	4	40	1.2	4	—
Shredded wheat, biscuit	1	28	100	3	23	.7	1	—
Waffles, ½ by 4½ by 5½"‡	1	75	240	8	30	.1	9	8
Wheat germ	1 cup	68	245	17	34	2.5	7	3
Wheat-germ cereal, toasted§	1 cup	65	260	20	36	2.5	7	3
Wheat-meal cereal, unrefined	¼ cup‖	30	103	4	25	.7	1	—
Wheat, unground, cooked	¾ cup	200	275	12	35	4.4	1	—
SOUPS, CANNED, AND DILUTED¶								
Bean soups	1 cup	250	190	8	30	.6	5	4
Beef and vegetable	1 cup	250	100	6	11	.5	4	4
Bouillon, broth, consommé	1 cup	240	24	5	0	0	—	—
Chicken or turkey	1 cup	250	75	4	10	0	2	2
Clam chowder, without milk	1 cup	255	85	5	12	.5	2	t
Cream soups (asparagus, celery, etc.)	1 cup	255	200	7	18	1.2	12	11
Noodle, rice, barley soups	1 cup	250	115	6	13	.2	4	3
Split-pea soup	1 cup	250	147	8	25	.5	3	3
Tomato soup, diluted with milk	1 cup	245	175	6	22	.5	7	6
Vegetable (vegetarian)	1 cup	250	80	4	14	—	2	2
DESSERTS AND SWEETS								
Apple betty	1 serving	100	150	1	29	.5	4	—
Bread pudding with raisins	¾ cup	200	374	11	56	.2	12	11

Linoleic acid grams	MINERALS					VITAMINS				
	Iron mg.	Calcium mg.	Phosphorus mg.	Potassium mg.	Sodium mg.	A units	B$_1$ mg.	B$_2$ mg.	Niacin mg.	C mg.
3	2	25	162	670	1,017	690	t	.1	2.1	13
2	2	45	135	407	955	830	t	t	1	15
—	1.5	35	98	577	790	1,260	t	t	1.7	15
—	1	13	122	116	1	0	t	t	1.3	0
1	1.4	124	150	114	327	310	.1	.2	1.1	0
3	5.5	57	744	550	5	0	1.4	.5	3.1	0
3	4.9	32	722	630	1	110	1.6	.9	4.1	0
—	1.1	15	130	126	1	0	.2	.1	1.4	0
—	1.6	40	400	174	1	0	.1	.1	4.8	0
t	2.8	95	254	445	1,007	260	t	t	1	2
t	.8	12	50	165	1,067	1,100	t	t	1	—
—	1	2	32	129	780	0	t	t	1	0
t	.5	20	75	—	751	0	t	.1	1.5	0
1	1	36	49	225	1,099	1,070	t	t	1	0
t	.5	217	157	295	1,058	200	t	.2	.1	0
1	.2	82	45	69	1,224	30	t	t	.7	0
t	1.4	31	152	275	959	450	.2	.2	1.4	0
t	.7	167	155	417	1,055	1,200	t	.2	1.2	0
t	.8	32	40	170	855	2,900	t	t	1	8
—	.7	14	36	100	152	100	t	t	.4	1
t	2.2	218	228	430	400	600#	.1	.3	.2	0

* Includes oleic acid.
† With tomatoes.
t Indicates trace only.
— No data available.
‡ Containing 4% milk solids.

§ Malt added.
|| Measured before cooking.
¶ No data available on soups prepared at home.
# If made with butter or fortified margarine.

FOOD	Approximate measure	Wgt. in grams	Calories	Protein grams	Carbohydrate grams	Fiber grams	Fat grams	Saturated fatty acid* grams
DESSERTS AND SWEETS (Continued)								
Cakes, angel food	1 slice	40	110	3	23	0	t	—
Chocolate cake, fudge icing	1 slice	120	420	5	70	.3	14	12
Cupcake with icing	1	50	160	3	31	t	3	2
Fruit cake, 2 by 2 by ½"	1 slice	30	105	2	17	.2	4	3
Gingerbread, 2" cube	1 piece	55	180	2	28	t	7	6
Plain cake, without icing	1 slice	55	180	4	31	t	5	4
Sponge cake, without icing	1 slice	40	115	3	22	0	2	2
Candy, caramels	5	25	104	t	19	0	3	3
Chocolate creams	2	30	130	t	24	0	4	4
Fudge, plain, 1" square	2 pieces	90	370	t	80	.1	12	11
Hard candies	1 oz.	28	90	t	28	0	0	0
Marshmallows, large	5	30	98	1	23	0	C	0
Milk chocolate	2-oz. bar	56	290	2	44	.2	6	6
Chocolate syrup	2 T.	40	80	t	22	0	t	t
Doughnuts, cake type	1	33	135	2	17	t	7	4
Gelatin, made with water	1 cup	239	155	4	36	0	t	t
Honey, strained	2 T.	42	120	t	30	0	0	0
Ice cream, see Dairy products								
Ices, lime, orange, etc.	1 cup	150	117	0	48	0	0	0
Jams, marmalades, preserves	1 T.	20	55	0	14	t	0	0
Jellies	1 T.	20	50	0	13	0	0	0
Molasses, blackstrap	1 T.	20	45	0	11	0	0	0
Cane, refined	1 T.	20	50	0	13	0	0	0
Pie,§ apple, ½ of 9"-diam. pie	1 slice	135	330	3	53	.1	13	11

Lino-leic acid grams	MINERALS					VITAMINS				
	Iron	Cal-cium	Phos-phorus	Potas-sium	Sodium	A	B₁	B₂	Niacin	C
grams	mg.	mg.	mg.	mg.	mg.	units	mg.	mg.	mg.	mg.
—	.1	2	40	40	113	0	t	t	.1	0
1	.5	118	162	184	282	140†	t	.1	.3	0
t	.2	58	54	72	150	50	t	t	.1	t
t	.8	29	38	165	52	50†	t	t	.3	t
t	1.4	63	33	222	119	50†	t	t	.6	0
t	.2	85	50	40	150	70	t	§	.2	0
t	.6	11	49	32	70	210	t	t	.1	0
t	.8	40	22	48	55	40	t	t	t	0
t	.2	18	16	30	63	t	0	0	t	0
t	.1	13	72	132	180	50	t	t	t	0
0	0	0	0	0	8	0	0	0	0	0
0	0	0	2	2	13	0	0	0	0	0
0	.6	72	115	192	47	100	0	0	0	0
0	.5	0	36	120	20	0	0	0	0	0
3‡	.4	23	63	26	80	40	t	t	.4	0
0	0	0	0	0	122	0	0	0	0	0
0	.4	2	2	22	2	0	t	t	t	2
0	0	t	t	5	8	0	0	0	0	8
0	.1	14	t	19	3	t	t	t	t	1
0	.1	13	t	15	3	t	t	t	t	1
0	2.3	116	14	585	19	0	t	t	t	0
0	.9	30	9	185	3	0	0	0	0	0
1	.5	9	29	106	400	220	t	t	.3	1

* Includes oleic acid.   † If made with butter or fortified margarine.
t Indicates trace only.   ‡ If fried in oil.
— No data available.   § Crusts prepared with refined flour and hydrogenated fat.

FOOD	Approximate measure	Wgt. in grams	Calories	Protein grams	Carbohydrate grams	Fiber grams	Fat grams	Saturated fatty acid* grams
DESSERTS AND SWEETS (Continued)								
Cherry	1 slice	135	340	3	55	.1	13	11
Custard	1 slice	130	265	7	34	0	11	10
Lemon meringue	1 slice	120	300	4	45	.1	12	10
Mince	1 slice	135	340	3	62	.7	9	8
Pumpkin	1 slice	130	265	5	34	.8	12	11
Puddings, milk, custard,† rice, bread‡								
Sugar, beet or cane	1 cup	200	770	0	199	0	0	0
3 teaspoons or	1 T.	12	50	0	12	0	0	0
Brown, firm-packed, dark	1 cup	220	815	0	210	0	0	0
Syrup, maple	2 T.	40	100	0	25	0	0	0
Table blends	2 T.	40	110	0	29	0	0	0
Tapioca cream pudding	1 cup	250	335	10	42	0	10	9
NUTS, NUT PRODUCTS, AND SEEDS								
Almonds, dried	½ cup	70	425	13	13	1.8	38	28
Roasted and salted	½ cup	70	439	13	13	1.8	40	31
Brazil nuts, unsalted	½ cup	70	457	10	7	2	47	31
Cashews, unsalted	½ cup	70	392	12	20	.9	32	28
Coconut, shredded, sweetened	½ cup	50	274	1	26	2	20	19
Peanut butter, commercial‖	⅓ cup	50	300	12	9	.9	25	17
Peanut butter, natural	⅓ cup	50	284	13	8	.9	24	10
Peanuts, roasted	⅓ cup	50	290	13	9	1.2	25	16
Pecans, raw, halves	½ cup	52	343	5	7	1.1	35	25
Sesame seeds, dry	½ cup	50	280	9	10	3.1	24	13
Sunflower seeds	½ cup	50	280	12	10	1.9	26	7
Walnuts, English, raw	½ cup	50	325	7	8	1	32	7
BEVERAGES								
Alcoholic, beer (4% alcohol)	2 cups	480	228	t	8	0	0	0
Gin, rum, vodka, whiskey (86 proof)	1 oz.	28	70	0	t	0	0	0

| Lino-leic acid grams | MINERALS | | | | | VITAMINS | | | | |
	Iron mg.	Cal-cium mg.	Phos-phorus mg.	Potas-sium mg.	Sodium mg.	A units	B₁ mg.	B₂ mg.	Niacin mg.	C mg.
1	.5	14	33	140	405	520	t	t	.3	2
1	1.6	162	151	182	382	300	t	.2	.4	0
1	.6	24	65	66	337	210	t	.1	.2	1
1	3	22	50	236	600	10	t	t	.5	0
1	1	70	92	219	285	2,480	t	.1	.4	8
0	0	0	0	0	0	0	0	0	0	0
0	0	0	0	0	0	0	0	0	0	0
0	5.7	167	38	688	60	0	0	0	0	0
0	.6	41	3	70	4	0	t	t	t	0
0	.3	2	1	10	1	0	0	0	0	0
1	1	262	265	337	390	580	.1	.4	.2	0
8	3.3	163	353	541	2	0	.2	.6	2.4	0
8	3.3	163	353	541	140	0	t	.6	2.4	0
12	2.3	124	464	476	1	t	.6	.1	1	0
2	2.9	29	242	325	40§	70	.3	.1	1.2	0
t	1	8	56	176	0	0	t	t	.4	1
7	.9	29	154	309	300	0	.3	.1	6.2	0
7	1	30	204	337	2	0	.5	.1	7.9	0
7	1	37	200	337	2§	0	.2	.1	8.6	0
7	1.2	36	144	300	t§	60	.4	.1	.4	1
10	5.2	580	308	360	30	15	.4	.1	2.7	0
15	3.5	60	418	460	15	0	1.8	.2	13.6	0
20	1.5	50	190	225	1	15	.1	.1	.4	1
0	t	10	60	50	14	0	t	t	1	0
0	0	0	0	t	t	0	0	0	0	0

* Includes oleic acid.   t Indicates trace only.
† See Dairy products.   § Add 200 mg. for salted nuts.
‡ See Grain products. || Sugar and hydrogenated fat added.

FOOD	Approximate measure	Wgt. in grams	Calories	Protein grams	Carbohydrate grams	Fiber grams	Fat grams	Saturated fatty acid° grams
BEVERAGES (Continued)								
Wines, dessert								
(18.8% alcohol)	½ cup	120	164	t	9	0	0	0
Table								
(12.2% alcohol)	½ cup	120	100	t	5	0	0	0
Carbonated drinks								
Artificially sweetened	12 oz.	346	0	0	0	0	0	0
Club soda	12 oz.	346	0	0	0	0	0	0
Cola drinks, sweetened	12 oz.	346	137	0	38	0	0	0
Fruit-flavored soda	12 oz.	346	161	0	42	0	0	0
Ginger ale	12 oz.	346	105	0	28	0	0	0
Root beer	12 oz.	346	140	0	35	0	0	0
Coffee, black, unsweetened	1 cup	230	3	t	1	0	0	0
Tea, clear, unsweetened	1 cup	230	4	0	1	0	t	0
SUPPLEMENTARY FOODS								
Bone meal or powder	½ t.	2.5	0	0	0	0	0	0
Calcium gluconate	7½ t.	11	—	0	0	0	0	0
Calcium lactate	3½ t.	5	—	0	0	0	0	0
Dicalcium phosphate	1 t.	4	0	0	0	0	0	0
Desiccated liver, defatted†	¼ cup	37	120	28	3	1.6	t	—
Lecithin, granular	2 T.	15	105	0	0	—	11	9
Powdered yeast, brewers' debittered	¼ cup	33	91	13	12	.6	t	t
Primary, grown on molasses‡	¼ cup	33	115	16	11	2.3	4	—
Torula	¼ cup	40	148	20	10	.2	3	t
Torula, calcium-fortified§	¼ cup	40	148	20	10	.2	3	t

Lino-leic acid grams	MINERALS					VITAMINS				
	Iron mg.	Calcium mg.	Phos-phorus mg.	Potas-sium mg.	Sodium mg.	A units	B_1 mg.	B_2 mg.	Niacin mg.	C mg.
0	t	4	t	37	2	0	t	t	.1	0
0	.5	10	12	100	6	0	t	t	.1	0
0	0	0	—	—	—	0	0	0	0	0
0	0	0	—	—	—	0	0	0	0	0
0	0	0	—	—	—	0	0	0	0	0
0	0	0	—	—	—	0	0	0	0	0
0	0	0	—	—	—	0	0	0	0	0
0	0	0	—	—	—	0	0	0	0	0
0	.2	9	9	40	2	0	0	t	.6	0
0	t	t	t	58	t	0	0	t	t	0
0	1.8	1,000	516	t	t	0	0	0	0	0
0	0	1,000	0	0	0	0	0	0	0	0
0	0	1,000	0	0	0	0	0	0	0	0
0	0	1,000	778	0	0	0	0	0	0	0
—	6	10	600	480	140	0	.2	4.4	11.3	70
1.2	t	t	500	t	t	—	—	—	—	—
t	5	70	584	631	40	t	5.2	1	12.9	0
—	2.5	82	231	690	165	0	8	8	33	0
2	7	90	600	800	6	0	6	6	40	0
2	7	600	600	800	6	0	10	10	100	0

° Includes oleic acid.
t Indicates trace only.
— No data available.
† Supplies 370 milligrams of cholin, 74 of Inositol, 5.5 of pantothenic acid, and 18.5 micrograms of vitamin B_{12} as well as other B vitamins.
‡ One-half cup of flake yeast has the same nutrients as ¼ cup powdered.
§ Fortified with calcium and magnesium, as directed on page 220.

whole wheat in loss of nutrients, 254-55; adding of
"caramel coloring" to white,
255-56; labeled as "wheat,"
255-56
Bread-making, 101, 265
Breadstuffs, former value of, 63
Breakfast: importance of, 20-28;
studies of, 21-23; of coffee,
21; typical American, 22, 23;
relation of, to well-being during afternoon, 22; on Indiana
farm, 25; buffet, 25; Scandinavian, 25-26; suggestions for,
220-21
Breath, shortness of, 78, 96,
103, 117, 178
Brewers' yeast, see Yeast
Bromfield, Louis, 206
Bromide poisoning, vitamin C
and, 129
Bromine in human blood, 201
Bronchial tubes, 56
Bruise: relation of, to vitamin-C
intake, 123, 136; as danger
signal, 128
Buerger's disease, 161
Bulk, sources of, 219
Burns: sprayed with solution of
vitamin C, 136; treatment of,
with vitamin E, 155, 156
Burr, George O., 43-44
Bursitis, 132, 155, 171
Butter, 43; vitamin A in, 46, 53,
58; rancidity of, 47; compared
to margarine, 48
Buttermilk, 34, 217; protein con-
tent of, 39; churned; cultured, calcium in, 167, 168,
169; value of, in iron absorption, 179

Cabbage, 122, 127
Cactus juice, fermented, 244
Cake mixes, 47, 255
Calcium: diet supplemented
with, 97; relation of, to phosphorus, 107, 140, 166, 168;
gluconate, 107, 166, 167, 168;
lactate, 107, 167, 168, 217;
relation of, to vitamin C, 123,
125, 131; importance of, in
healing, 125; absorption of,
138, 140, 143, 146, 164, 165,
167, 168; relation of, to vitamin D, 138, 140, 168; extent
of deficiencies of, 140, 166-67;
losses of, from body, 140, 168;

solubility of, 140, 164; reaction with acids, 143; relation
of, to nervousness, 143, 144,
163, 164, 165; effect of, on
menopause symptoms, 143;
salivary, 143-44; effect of, on
dental health, 144, 166; importance of, in arresting pyorrhea, 144; daily intake of, 146;
deposits, from cell breakdown,
152-53; effect of, on relation,
163, 164, 166, 210; relation
of, to air swallowing, 163-64;
deficiency of, as cause of "indigestion," 164; milk as only
source of, 164, 167; relation
of, to cramps, 164; tablets, for
relief of insomnia, 164; tablets, for relief of menstrual
cramps, 165; use of, in reliev-
ing pain, 165-66; relation of,
to vitamin D, 165; importance
of, in maintaining skeletal
health, 166; effect of, on
muscle tone, 166; tablets of,
for arthritis, 166; tablets of,
for dental pain, 166; tablets
of, for headaches, 166; tablets of, for pain of childbirth,
166; tablets of, for itching of
hives, 166; value of, in clotting
blood, 166; effect of candy on,
167; salts of, 167, 168; sources
of, 167, 219; amount of, in
blood, 168, 169; removal of,
from bones, 168, 169; storage
of, 168, 169; quantities of,
supplied by milk, 169; daily
need of, in blood, 169; deposits of, in soft tissues,
171-72; relation of, to magnesium, 171, 172, 174, 175, 176;
relation of, to bone development, 174; losses of, 174; see
also Blood calcium
Calories: derived from fat, 42;
amount of, from refined foods,
63; former vs. present consumption of, 63
Cancer, 244; growth of, in biotin
deficiency, 69; and vitamin E,
160; thyroid, 182, 185; from
fallout, 185; produced by arsenic, 204; freedom from, 243,
244; per cent of, among African natives, 244-45; in babies
and children, 247; expected
increase in, 247

of carotene, 53, 58, 59-60; absorption of carotene from, 59; effect of growing conditions on, 59, 205; green, as source of folic acid, 77; green, as source of pantothenic acid, 79; leafy, vitamin B2 in, 90; effect of chopping on, 126; effect of peeling on, 126; effects of soaking on, 126; effect of boiling on, 126; as source of vitamin C, 127; leafy; as source of magnesium, 175; leafy, iron in, 179; as source of potassium, 187; leafy, as source of copper, 198; leafy, as source of manganese, 199; leafy, as source of zinc, 199; deficiency symptoms of, 201; relation of soil to flavor of, 202, 204, 205; daily need of, 217, 218

Vegetarians, 77, 78; diet of, 243

Veins, function of, 211

Vietnam War, statistics on army rejections, 245

Vigor, retention of, 38

Vincent's disease, 87

Violence, relation of, to niacin deficiency, 87

Viosterol, 138, 141

Virus, 123, 129, 132

Vision: day, 53, 54; night, 53-54, 57; dim, and vitamin-A deficiency, 53-55, 57; blurred, from excess vitamin A, 60; failing, 94; relation of cholesterol to problems of, 116

Visual purple, 53

Vitality: lack of, 178; increased by pep-up drink, 220

Vitamin A: absorption of, 46; mineral oil and, 46; animal fats as sources of, 46; in fish-liver oils, 46, 58; destruction of, by rancid fats, 47; added to margarine, 48; how formed, 53; functions of, 53-57; deficiencies of, 53; relation of, to vision, 53-55, 60; relation of, to skin, 55, 60; relation of, to bacterial growth, 55-57; relation of, to mucous membrane, 55-57; relation of, to infections, 56-57; relation of, to bones, 57, 60; relation of, to teeth, 57; relation of, to warts, 57; correcting deficiencies of, 57; sources of, 58,

217, 218; recommended daily allowances, 58, 60-62; storage of, 59, 60, 61; influence of vitamin E on, 59, 62, 160; soil influence on, 59, 62; amounts used to correct deficiencies of, 60-61; toxicity to over-dosage of, 60; variations in requirements of, 61; food handling influence on, 62; relation of, to gums, 124

Vitamin B, *see following headings, also* B vitamins

Vitamin B1: beriberi and, 65; cheapness of, 90, 95; deficiency of, in humans, 95-97; "enriching" foods with, 95; danger of taking alone, 95; sources of, 96; primary function of, 97-98; recovery from deficiency of, 97-98; energy production and, 98, 99; mental alertness and, 98; digestive disturbances and, 98; constipation and, 99; heart abnormalities and, 99; neuritis and, 99; tablets of, 109, 110; proportion of, to other B vitamins, 109; importance of, in maintaining metabolic rate, 182; as part of enzymes, 209

Vitamin B2: tongue changes, and deficiency of, 66; sources of, 90; cheapness of, 90; symptoms of deficiency of, 90-91; extent of deficiencies of, 90, 93; lip changes, and deficiency of, 90-91; formation of blood vessels and deficiency of, 91-92; eye symptoms, and deficiency of, 91-93; milk sugar intake, and deficiency of, 94; tablets of, 109, 110; proportion of, to other B vitamins, 109; enzymatic action of, 209

Vitamin B3, 86

Vitamin B6: sources of, 81-82; symptoms of deficiency of, 82-83; eczema relieved by, 82; functions of, 83; as necessary for normal functioning of brain, 83; relation of, to magnesium, 83, 85, 173, 174; epilepsy treated with, 83; absorption of, 84; tremors relieved by, 84; tics relieved by, 84; daily requirement of, 85; pro-